J. A. Sturm (Ed.)

Adult Respiratory Distress Syndrome

An Aspect of Multiple Organ Failure
Results of a Prospective Clinical Study

Contributors
H. Bartels · M. Behrmann · U. Böhme · J. Bruch
H. Creutzig · A. Dwenger · M. Funck · R. Funk · K.F. Gratz
M. Jochum · E. Jonas · Th. Joka · C.-J. Kant · M. Kirschfink
J. Knöller · W. König · E. Kreuzfelder · U. Lehmann
J. Lindena · B. Lueken · W. Machleidt · M. Maghsudi
J. Mirkhani · M.L. Nerlich · H. Neuhof · B. Neumann
C. Neumann · U. Obertacke · H.-J. Oestern · H.-C. Pape
U. Pison · T. Pohlemann · E. Reale · G. Regel · M. Reuter
G. Röllig · U. Rother · K.P. Schmit-Neuerburg
W. Schönfeld · W. Schramm · G. Schweitzer · W. Seeger
A. Seekamp · J. Seidel · M. Spannagl · W. Stangel
J.A. Sturm · N. Suttorp · O. Thraenhart · H. Tscherne
D.H. Wisner · G. Zilow

With 178 Figures

Springer-Verlag
Berlin Heidelberg New York London Paris
Tokyo Hong Kong Barcelona Budapest

Professor Dr. J. A. STURM
Department of Trauma Surgery
Hannover Medical School
Konstanty-Gutschow-Str. 8
W-3000 Hannover 61, FRG

ISBN-13: 978-3-540-52180-8 e-ISBN-13: 978-3-642-84098-2
DOI: 10.1007/ 978-3-642-84098-2

Typesetting: Best-set Typesetters Ltd., Hong Kong
24/3130-543210 – Printed on acid-free paper

Contents

IV Activation of Inflammatory Cells

V Endothelial and Epithelial Mechanisms of Injury

VI Experimental Studies

List of Contributors

You will find the addresses at the beginning of the respective contribution

Introduction

J.A. Sturm

In modern society, trauma remains the number one cause of death in people under 50 years, but, despite this, very little attention has been paid to trauma care compared with other diseases such as malignancy or myocardial infarction (Table 1). The efforts that have been made in medical care, however, have showed some success; for example although the frequency of traffic accidents in the Federal Republic of Germany has remained constant over the years, the number of deaths resulting from them has decreased (Fig. 1). The results of improvements in rescue systems, surgical techniques, and intensive care are evident, as shown by a review of the statistics of about 3000 multiple trauma patients treated in the last 15 years at the trauma department of Hannover Medical School which reflects the progress that has been made in medical care.

After the problem posed by posttraumatic kidney failure had been solved in the 1960s and 1970s, the adult respiratory distress syndrome (ARDS) became the biggest problem in the 1970s and 1980s (Fig. 2). ARDS as a single entity disappeared in the literature in the early 1980s and was replaced by the so-called multiple organ failure (MOF) syndrome. Between 1985 and 1990 35% of the patients in our intensive care unit developed MOF, and 70% of them died. Overall MOF mortality has remained constant since 1985 at about 20% (Fig. 3). The term MOF is actually somewhat misleading, because the organs do not usually fail completely; it is rather the summation of disturbances in all organs which finally leads to a breakdown of the circulatory system. A common finding at autopsy is increased weight in all organs which is due to interstitial edema, and electromicroscopic studies often show the presence of an intracellular edema. The substrate of the protein-rich interstitial edema, formerly described in isolated as ARDS, cases is pathological due to permeability damage to the cellular and endothelial membranes. This permeability results in a loss of cellular integrity and a breakdown in organ function.

Department of Trauma Surgery, Hannover Medical School, Konstanty-Gutschow-Str. 8, W-3000 Hannover 61, FRG

J.A. Sturm (Ed.)
Adult Respiratory Distress Syndrome

Table 1. Comparison of various causes of death

Cause of death (place/time period)	Age distribution (years)				
	0–15 (%)	15–25 (%)	25–45 (%)	45–65 (%)	65 (%)
Polytraumatized patients (*Hannover Medical School*/1972–1988)	7	32	35	18	7
Car accidents (FRG/1988)	5	34	24	14	21
Malignant tumors (FRG/1988)	0.2	0.32	3.1	16	70
Myocardial infarction (FRG/1988)	–	0.01	1.3	21	88

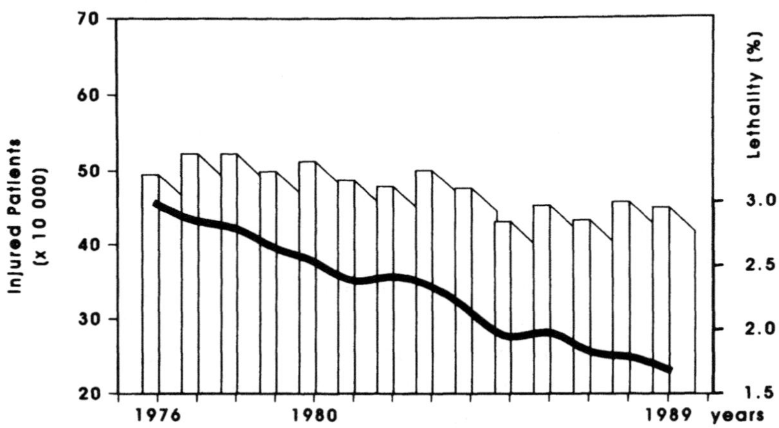

Fig. 1. Number of patients injured in road accidents (*Blocks*) between 1976 and 1989 in the Federal Republic of Germany. *Black line* indicates the percentage of mortality in these patients

Despite the extensive trials carried out during the past few years, no therapeutic breakthrough was achieved. It is not even completely clear at what time this generalized cell damage occurs: Is it directly related to trauma and shock, or are later complications such as posttraumatic sepsis responsible for the permeability damage? The nature of the clinical findings led to the general belief for a long time that sepsis played a major role. The symptoms seen, i.e., a hyperdynamic circulatory status, fever, and leukocytosis, are also all found typically in clinical sepsis. Another argument for sepsis as a cause of the described pathomechanisms is the lack of time between trauma and the onset of organ function loss. First signs of MOF develop during the 3rd or 4th day after trauma and are accompanied by the onset of clinical "sepsis". Therefore, research and therapy focused on, for example, improving hygenic measures or the effective use of antibiotics.

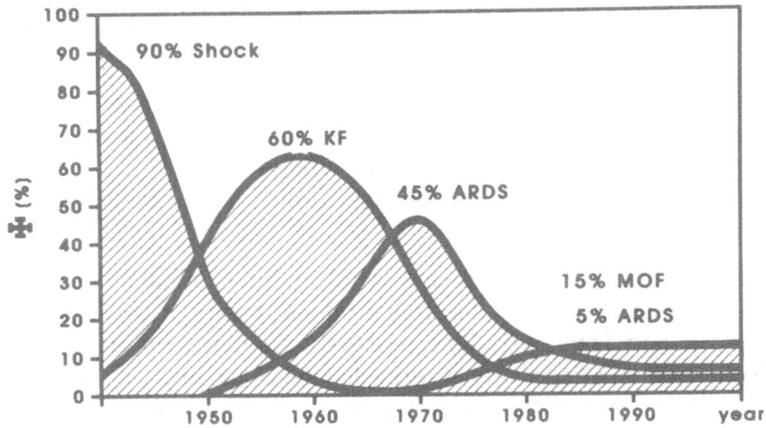

Fig. 2. Comparison of major causes of death between 1940 and 1990 in the Federal Republic of Germany (*KF*, kidney failure; *MOF*, multiple organ failure; *ARDS*, adult respiratory distress syndrome)

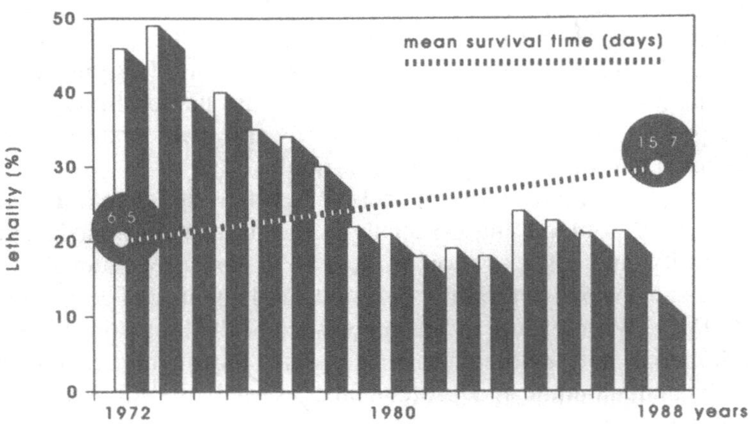

Fig. 3. Mortality in multiple trauma patients treated between 1972 and 1988 in the Hannover Medical School (n = 3074)

Nothing has so far, however, proved to be effective. Therefore, the discussion of the theory of an abacterial or endotoxic origin has been revived. Experimental results in particular have shown that inflammatory abacterial pathomechanisms cause the clinical signs of MOF; in some cases, major changes were seen in the lungs, causing an ARDS-like entity. In patients with multiple trauma, clinical data show that there are significant differences very early on in the pulmonary parameters of those patients who eventually survive and those who do not, thereby supporting the idea that even the "delayed" reactions are also directly dependent on trauma and hemorrhagic shock. Therefore, we undertook a clinical study to answer the following questions:

1. When does the permeability or cell damage after trauma occur?
2. What is the effect of this damage and how can we measure the manifestation and extent of cell and permeability damage?
3. What is the pathogenesis of this damage (time course, mediators, cell factors, etc.)?

Between 1983 and 1987, 84 patients with multiple trauma entered a multicenter prospective study at the trauma departments of the University Hospitals Essen and Hannover. The prospective study tried to minimize individual variation by using a very strong selection of patients on the basis of a strict protocol of treatment and measurements. We made a great effort to judge the severity of injuries accurately. The scoring and clinical judgment were performed by a small group of physicians only. The selected patients had an expected mortality of 50% and the likelihood of MOF development was high (see chapter "I").

All further efforts concentrated on elucidating the unknown pathomechanisms. In the chapter "III" the activation of cellular components is discussed. Phagocytes seem to be the effector cells of the inflammatory reaction at the endothelial membrane of all capillary systems. This theory was confirmed in our study since a severe disturbance of this humoral-phagocytic axis could be proved, to which mainly neutrophils and macrophages of the reticuloendothelial and alveolary systems contribute.

We paid special attention to the role of certain inflammatory cell mediators appearing in blood and especially in the bronchoalveolar lavage. The origin, identity, and concentration of these mediators after trauma seem to be essential factors which determine the quality and quantity of destruction (see chapter "IV"). With respect to the importance of the lung injury in this context, endothelial and epithelial damage were thoroughly examined. Changes in alveolar albumin and protein flux, as well as disturbances of surfactant function were documented. These results showed that both early and late ultrastructural changes take place as a consequence of multiple trauma (see chapter "V").

The results summarized in this book lead us to believe that ARDS is the first consequence of a generalized inflammatory reaction at the endothelial membrane seen after trauma. It leads to a loss of cell integrity and an increase in permeability and ends in a subsequent failure of all organ systems, i.e., MOF. The damage is strongly related to trauma and shock, and all therapeutic efforts should therefore be concentrated in the very early phase after trauma.

I Clinical Aspects

Study Protocol

H.-C. Pape and C.-J. Kant

For comparison purposes the selection of patients was made according to strictly defined criteria. This was also applied for the types of parameter and time table. If the criteria set up could not be maintained, the patient was excluded from the study.

Definition of Polytrauma

The following definition of polytrauma was applied: two or more injuries, one of which must be life-threatening. The severity of injury was graded according to the PTS (Hannover Polytrauma Score)

Criteria for Inclusion in the Study

a. Severity of injury: PTS grade III or IV.
b. Severity of head injury. If GCS was smaller than 8 points within the first 6 after admission, the patient was excluded.
c. Only patients from 15 to 65 years were included.
d. The maximum time allowed between trauma and primary care was 60 min, between trauma and admission 120 min.
e. If the therapy regimen or time table in the prehospital phase was not maintained, the patient was excluded.
f. Patients transferred from another hospital or treated with steroids or colloidal solutions were excluded.
g. The decision for inclusion had to be made by a member of the "shock research team".

Department of Trauma Surgery, Hannover Medical School, Konstanty-Gutschow-Str. 8, W-3000 Hannover 61, FRG

J.A. Sturm (Ed.)
Adult Respiratory Distress Syndrome

Primary Care (Place of Accident, Transfer to Trauma Center)

1. Volume therapy.
   a. Cristalloid solutions in quantities of 2000 ml each
   b. No dextrane, no colloidal solutions
   c. Gelatinous solutions (only after blood has been drawn) in quantities of 1000 ml.
2. Initial blood sampling.
   a. Sampling only before protein-containing solutions have been given.
   b. Amount sampled did not exceed 120 ml.

Hospital Phase [Admission and intensive care unit (ICU) Stay]

Timetable

a. Setting up the measurement equipment must not take place more than 6 h after trauma.
b. Days 1 and 2 count exactly from the time of accident (48 h). Blood sampling every 6 h.
c. Day 3 is a gap day of variable length to account for the different time of the accident.
d. After day 4 has passed, measurements are done at 8:00 A.M. every day and every 12 h afterwards.
e. Cell function studies are performed on admission, 12 h post admission, and on days 2, 4, 6, and 12.

Parameters

a. Hemodynamics

1. Femoral artery catheter (systolic, diastolic, and mean blood pressure).
2. Pulmonary artery catheter (Swan-Ganz) (systolic, diastolic, mean pulmonary artery pressure, and end expiratory and mean wedge pressure).
3. Central venous pressure (mean).
4. Cardiac output measured using Edward's computer (0.9% NaCl) or Edward's lung water computer (Cardio-Green solution). Solutions at 4°C in iced water. This is injected at end expiration. The mean of three measurements is calculated.
5. Calculation of pulmonary shunt.
6. Temperature: peripherally and rectally.

b. Ventilation

1. Respiratory parameters: respiratory rate, tidal volume/minute, positive end expiratory pressure (PEEP), mean airway pressure, plateau pressure, inspiratory oxygen concentration, expiratory CO_2 concentration
2. Calculation of $AaDo_2$, dead space ventilation, and compliance
3. Blood gas analysis of arterial and mixed venous blood

c. Renal monitoring

1. Urinary output 12-hourly and fluid balance
2. Creatinine clearance
3. Urine electrolytes

d. Further monitoring

1. SMA-6
2. Differential blood count (daily)
3. Coagulation studies
4. Electrolytes, serum urea, and creatinine

Therapeutic Concepts

a. Volume substitution

1. Cristalloid solutions only (according to central venous pressure (CVP) pulmonary artery pressure, cardiac output, and urinary output)
2. Blood substitution in the ICU only with red blood cell concentrations of hemoglobin (Hb) below 10 g/100 ml. In case of coagulation disorders, fresh blood are used in preference.
3. Blood products. Fresh frozen plasma should be used if total protein is below 3.0 g/100 ml or after 10 units of blood have been given.
4. Albumin must not be given, fresh frozen plasma should be used in preference.

b. Medication

1. Vasoactive substances
   a. Dopamine is mandatory from the beginning of the study up to 14 days [3–5 µg/kg body weight (BW)].
   b. Nitroglycerine if temperature difference exceeds 1.5°C.
   c. Hydergine, 30 mg (indication: see b.).
   d. Phentolamine is not recommended.

2. Cardiac drugs, diuretics
   a. Digitalis, only if it has been given previously or if heart failure is present.
   b. Furosemide only in the case of renal failure of cardiac lungg edema.

3. Further drugs
   a. Cimetidine 1200 mg/day
   b. Heparin After 12 h post trauma, then s.c. at 3 × 5000 IU

4. Parenteral nutrition
   a. For the first 24 h after trauma only electrolyte solutions, then 10%–20% glucose. From day 2, 30 cal/kg Xylite (LGX solution) must not be used.
   b. Amino acids: 8%–10%, 1 g/150 cal. Daily weight control of the patients.

5. Ventilation therapy
   Nasotracheal intubation should be done as soon as possible. Respiratory setting should be as follows:

   - Inspiration/Expiration 1:2–1:0.8
   - PEEP + 5 cm H_2O initially
   - Breathing frequency 12–16/min
   - Tidal volume > 10 ml/kg BW. In the case of hypoxemia, PEEP is augmented firstly, then inspiratory oxygen concentraion.

Extravascular Lung Water: Clinical Methodology

A. Seekamp[1], U. Obertacke[2], and J.A. Sturm[1]

Introduction

The adult respiratory distress Syndrome (ARDS) is characterized by low-pressure interstitial lung edema due to an increase of capillary permeability. Different methods have been established to measure the extravascular lung water (EVLW) for diagnostic and therapeutic purposes.

The most reliable measurements have been obtained by the gravimetric method described by Pearce et al.[14]. The total water content is determined in a lung tissue specimen. Total blood volume is measured separately using C_{51}-marked erythrocytes. After calculating the water content of blood in the lung, the difference between it and the total lung water content reflects the EVLW. As this method can only be performed postmortem or at the end of a study, it has become more important as a reference than as a clinical method.

In patients ARDS is more often diagnosed by interpreting physical signs such as arterial blood gases, pulmonary dynamics, and chest X-ray, Pulmonary edema is known to cause an increase of the pulnonary shunt, but Said et al. [16] have reported that it increases by only 25% when the edema doubles. The arteriolveolar difference in oxygen saturation is also increased in pulmonary edema, but depends very much on cardiac output and oxygen-binding capacity. Of the pulmonary dynamics, compliance in ARDS patients has been reported to decrease linearly with the increase in interstitial fluid. In contrast, Cook et al. [4] noted that the decrease in compliance is more dependent on the tension of the alveolus surface than on an interstitial edema. Therefore, especially the initial perivascular edema does not cause any change in pulmonary compliance.

The chest X-ray is the most frequently performed method of estimating pulmonary interstitial fluid. As only a small increase in EVLW has been

[1] Department of Trauma Surgery, Hannover Medical School, Konstanty-Gutschow-Str. 8, W-3000 Hannover 61, FRG
[2] Department of Trauma Surgery, University Medical School, Hufelandstr. 55, W-4300 Essen 1, FRG

J.A. Sturm (Ed.)
Adult Respiratory Distress Syndrome

recognized by the Kerley lines in a chest X-ray, this method is quite sensitive to the onset of pulmonary edema. According to Snashall [17], in the case of severe edema quantification is no longer possible.

To determine the EVLW directly a double-indicator dilution method is needed. This technique was first proposed by Chinard and Enns in 1954 [3], using iodinated albumin as an indicator for the intravascular space and tritiated water as the indicator for the total intra- and extravascular water space. Although this technique was improved during the subsequent 10 years, only 50%–70% of true water content was detected compared with the gravimetric EVLW measurement. In 1965 Pearce and Beazell [3] reported the use of a thermal indicator to detect the water content. A thermal bolus was injected into the right atrium and detected with a thermistor placed in the distal airways. With this technique, measured extravascular thermal volume (EVTV) was twice as large as the EVLW measured by radioactively labeled indicators. The first to use a thermal indicator in combination with indocyanine green dye was Gee et al. in 1971 [5]. Indocyanine is binded to plasma protein immediately after injection and therefore distributed only in the intravascular space [6]. With this method, almost 90% of the true water content was detected. Holcroft and Trunkey [8] improved the technique and achieved a correlation coefficient of 0.93 between thermal dilution dye and gravimetrically measured EVLW. Since Lewis and Elings [9] have employed a microprocessor for mathematical analysis of the transit time curves, the thermal dilution dye technique has become very convenient.

Method

To prepare the dye indicator, 50 mg indocyanine green dye is dissolved in 10 ml saline solution and then diluted in 70 ml 5% dextrose. The thermal indicator is a 10-ml aliquot of the prepared iced dextrose solution. So both indicators are combined in one syringe. The patient is provided with a central venous catheter and a special aortic catheter, which is placed in the femoral artery and is 10 cm in length and 1.6 mm in diameter, with an attached thermistor proximal to the distal end.

The indicator is injected into or proximal to the right atrium. Simultanously blood is withdrawn at a flow rate of 30 ml/min using a 50-ml syringe and the lung water computer is started. The thermal indicator is then detected by the thermistor and recorded by the computer while green dye is sampled by a densitometer with a small cuvette placed external to the catheter but in series with it. After the computer has finished one measurement, all blood is reinfused and the catheter is flushed with saline before the next run is started. At least three consecutive injections should be made and the results averaged.

Mathematical Analysis

Calculation of the EVLW is based on the different transit times of a diffusible and a nondiffusible indicator. The volume of distribution of each of these indicators between the point of injection and the point of sampling in the circulation is given by the product of the flow rate, i.e., cardiac output, and mean transit time of each indicator. Intravascular volume and total thermal volume are defined as:

$$V_{intravasc} = Q \times MTT_{dye}$$
$$V_{total} = Q \times MTT_{thermal}$$

$V_{intravasc}$ = intravascular blood volume between injection and sampling
V_{total} = total thermal volume (EVTV) between injection and sampling
Q = cardiac output
MTT_{dye} = mean transit time of indocyanine green dye
$MTT_{thermal}$ = mean transit time of thermal indicator

The space only detected by the thermal indicator is called the extravascular thermal volume (EVTV) and defined as:

$$\text{EVTV} = V_{total} - V_{intravasc}$$
$$= Q \times (MTT_{thermal} - MTT_{dye})$$

which is directly equal to EVLW. Although the mean transit time is a summation of the appearance time and the time of dilution, the former does not have to be considered, as cardiac output and injection flow rate are the same for both indicators. For calculating the EVLW only the dilution times of both indicators are important:

$$\text{EVLW} = Q \times (MT_{thermal} - MT_{dye})$$

The microprocessor calculation according to Lewis [9] is based on the following technical and mathematical factors (Fig. 1):

- Inputs from dye and thermal detection systems are accepted simultaneously at a rate of 7/s and stored as analog data. After the indicator dilution curves rise to a peak and fall again to 25% of that peak value, the calculation is started.
- The starting point of each curve for integration ($t = 0$) is determined by a back to baseline extrapolation of a straight line defined by the points of 25% and 50% of the peak value on the upsweep part of the curve.
- Baseline concentrations of the indicators are defined as a 2-s average of the indicator dilution starting at $t = 0$ minus 4 s.
- The integrals for the calculation are determined by data measured from $t = 0$ to the 30% of peak point on the down slope of the curve.
- To determine the integrals beyond the 30% of peak point, an exponential

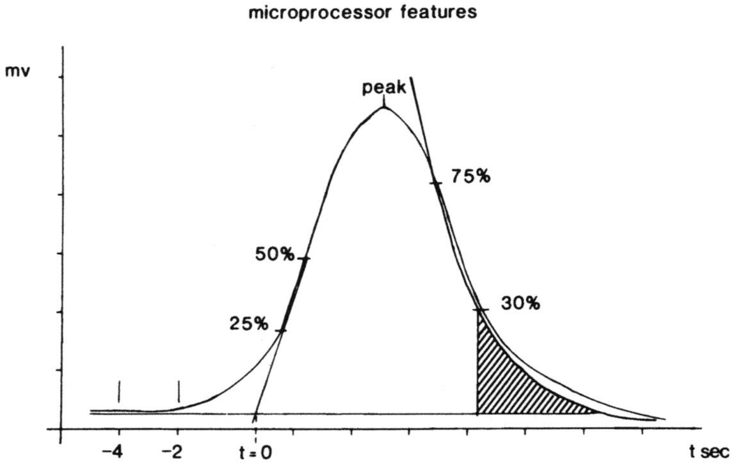

Fig. 1. Microprocessor analysis of the measured data. The starting point is defined by time whereas the end point is defined by extrapolation of the descendant part of the curve

curve is fitted to the data between the 75% and 30% of peak points and extrapolated to infinity.

Discussion

In order to evaluate the method of EVLW measurement, Lewis et al. [10] calculated a linear regression for EVLW data measured by the double-indicator dilution technique and determined by the gravimetric method in dogs. The correlation coefficient was 0.95. This correlation was also found by Sturm et al. [18], who performed these measurements in patients. As it seems that EVLW most reliably reflects an interstitial pulmonary edema, we were interested whether clinical parameters which are supposed to represent the state of oxygen diffusion also correlate with the EVLW data (Neumann et al., this volume).

As there is good evidence that the double-indicator dilution method is the most sensitive technique for measuring pulmonary edema, the likelihood and disadvantages of false measurements also need to be discussed. The thermal indicator is most likely influenced by the tissue through which it is passing. The heat capacity of, e.g., heart muscle, bronchioli, and lung parenchyma, will cause an overestimation of EVLW [11]. Less important is a shift in body temperature during the sampling time, as long as there is not a big difference between intrapulmonary and thermistor blood temperature. Otherwise values would again be overestimated.

Indocyanine green (ICG) indicator is supposed to be lost into the interstitium in the case of capillary leak syndrome. But even when the endothelial membrane is totally freely permeable for protein, Pfeiffer and Eimmermann [15] reported the loss of ICG during the sampling time to be less than 1%.

Besides the effects that only influence the measurement of one indicator, circumstances may also occur which effect both indicators simultaneously but in different ways. The question of whether the thermal-dye dilution technique depends on the cardiac output has been discussed repeatedly. In a study on dogs, Lewis et al. [10] reported that only in 7 of 46 observations was a significant decrease of EVLW after an increase of cardiac output noted. Holecroft and Trunkey [7], using a similar protocol, did not find an effect on EVLW after changing cardiac output. A reasonable explanation was given by Pfeiffer and Eimmermann [15], who reported that the main problem is the difference in response time and in sampling location of both indicator systems. The thermistor records a temperature at a given time concentration of ICG. If cardiac output then which does not correspond directly to the increases, both systems give different signals. Therefore whether one finds a positive or a negative correlation between the EVLW measurement and cardiac output depends on which system has the longer response time. As the different response times can be considered in the calculation, the influence of cardiac output on the EVLW measurement is minimized.

The most important limitation of the thermal-green dye indicator dilution method is the occlusion of pulmonary capillaries. Edema in nonperfused areas will not be detected or at least not totally. Different studies with induced micro- and macroembolism have given contradictory results [1, 2, 12]. So far it has not been clearly shown what range of occlusion would influence the distribution of the indicators. A corresponding problem is that in some lung areas P_{alv} is higher than P_{art} [19]. This is even more important in patients with high positive and expiratory pressure (PEEP) ventilation. So in real critical patients EVLW might be underestimated more than in patients without pulmonary edema.

In conclusion the thermal-green dye method is the most directly and practical way of measuring pulmonary edema. In spite of all the possible mistakes, the measurement is capable of providing frequent information for diagnostic and therapeutic purposes.

References

1. Allison RC, Parker JC, Duncan CE, Taylor AE (1983) Effect of air embolism on the measurement of extravascular lung thermal volume. J Appl Physiol 54:943
2. Beckett RC, Gray BA (1954) Effect of atelectasis and embolization on extravascular thermal volume of the dog. J Appl Physiol 178:197

3. Chinard FP, Enns T (1954) Transcapilary pulmonary exchange of water in the dog. Am J Physiol 178:197.
4. Cook CD, Mead J, Schreiner GL, Frank NR, Craig JM (1969) Pulmonary mechanisms during induced pulmonary edema in anesthetized dogs. J Appl Physiol 14:197
5. Gee MH, Miller PD, Stage AF, Banchero N (1971) Estimation of pulmonary extravascular fluid volume by use of thermodilution. Fed Proc 30:379
6. Gilly H (1984) Flow- und Volumenbestimmungen mittels Dilutionsverfahren. In: Bergmann H, Gilly H, Steinbereithner K, Sturm JA (eds) Lungenwasserbestimmung. II. Klinische Bedeutung. Maudrich, Vienna
7. Holcroft JW, Trunkey DD (1973) Extravascular lung water following hemorrhagic shock in the baboon. Ann Surg 34:508
8. Holcroft JW, Trunkey DD, Carpenter MA (1978) Excessive fluid administration in resuscitating baboons from hemorrhagic shock, and an assessment of the thermodye technic for measuring extravascular lung water. Am J Surg 135:412
9. Lewis FR, Elings VB (1978) Microprocessor determination of lung water using thermal-green dye double indicator dilution. Surg Forum 29:182
10. Lewis FR, Elings VB, Hill SL, Christensen JM (1982) The measurement of extravascular lung water by thermal-green dye indicator dilution. Ann NY Acad Sci 384:394
11. Lewis FR, Elings VB, Christensen JM (1984) The use of thermal-green dye indicator dilution to determine extravascular lung water. In: Bergmann H, Gilly H, Steinbereithner K, Sturm JA (eds) Lungenwasserbestimmung. II. Klinische Bedeutung. Maudrich, Vienna
12. Oppenheimer L, Elings VB, Lewis FR (1979) Thermal-dye lung water measurements. Effects of edema and embolization. Surg Res 26:504
13. Pearce ML, Beazell JW (1966) The measurement of pulmonary parenchymal Circ by thermal indicator dilution. Clin Res 14:182
14. Pearce ML, Yamashita J, Beazell J (1965) Measurement of pulmonary edema. volume Res 16:482
15. Pfeiffer U, Zimmermann G (1984) Fehlermöglichkeiten und Grenzen der Lungenwasserbestimmung mit der Thermo-Dye-Technik. In: Bergmann H, Gilly H, Steinbereithner K, Sturm JA (eds) Lungenwasserbestimmung. II. Klinische Bedeutung. Maudrich, Vienna
16. Said SI, Longacher JW, Davis RL, Woodell WL (1964) Pulmonary gas exchange during induction of pulmonary edema in anesthetized dog. J Appl Physiol 19:403
17. Snashall PD (1981) The radiographic detection of actue pulmonary edema. A comparison of radiographic appearances, densitometry and lung water in dogs. Br J Radiol 54:277
18. Sturm JA, Oestern HJ, Maghsudi M, Pfeiffer O, Joachim H (1982) Die gravimetrische Überprüfung der klinischen Lungenwassermessung. Langenbecks Arch [Suppl] 49:32
19. West JB, Dollery CT, Naimark A (1964) Distribution of blood flow in isolated lung, relation to vascular and alveolar pressures. J Appl Physiol 19:713

Bronchoalveolar Lavage

U. Obertacke, Th. Joka, M. Reuter, and K.P. Schmit-Neuerburg

Introduction

Diseases of the lung interstitium characterized by inflammatory processes in the area of the alveoli and the alveolar interstitium (alveolitis) can be noninvasively diagnosed or assessed only by radiological procedures or pulmonary function analysis. Lung biopsy as an invasive investigational procedure is not always representative, due to the multifocal alterations and dynamics of morphological processes in the alveolitis. Furthermore, the limited opportunity for repetition restricts the necessary follow-ups. In order to obtain alveolar cytological as well as pathobiochemical findings in the course of acute and chronic diseases of the lung interstitium, bronchoalveolar lavage (BAL) is an option. The endoscopic method as practised today was described by Reynolds and Newball in 1974 [7]. Extensive preliminary research [1, 2] demonstrated the possibilities of employing BAL in obtaining representative alveolar cytology in the course of alveolitis. It was proved that the cellular parts and the fluid components located in the epithelial surface (alveolus) reflect the inflammatory processes of the lower respiratory tract.

Following extensive early applications in chronic interstitial lung affections (sarcoidosis, idiopathic fibrosis), BAL has been used since 1981 [1, 6] for the investigation of alveolar reactions in the adult respiratory distress syndrome (ARDS).

Examination

Bronchoalveolar lavage is conducted with the aid of a bronchofiberscope. In the study-patients who have been ventilated for a long period, BAL is carried out with a bronchoscope (maximal outer diameter, 5.8 mm) through

Department of Trauma Surgery, University Medical School, Hufelandstr. 55, W-4300 Essen 1, FRG

J.A. Sturm (Ed.)
Adult Respiratory Distress Syndrome

the endotracheal tube (minimal inner diameter, 8.0 mm). This takes place with controlled maintenance of the suspended tidal volume and continuation of the prevailing analgesia. After inspecting the bronchial tree, the tip of the bronchofiberscope is positioned in a segmental ostium (lingula or right middle lobe). The intubated end of the bronchoscope should not completely occlude the segmental ostium. Then, 10 × 10 ml sterile NaCl 0.9% at body temperature is instilled and immediately retracted with light suction. The lavage time must not exceed 90 s to prevent the occurrence of diffusion processes. "Recovery" depends on the technique used and possibly on any lung alterations which are present. As a rule, 60% of the instilled volume can be recovered. A much lower recovery, as well as findings of bronchial epithelial cells in the BAL smear, indicates inadequate technique.

The aspirated fluid is collected in receptacles, is freed from mucous residues, and is examined separately for humoral and cellular components:

1. Cells: differential count, chemoluminescence response
2. Soluble components:
   a. Proteins: total protein, albumin, transferrin, α_1-proteinase inhibitor (α_1-PI) α_2-macroglobulin (α_2-MG), IgG, IgA, etc.
   b. Mediators: neutrophil elastase, C3a, LTC4, etc.
   c. Surfactant: phospholipid profile, alteration of function

For the collective study of patients with multiple injuries, the BAL was first carried out within 6 h after the trauma, and again at 8 a.m. the following days.

Epithelial Lining Fluid

In order to relate the alterations of cellular and humoral components in the lavage fluid to a reference value which is independent of the instilled or rather the recovered NaCl liquid volume, we used the epithelial lining fluid (ELF) as specified by Rennard et al. [5]. The ELF represents the part of the epithelial surface film obtained through BAL (Fig. 1) that was washed out in the "recovery." Because of the anatomic structures and the small molecular size (60 daltons), free diffusion of urea occurs. Therefore, the same urea concentrations are present in the plasma, interstitium, and alveoli. Under the assumption that urea ELF = urea PL, the theoretical volume of ELF is calculated as follows (Fick's principle):

$$\text{ELF (ml)} = \frac{\text{BAL urea concentration (mg/ml)} \times \text{Recovery (ml)}}{\text{Plasma urea concentration (mg/ml)}}$$

The conversion of a value, or rather concentration, found in the BAL to the concentration per milliliter ELF is as follows:

$$\frac{X\ \text{(mg/ml)}}{\text{ml ELF}} = \frac{X\ \text{(mg/ml)} \times \text{Plasma urea concentration} \times \text{Recovery}}{\text{Recovery} \times \text{BAL urea concentration}}$$

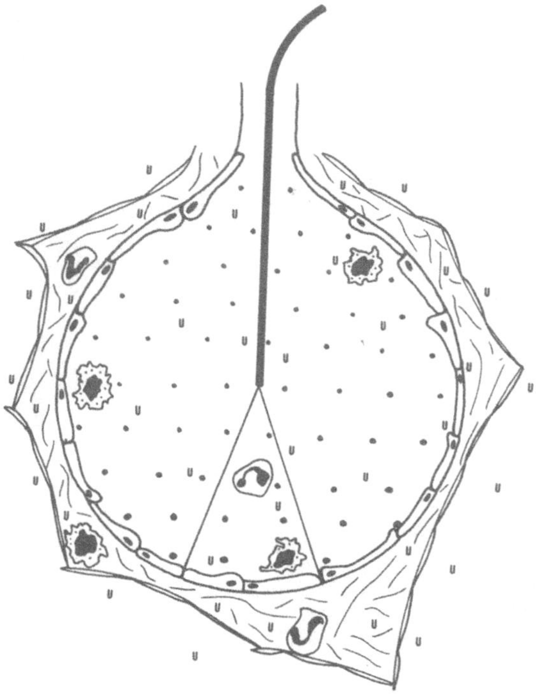

Fig. 1 Effect of BAL: a representative "part" of the alveolar lining layer is collected (including proteins, cells, and surfactant components)
U = urea; • = alveolar proteins

To relate an obtained value to the ELF, it is sufficient to multiply this stated value by:

$$\frac{{}^{\mathrm{Urea}}\,\mathrm{PL}}{{}^{\mathrm{Urea}}\,\mathrm{BAL}}$$

The limits of these ELF calculations lie within the urea diffusion from the plasma to the alveolus *during* the course of the BAL examination. This fundamental error, which was described by Marcy et al. in 1987 [4], also appears in small BAL volumes of about 30 ml. These small volumes are not useful in any case, because of the small yield of proteins and cells. Lavage quantities of 300 ml show values for urea diffusion during the examination that no longer enable an ELF calculation to be carried out. An acceptable lavage quantity with negligible error in the ELF calculation is stated as being 100 ml, especially when the lavage time is clearly below 2 min (4).

Determination of the Normal Values

Normal values for BAL were first specified for 23 patients who had previously been informed about BAL and had given their consent to it. This was per-

Table 1. Normal BAL content.
ELF volume = 1.2 ml ± 0.08 (100 ml lavage)

1. Cells (%)	
AM/PMN/L 85/2/12	
2. Surfactant	
Total phospholipids	3.5 mg/ml ELF
% PC	62 ± 3
SPA	20–60 μg/mg protein
3. Proteins (ELF)	
Total protein	<10 mg/ml ELF
Albumin	<3 mg/ml ELF
Transferrin	<0.3 mg/ml ELF
α_1-PI	<0.25 mg/ml ELF
α_2-MG	<0.05 mg/ml ELF
Ceruloplasmin	<0.03 mg/ml ELF
IgA	<0.2 mg/ml ELF
C3a	<2 μg/ml ELF
Elastase-α_1-PI	<1 μg/ml ELF

AM, alveolar macrophage; PMN, polymorph nucl. neutrophil; L, lymphocyte; PC, phosphatidylcholine; SPA, surfactant protein A; α_1-PI, α_2-proteinase inhibitor; α_2-MG, α_2-macroglobulin

formed with patients under general anesthesia during removal of the implant after osteosynthesis.

One investigator lavaged the same lung segment (LB4) of ten more probands, each for three consecutive days, to quantity further the influence of serial BAL on the alveolar environment [3]. The ten probands were bronchoscoped under local anesthesia.

Table 1 summarizes the cellular and humoral components found in healthy probands. The molecular weight of proteins that usually appear in relevant concentrations in the alveoli lies in the range of 80 000–100 000 (e.g., transferrin). Proteins of high molecular weight (α_2-macroglobulin) and inflammatory mediators (elastase, $C3_a$) are detectable only in minimal concentrations, or rather within the limits determined by the methods. A relevant increase, therefore, can certainly be interpreted as a pathological sign.

Complications/Side Effects

Serious complications did not arise in over 600 BAL examinations, over 250 of them conducted within the scope of the study. Decreases of more than 20% of the initial value of the PaO_2 only occurred in 2% of the examinations. In the collective study of patients with multiple injuries, the described general reactions like fever and changes in blood count could not be related to the

BAL. They did not appear in normal persons, or rather in the probands. There is agreement in the international literature that complications with BAL are extremely rare and never dangerous [1, 6] After BAL was performed three times in the same segment, probands suffered chemotaxis of the polymorphonuclear (PMN) granulocytes. However, signs of further phagocyte activity could not be found [3].

Conclusion

For the investigation of the basic mechanism of posttraumatic lung failure, BAL presents the following advantages:

1. For patients with multiple injuries, serial BAL enables immediate and continuous assessment of local alveolar reactions to be made.
2. In addition to the determination of alveolar cytology and the release of mediators, the composition and function of the normal and the altered surfactant can be described only by BAL examination.

References

1. Crystal RG, Reynolds HY, Kalica AR (1986) Bronchoalveolar lavage. The report of an international conference. Chest 89:122
2. Hunninghake GW, Gadek JE, Kawanami O, Ferrans VJ, Crystals RG (1979) Inflammatory and immune processes in the human lung in health and disease: evaluation by bronchoalveolar lavage. Am J Pathol 97:149
3. Joka T, Nakhosteen J, Obertacke U, Herrmann J, Coenen T, Brand M, Jochum M, Zilow G, Dwenger A, Kreuzfelder E (1988) Does bronchoalveolar lavage exercise an influence on the milieu in the alveoli? Prax Klin Pneumol 42:705
4. Marcy TW, Merrill WW, Rankin JA, Reynolds HY (1987) Limitations of using urea to quantify epithelial lining fluid recovered by bronchoalveolar lavage. Am Rev Respir Dis 135:1276
5. Rennard SI, Basset G, Lecossier D, O'Donnell KM, Pinkston P, Martin PG, Crystal RG (1986) Estimation of volume of epithelial lining fluid recovered by lavage using urea as marker of dilution. J Appl Physiol 60:532
6. Reynolds HY (1987) State of art: bronchoalveolar lavage. Am Rev Respir Dis 135:250
7. Reynolds HY, Newball HH (1974) Analysis of proteins and respiratory cells obtained from human lungs by bronchial lavage. J Lab Clin Med 84:559

Morphometric Description of the Study Population

Th. Joka[1], J.A. Sturm[2], U. Obertacke[1], and G. Regel[2]

Introduction

Clinical and laboratory data of 57 patients from two study centers (Hannover, 32; Essen, 25) who complied with the criteria of entry for the study described above (see Sect. "Protocol of the Study") were evaluated. This joint group of patients was distributed homogeneously. Comparison of the two study centers showed both groups to be nearly identical morphometrically (Table 1). The patients were distributed as follows: 40.3% car passengers, 26.4% pedestrians, 16.6% motorcyclists, and 16.7% victims of falls. The average number of single injuries per patient was 8.2. Injuries to the extremities were the commonest, occurring in 97% of patients (Table 2). Furthermore, the majority of patients (83% and 78%, respectively) also suffered injuries to the head and the organs of the thorax. Because severe skull brain injuries were excluded from the study, the head injuries (skull brain trauma, face skull injury) studied were of limited severity. There were no relevant differences between patients from both centers regarding the severity of injuries and injured regions.

The preclinical phase, consisting of first aid to the patients, had an average therapy-free interval (length of time between the accident and the arrival of an ambulance or rescue helicopter) of 16.4 min. The range was relatively small for the joint cohort of the study and no relevant difference was found between both centers.

The duration of the rescue (from the arrival of an emergency doctor until the arrival in the clinic) totaled 1 h on the average, with a relatively large range. This span was due to the number of patients who were admitted to our own clinic only after having received emergency care in another hospital. The time of preclinical endotracheal intubation shows a greater range than for the time lapse following the accident. It ranges in both centers from

[1] Department of Trauma Surgery, University Medical School, Hufelandstr. 55, W-4300 Essen 1, FRG
[2] Department of Trauma Surgery, Hannover Medical School, Konstanty-Gutschow-Str. 8, W-3000 Hannover 61, FRG

J.A. Sturm (Ed.)
Adult Respiratory Distress Syndrome

Table 1. Patient data. $n = 57$ (Hannover, 32; Essen, 25)

Male 45	
Female 12	
Age 36 ± 17 years	
Development of ARDS	25 (Hannover, 15; Essen, 10)
Lethal outcome	21 (Hannover, 12; Essen, 9)
ARDS	17
No ARDS	4

Table 2. Severity of injury [polytrauma score (PTS)]

PTS_{head}	6 ± 4	(83% of all patients)
PTS_{chest}	9 ± 7	(78% of all patients)
$PTS_{abdomen}$	8 ± 8	(52% of all patients)
$PTS_{pelvis/spine}$	6 ± 7	(59% of all patients)
$PTS_{extremities}$	17 ± 10	(97% of all patients)
Mean PTS	47 ± 13	

Table 3. Preclinical treatment

Time without therapy (accident → emergency doctor)	16.4 ± 10.3 min
Time of rescue (emergency doctor → hospital)	61.2 ± 32.5 min
Time of endoctracheal intubation (time after accident)	49.2 ± 41.5 min

early intubations at the scene of the accident, just a few minutes after its occurrence, to intubation and start of respiration after admission to the clinic (Table 3).

Both centers also do not show a difference in the quantities of infusions and transfusions necessary within the first 24 h to achieve primary stabilization. An average of 16 l crystalloid solutions and 9 l blood transfusions were needed in each case.

The surviving patients spent an average of 25 days in the intensive care unit and were sustained on a respirator for an average of 14 days. The number of patients developing adult respiratory distress syndrome (ARDS) and the number of patients who died were the same in both centers. The incidence of ARDS was 44%. The total lethality rates were 36% for the Essen group and 37.5% for the Hannover group. Out of 21 patients, 17 died from ARDS, and only 4 out of the Essen group died from another organ failure (Table 4).

Table 4. Lethal outcome

		"Early" ≤12th day	"Late" >12th day	
ARDS	Essen	1	4	17
	Hannover	10	2	
Non-ARDS	Essen	1	3	4
	Hannover	–	–	
		12	9	21

Summary

Comparison of the patients on an individual basis and on a group basis, the latter depending on the study center to which they were admitted, revealed no significant differences. Patient age, distribution of single injuries, degree of severity of the injury according to polytrauma score (PTS), preclinical therapy, clinical first aid administered, and total lethality rates were nearly the same in both centers. There were great differences, however, with regard to reason for death. Therefore, the joint group appears to be homogeneous according to the introductory criteria, as well as in relation to the morphological data and the patient's course in both centers. It was not possible to establish a correlation between the basic morphometric data and the lethality. Neither was the distribution of injuries in different regions of the body correlated with the appearance of lung failure. However, the severity of injury could be linked with subsequent development of ARDS ($p < 0.001$). The lung contusion documented in the diagnostic sheet showed an ARDS incidence of over 50% for each of the two study centers, as well as on the whole.

Reference

1. Oestern HJ, Tscherne H, Sturm J, Nerlich M (1985) Klassifizierung der Verletzungsschwere. Unfallheilkd 88:465–472

Development of a Linear Scoring System

U. Obertacke[1], Th. Joka[1], and C. Neumann[2]

Introduction

Adult respiratory distress syndrome (ARDS) was first defined as a clinical entity in 1967 by Ashbaugh et al. [1] using the following clinical parameters: severe dyspnea, tachypnea, cyanosis, refractoriness to O_2-therapy, loss of lung compliance, and diffuse alveolar infiltration (X-ray). The precondition for a diagnosis of ARDS was the absence of any pulmonary disease in the patient's history. Of the 12 patients Ashbaugh et al. [1] based his definition of ARDS on, 4 sustained multiple injury and 1 later had respiratory distress syndrome which was caused by a blunt pulmonary contusion.

In 1982 Petty and Fowler [4] introduced the following definite parameters and limits for the definition of ARDS: exclusion of chronic pulmonary disease and left ventricular failure in the clinical history of a catastrophic event, tachypnea > 20/min, diffuse pulmonary infiltrates (X-ray), $PaO_2 < 50\,mmHg/FiO_2 > 0.6$, total respiratory compliance $\leq 50\,ml/cm\ H_2O$, increased shunt fraction, and increased dead space ventilation. Beside clinical and technical measurements of the ventilatory mechanics and gas exchange, Petty and Fowler required an increase in both shunting and deadspace volume for the definition of ARDS.

There has been general agreement on the *clinical* definition of ARDS: It is a pulmonary failure refractory to oxygen without preexisting pulmonary diseases and without an existing restriction of cardial function ("noncardiogenic edema").

The pathophysiological changes in ARDS influence the gas exchange between the alveoli and capillaries, ventilatory mechanics, pulmonary blood flow, and pulmonary interstitium. These pathophysiological processes can be measured by clinical and technical parameters (Fig. 1).

[1] Department of Trauma Surgery, University Medical School, Hufelandstr, 55, W-4300 Essen 1, FRG
[2] Department of Trauma Surgery, Hannover Medical School, Konstanty-Gutschow-Str. 8, W-3000 Hannover 61, FRG

J.A. Sturm (Ed.)
Adult Respiratory Distress Syndrome

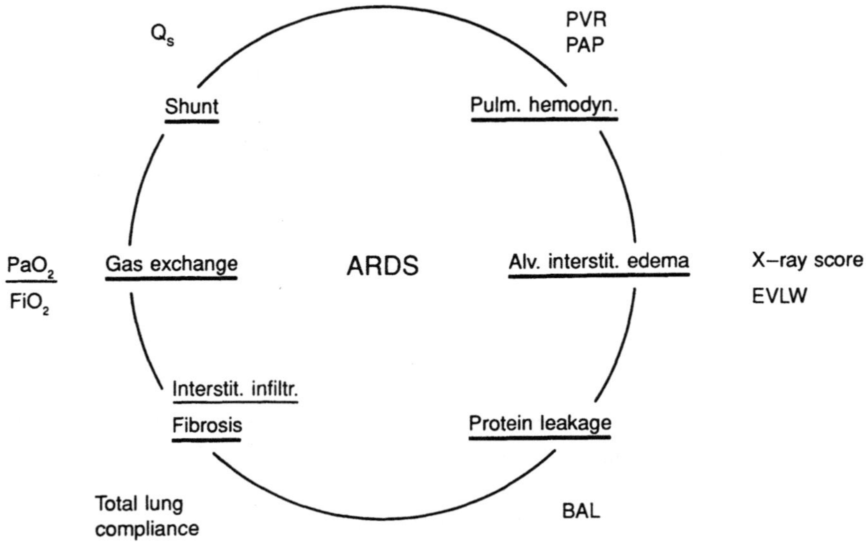

Fig. 1. Adult respiratory distress syndrome: pathophysiological processes (*inner circle*) and clinical parameters and measurements

Methods

Based on these existing criteria and definitions, the patients in Essen were classified according to severity of pulmonary failure daily using steps of 0.1, from 0 (= normal pulmonary function) to 1 (= complete ARDS). The mean value of the daily classification was used as a criterion to differentiate between two groups of patients, on one hand those with ARDS and on the other hand those with MPD (minimal pulmonary dysfunction) (Fig. 2). The dividing line between these groups was defined retrospectively as 0.6. Then a

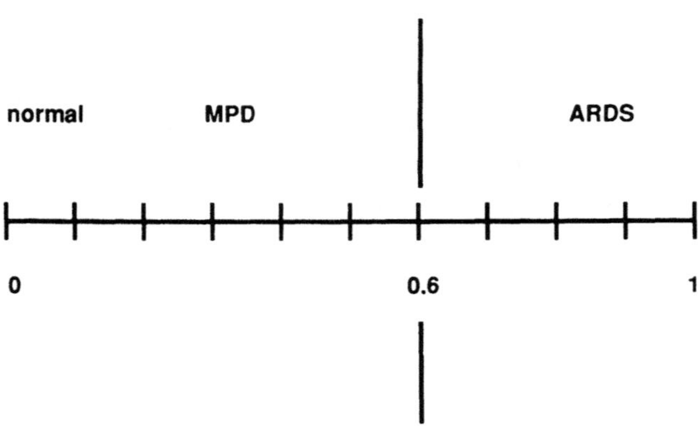

Fig. 2. Subjective classification of "severity of pulmonary failure" from 0 to 1

Table 1. Chest X-ray score [5]

Score	Chest roentgenogram
0	Normal
1	Moderately increased interstitial marking
2	Markedly increased interstitial marking
3	Patchy air-space consolidation
4	Extensive air-space consolidation

stepwise multifactor regressive analysis of all the parameters describing the pulmonary function and mechanical ventilation was performed. This produced the linear score:

$$Y = \sum_{i=1}^{n} a_i x_i + a_0$$

Four unknowns were left: Alveolar-arterial oxygen quotient $(PAO_2 - PaO_2)/PAO_2$ (OQ), chest X-ray score (Suter [5], Table 1) (X-ray), mean pulmonary artery pressure (PAPm), and total static pulmonary compliance (C). Extravascular lung water (EVLW) and positive end expiratory pressure (PEEP) did not contribute to the explanation of this model.

Results

The arrived linear score was:

$$0.108 + 0.62081\,\mathrm{OQ} + 0.1512\,\text{X-ray} + 0.00725\,\mathrm{PAPm} - 0.00416\,\mathrm{C}. \qquad [2a]$$

The R^2 for this model was 0.75, i.e., 75% of the variability of the ARDS score was explained by the clinical and technical parameters. The coefficient of correlation (Spearman's) of this score to the severity of pulmonary failure was 0.86 ($p = 0.001$) (Fig. 3).

To check the quality of this ARDS scoring system we had to answer three questions:

1. How stable is the model if mean values over a shortened period (less than 14 days) are introduced as parameters to the model?
2. What effects can be seen if only a selection of patients are used to arrive at the score?
3. What are the results for other patients who were not classified by our team?

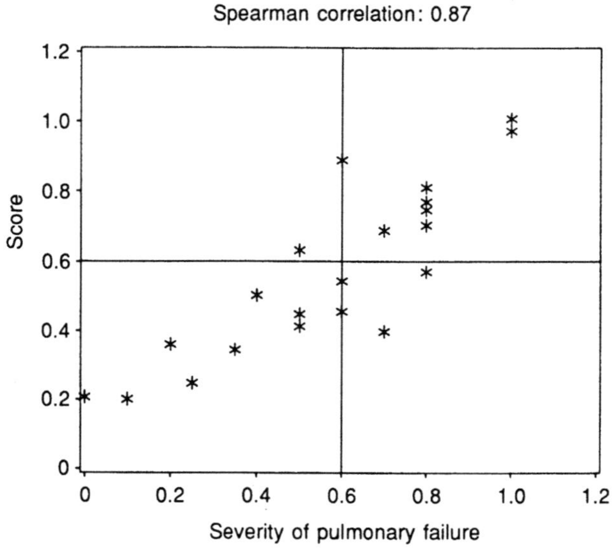

Fig. 3. Corrélation between ARDS score and severity of pulmonary failure in the Essen group

Considering the first two questions we were able to demonstrate that the model had sufficient stability: No more than four patients were classified differently by ARDS/MPD using the scoring system with a smaller number of patients or shorter periods (≥48 h) for the observation.

For the third question we tested the model with the group of patients from Hannover. We found a Spearman's correlation of 0.72 for the classification, a sensitivity of 0.88, and a specificity of 0.76 (Fig. 4).

Conclusions

The score is valid because it is based only on criteria for the definition of ARDS, and thus a classification of patients with ARDS/MPD based on objective measurable parameters is possible. Score values of >0.6 in an observation period of 48 h from one single patient are sufficient for the determination of ARDS.

Murray et al. [2] and Petty [3] in 1988 demanded improved definition and diagnostic detection of ARDS:

The need for an ARDS scoring system was stressed, and a lung injury score with the parameters X-ray, OQ, PEEP, and C was also suggested, from which the extend of pulmonary failure could be classified as "mild," "moderate," or "severe."

The scoring system we have introduced, in addition to this, demonstrates the parameters influencing ARDS, with one factor for each parameter, which

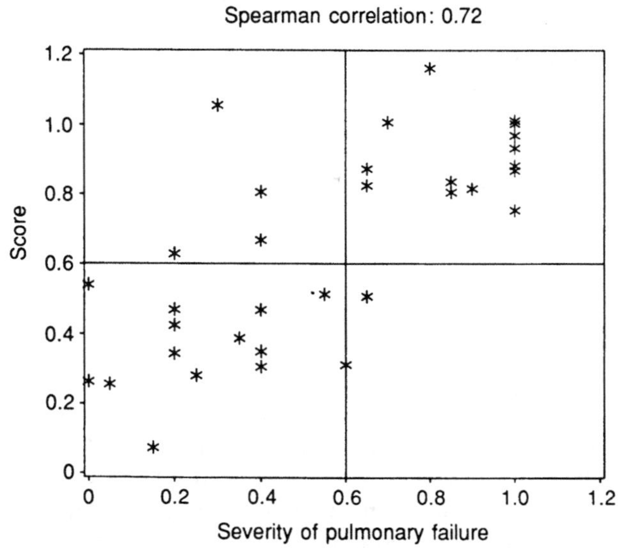

Fig. 4. Correlation between ARDS score and severity of pulmonary failure in the Hannover group

should determine the relevance of each parameter for the pathogenesis of ARDS. Using multifactor regressive analysis nonrelevant parameters for the definition and numerical measurement of ARDS were omitted.

References

1. Ashbaugh DG, Bigelow DB, Petty TL, Levine BE (1967) Acute respiratory distress in adults. Lancet 2:319
2. Murray JF, Matthay MA, Luce JM, Flick MR (1988) An expanded definition of the adult respiratory distress syndrome. Am Rev Respir Dis 138:720

2a. Obertacke U, Kulotai J, Coenen Th, Joka Th, Schmit-Neuerburg KP (1988) Ein linearer ARDS – Schweregradscore. Intensivmed 25:264

3. Petty TL (1988) ARDS: refinement of concept and redefinition. Am Rev Respir Dis 138:724
4. Petty TL, Fowler AA (1982) Another look at ARDS. Chest 82:98
5. Suter PM (1987) Adult respiratory distress syndrome: a scoring system for the estimation of the gravity of pulmonary disease and comparison of patient populations. In: Kox W, Bihari D (eds) Shock and the adult respiratory distress syndrome. Springer, London, p. 220

Clinical Definition of ARDS
An Index Based on Bedside-Derived Parameters*

C. Neumann, J.A. Sturm, and G. Regel

Introduction

In the present study one of the major problems was classification of patients into groups with or without adult respiratory distress syndrome (ARDS). The pathomorphologic substrate of ARDS is an interstitial edema showing high protein concentrations, which can be measured as extravascular lung water (EVLW). Therefore the primary parameter for determining ARDS and EVLW. Clinical definitions of ARDS as found in the literature are mostly unspecific, simply requiring "respiratory failure" with ventilation. Some definitions require certain values of respiratory parameters in conjunction with low left atrial filling pressures to exclude left pulmonary insufficiency due to left ventricular failure [1]. But these definitions have shown to be too unspecific for the purpose of the present study, which describes the development of an ARDS index to assess ARDS by clinical parameters and validation of ARDS grouping by EVLW.

Methods

To derive the ARDS index, 75 patients with a total of 152 lung water measurements and documentation of pulmonary function [dynamic compliance, $AaDO_2$, oxygenation index ($AaDO_2$/alveolar pO_2 + 0.0014 × PEEP) [2], Shunt] and hemodynamics [mean arterial pulmonary pressure (PPAM) capillary wedge pressure (PCWP)] during their course in the intensive care unit were investigated retrospectively. Due to the skewness of compliance data, compliance was entered in the analysis as 1/compliance.

Clinical parameters were correlated with EVLW, and stepwise multiple linear regression performed. The parameters with the best correlation were

---

* Supported by Deutsche Forschungsgemeinschaft Project No. TS 14/3–1; 2; 4.

Department of Trauma Surgery, Hannover Medical School, Konstanty-Gutschow-Str. 8, W-3000 Hannover 61, FRG

J.A. Sturm (Ed.)
Adult Respiratory Distress Syndrome

entered into discriminant analysis and the formula for an ARDS index derived. The criterion for this analysis was an EVLW value of 10 ml/kg body weight, which reflects the mean EVLW found in normal healthy patients plus twice the standard deviation [3]. The ARDS index was then prospectively tested on data of the present study. To predict a patient as being an ARDS patient, the ARDS index had to be positive at least three times. This criterion was tested against the ARDS classification by EVLW.

Results

Retrospective Analysis

The correlation of the clinical parameters with EVLW was poor (r about 0.5). Oxygenation index, compliance, and mean arterial pulmonary pressure were entered in stepwise performed multiple linear regression. Inclusion of more parameters did not further increase the significance of this analysis. Using discriminant analysis, the following formula was derived:

$$\text{ARDS index} = 4.71 \times \text{oxygenation index} + 36.5/\text{compliance} + 0.02\ \text{PPAM} - 5.83$$

Positive values indicate the prediction of EVLW higher than 10 ml/kg body wt., and negative values low EVLW. Sensitivity in this retrospective group of ARDS index measurements was 75% (out of 64 measurements with a high EVLW, 48 were predicted) and specificity was 81% (out of 88 measurements of low EVLW, 71 were predicted correctly).

Prospective Analysis

The prospective application of the ARDS index on all measurements of the present study is shown in Table 1. Sensitivity was not as high as found in the retrospective group. The time course of EVLW and the ARDS index is shown in Fig. 1. The ARDS index became positive about 48 h later than the point at which EVLW passed the 10 ml mark. Classification of patients by a three times positive ARDS index compared with classification by EVLW showed a sensitivity of 92% and a specificity of 100% (Table 2).

Discussion

Selection of parameters in the retrospective group by stepwise multiple linear regression was very interesting. Each parameter used described a different

Table 1. Prospective application of the ARDS index

		EVLW > 10 ml/kg	
		Yes	No
ARDS index	>0	155	55
	<0	101	552
		61%	91%

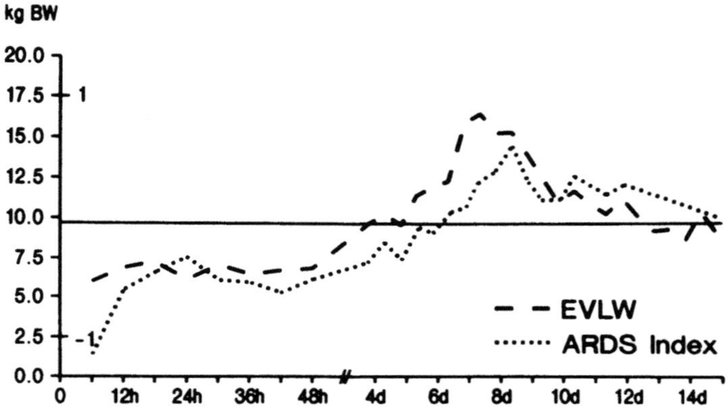

Fig. 1. Time course of the EVLW and ARDS indexes

Table 2. Classification of patients by a three times positive ARDS index

	Yes	No
Three times positive ARDS index	23	0
	2	31
	92%	100%

compartment of the lung. This provided an excellent fit to the clinical course of ARDS, which affects the alveolocapillary wall (oxygenation index), stiffness (compliance), and PPAM [4].

Application of the derived index to the present group showed an excellent prediction value of 82%, although sensitivity was much lower than specificity. This has to be explained by a delayed increase in index values compared with an increase in EVLW at about 48 h (Fig. 1). During this time high EVLW was not predicted, which resulted in lower sensitivity.

The overall classification by a three times positive ARDS index fits the actual classification by EVLW very well (Table 2).

Conclusion

The derived ARDS index detects high EVLW values very well in manifest ARDS although it fails to detect the initial EVLW increase. The classification by EVLW is confirmed by the ARDS index, i.e, the given classification is validated. All investigations comparing these groups have a solid statistical base.

References

1. Pepe PE, Potkin RT, Holtmann Reus D, Hudson LD, Carrico CJ (1982) Clinical predictors of adult respiratory distress syndrome. Am J Surg 144:124–130
2. Sturm JA, Oestern HJ, Maghsudi M (1992) Die gravimetrische Überprüfung der klinischen Lungenwassermessungen (Thermo-green-dye). Chir Forum 10:49–53
3. Benzer H, Koller W, Duma S, Mutz N, Pauser (1983) Ein Modell zur einheitlichen Behandlung und Therapieauswertung bei schwerem ARDS. Anästhesist 32:576–581
4. Lium B (1983) Adult respiratory distress syndrome (ARDS). Incidence, clinical findings, pathomorphology and pathogenesis. Nord Vet Med 35:38–47

Treatment and Clinical Course

TH. JOKA[1], U. OBERTACKE[1], J.A. STURM[2], and M.L. NERLICH[2]

Common Concept for Treatment

The 57 patients in this study (32/25) were treated at two centers, Essen and Hannover, following a common schematic protocol. All patients were included in all indicated types of therapy which fulfilled the requirements of this study.

Volume substitution was performed only with crystalloid solution (Fox's, Ringers lactate, NaCl 0.9%), blood components (whole blood, fresh whole blood, packed RBC), and plasma preparations. Protein solutions (fresh frozen plasma) were administered if the patient's total protein serum level fell below 3 g/l. The degree of volume substitution was controlled by the parameters urine output, central venous pressure, and cardiac output.

To exclude the influence of different remedies on the laboratory parameters measured, the two centers agreed on a list of drugs commonly used in intensive care with definite indications, including vasoactive drugs such as dopamine, dobutamine, glycerol, and digitalis, buffer solutions (lysine chloride/$NaHCO_3$), heparin (15000 IU/day), analgesic and sedative drugs (morphine/benzodiazepine), narcotics, and insulin for total parenteral nutrition. The administration of steroids, antihistamines (H1 blockers), barbiturates, and proteinase inhibitors was excluded. Parenteral nutrition was provided according to the uniform scheme shown in Table 1.

A precondition for the control of cardiac function was a cardiac index of 3 l/min. A constant decrease under this nominal value either caused – with respect to the underlying disturbance – volume substitution or necessitated the administration of vasoactive drugs. Guideline figures for respiratory function were a PaO_2 of 80–100 mmHg and a $PaCO_2$ of less than 40 mmHg.

[1] Department of Trauma Surgery, University Medical School, Hufelandstr. 55, W-4300 Essen, FRG

[2] Department of Trauma Surgery, Hannover Medical School, Konstanty-Gutschow-Str. 8, W-3000 Hannover 61, FRG

J.A. Sturm (Ed.)
Adult Respiratory Distress Syndrome

Table 1. Parenteral nutrition in the treatment of multiply injured patients

Time elapsed after trauma	Type of nutrition	Quantity (g/kg body wt)
Day 2/3	Carbohydrates	1.7
	Amino acids	1.0
Day 4/5	Carbohydrates	3.4
	Amino acids	1.4
After day 6	Carbohydrates	5.7
	Amino acids	1.4
As soon as possible	Nasoenteric tube feeding	

Management of respiratory and metabolic functions aimed to maintain a BE of −2 to +2 mVal/l. Defective oxygenation was treated by enhancement of positive endexspiratory pressure (PEEP) or manipulation of the relationship of inspiration to exspiration time (I:E), and not primarily by increase of FIO_2. Only after all ventilatory methods had been exhausted in regard to patient cardiac tolerance was stepwise increase of FIO_2 performed. Patients were removed from mechanical ventilation using the common methods of synchronized intermittent mandatory ventilations (SIMV) and continuous positive airway pressure (CPAP).

In spite of agreement on uniform therapy, small differences in therapeutic details occurred in both centers. A mean pulmonary artery pressure increase of over 30–35 mmHg was treated only in Essen with nitroglycerin. In Essen, ventilatory mechanics were regulated primarily by changes in PEEP, whereas in Hannover the I:E was usually changed with a constant PEEP.

Results

Reviewing all patient data, we found no major differences in volume substitution. The quantity of crystalloid infusion obtained within the first 48 h was up to 22000 ml/patient. The increment of fluid from 0–48 h was 23000 ml. In the second stage (3rd–7th day), the amount of crystalloid solution decreased to 4200 ml/patient, whereas in the third stage (>7th day) it increased again to over 10000 ml. The average high positive increments were mainly found in patients with prognostic severe course in all of the three stages.

To maintain hemoglobin at a level of 10–11 g/dl, 12000 ml blood was needed on average for each patient. The parameters for controlling adequate volume substitution (cardiac output, central venous pressure, urine output) and also the use of transfusions (hemoglobin) showed considerable agreement between both centers.

Operative Management

The operative treatment of the patients showed some differences between the two centers. These differences had no influence on the further course of the disease and the prognosis of the patient as far as the development of ARDS or lethality was concerned.

At Essen all life-saving procedures were carried out and fractures close to the trunk operated on within the first operative stage, with the aim of performing a primary and full treatment of most fractures. Treatment by traction in bone fractures was only given in exceptional circumstances. This resulted in 71.2% of all procedures being performed within 48 h, with a mean procedure length of 5 h. Between the 3rd and 7th day, 10.8% of procedures were performed, and only fractures of small bones, plastic procedures, and additional bone fixations were performed later (Fig. 1).

In Hannover, 64.2% of all procedures were performed during the first stage, within 48 h. Fractures close to the trunk were not operated on in the first 48 h, but treated by traction in the first stage. Consequently, the mean procedure length during the first stage was 3 h. Nineteen percent of the procedures were performed in the second stage (3rd–7th day). In the third stage (>7th day), further operative treatment was similar to that in Essen (Fig. 2).

The methods of operative treatment even of bone fractures were similar in both centers. The main difference was the preference for intramedullary nailing for femur or lower leg fractures in Hannover in comparison with the usual plate fixation at Essen. The complication rate of operative treatment showed no major differences between the two groups of patients. Repeated procedures on the body cavities and extremities had to be undertaken as

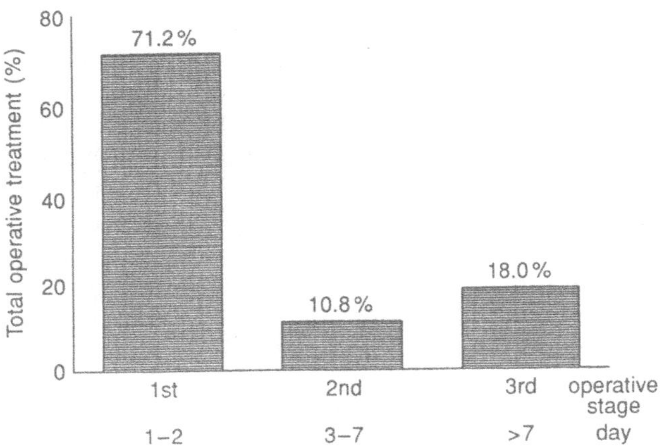

Fig. 1. Timing of operative treatment of multiply injured patients in Essen

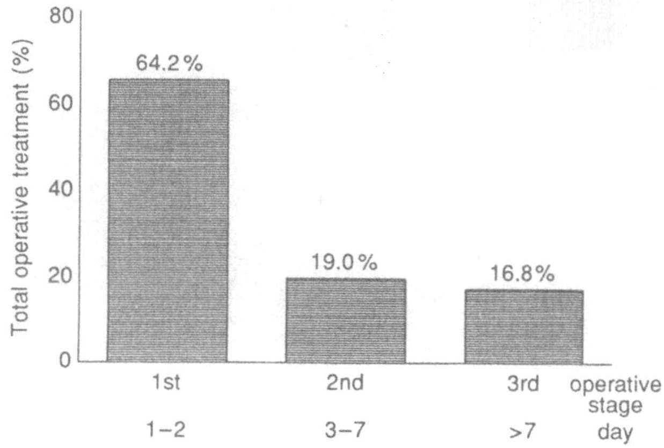

Fig. 2. Timing of operative treatment of multiply injured patients in Hannover

frequently in Essen as in Hannover. A total of 4.1 operative procedures were performed per patient in both centers.

The whole group of patients as well as the groups at each center proved to be homogeneous and comparable as far as treatment was concerned. Different nuances in cardiac/respiratory management and in the method or time of operative treatment chosen showed no influence on the development of ARDS, lethality, or mediator release.

Clinical Course

During the course of the 14-day study, a large body of clinical and laboratory data was recorded, reflecting the function of various organ systems.

Lung

The classic parameters for describing progressive pulmonary failure, used in the definition of ARDS, are compliance, oxygenation quotient (OQ), shunt fraction (Q_S/Q_T), mean pulmonary artery pressure (PAP_m), and extravascular lung water (EVLW). Within the first hours compliance separates patients with later development of ARDS from those without ($p = 0.05$). OQ data from the 12th h also showed a significant difference between the two groups of patients (ARDS/non-ARDS). The patients who developed ARDS had low OQs between the 12th h and 4th day, and on the 4th day a significant deterioration, with a drop in OQ of about 25%, occurred (Fig. 3).

A comparable picture was found in intrapulmonary right–left shunt (Q_S/Q_T). At the 18th h, there were significant and permanent differences between

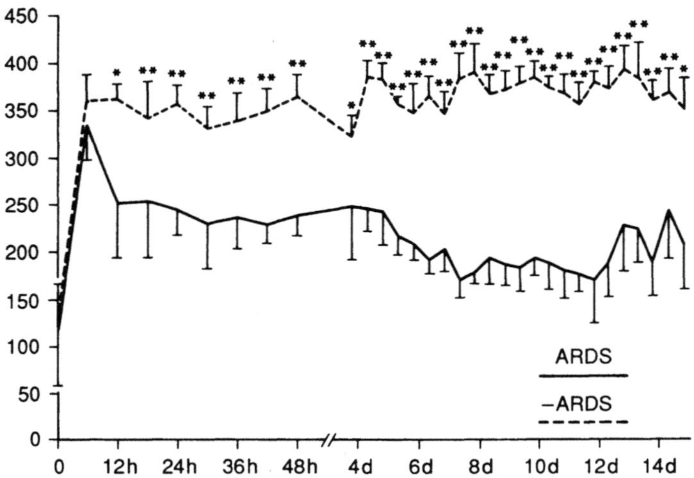

Fig. 3. 14-day course of the oxygenation quotient in both groups of patients (ARDS/non-ARDS). Level of significance: * <0.05; ** <0.01; *d*, day

the ARDS and non-ARDS group. The non-ARDS group had Q_S/Q_T of 10% after the 6th h, which was physiologically normal, whereas from the 4th day the ARDS group's Q_S/Q_T increased up to 20%, indicating a poor prognosis. The Hannover group was found to have an earlier and higher increase in Q_S/Q_T.

The course of PAP_m was significantly different between the ARDS and non-ARDS group from the 12th to the 24th h and also from the 4th day on throughout the whole study period. Prognostically poor values of over 30 mmHg were reached from the 4th day in the ARDS group. The greatest increase was found between the 24th and 36th h and during the 4th day after trauma. Patients at Essen were found to have permanently – sometimes significantly – lower values of PAP_m and pulmonary vascular resistance than the patients at Hannover. This correlated with the administration of nitroglycerin to lower blood pressure and pulmonary vascular resistance in the lesser circulation of patients at Essen.

Measurement of EVLW by the thermal-dye method showed a significant difference between the ARDS and non-ARDS group from the 4th to the 5th day after trauma, when the ARDS group had values around 10 ml/kg body weight, indicating a poor prognosis. The non-ARDS group had values around 6 ml/kg body weight over the whole of the measuring period. Thus, EVLW as an indicator of interstitial edema showed for the ARDS group the expected chronological order of the initial damage and increase in EVLW, because inflammatory changes in the lung interstitium and its alveolar structures must precede the development of an interstitial edema (Fig. 4).

Prognostic indexes like $PaO_2 \times Cl$ and $FIO_2 \times PAP_m$ have no predictive value for either group of patients and are unable to separate the two groups (ARDS/non-ARDS) at any time of the measuring period.

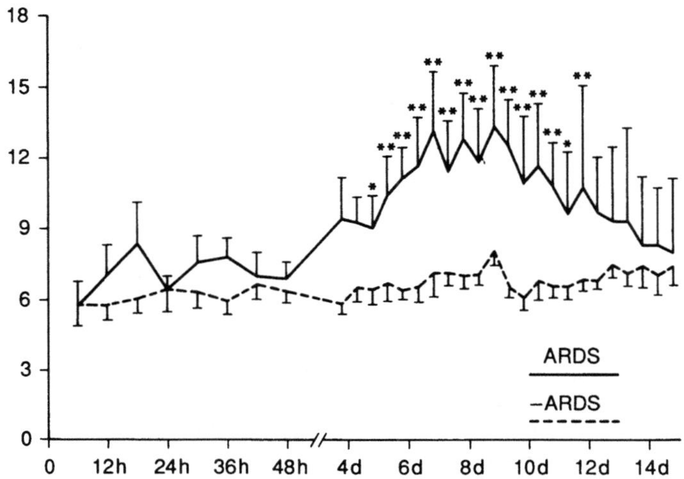

Fig. 4. 14-day course of the extravascular lung water (ml/kg body weight) as a marker of interstitial lung edema in both groups of patients (ARDS/non-ARDS). Level of significance: * <0.05; ** <0.01; *d*, day

Liver

The most remarkable parameter of liver function in the posttraumatic period is the level of bilirubin in human serum. During the clinical course, the two groups of patients (ARDS/non-ARDS) can be separated starting at the 7th day as far as the serum bilirubin level is concerned. By the 9th day there is a significant difference, which lasts for the whole study period (Fig. 5). The increase in serum bilirubin levels in the ARDS group also affects – although there were lower peak values – the survivors of ARDS in both centers. There was a highly significant correlation betwen γ-glutamyl-transferase (γ-GT) and

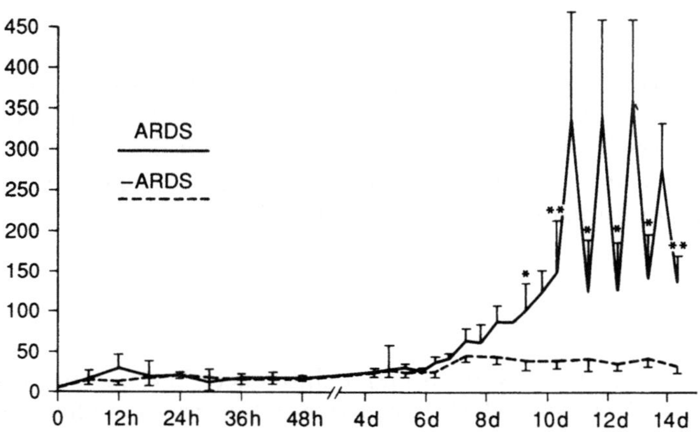

Fig. 5. 14-day course of serum bilirubin (μmol/l) in both groups of patients (ARDS/non-ARDS). Level of significance: * <0.05; ** <0.01; *d*, day

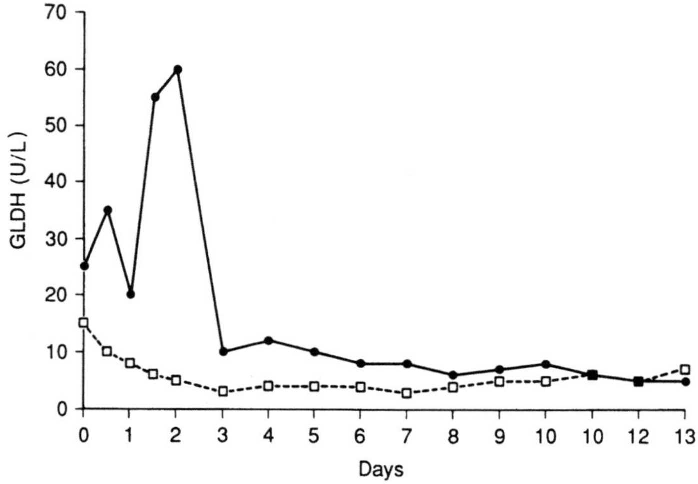

Fig. 6. 14-day course of the serum glutamat-dehydrogenase (U/I) in patients who survived (*broken line*) or died from multiple organ failure (*unbroken line*) later

prognosis: Starting with a noticeable difference by the 5th/6th day, from the 7th day γ-GT became a highly significant prognostic parameter in terms of survival or death in the ARDS group.

Serum glutamat-dehydrogenase (GLDH) also appeared to have a significant prognostic value in the first stage for the patients who died later. An early increase (24th h to 4th day) indicated extended damage of liver cells due to a higher incidence of liver trauma (Fig. 6).

To sum up, liver function parameters had prognostic value for the patients. In both groups we found frequent deaths from multiple organ failure (MOF) at a late posttraumatic stage after the study had finished.

Kidney

There were differences in endogenous clearance of creatinine (ECC) between ARDS and non-ARDS patients from the 12th h and lasting almost over the whole 14 days, although levels in the ARDS group did not decrease below 100 ml/min during this time. No clinically evident renal failure could be found in any of the patients during the study period (Fig. 7).

Circulation

The circulation parameters showed no major differences between the two groups of patients (ARDS/non-ARDS). Apparent differences in pulmonary capillary wedge pressure (PCWP) and the mean pressures in the lesser and

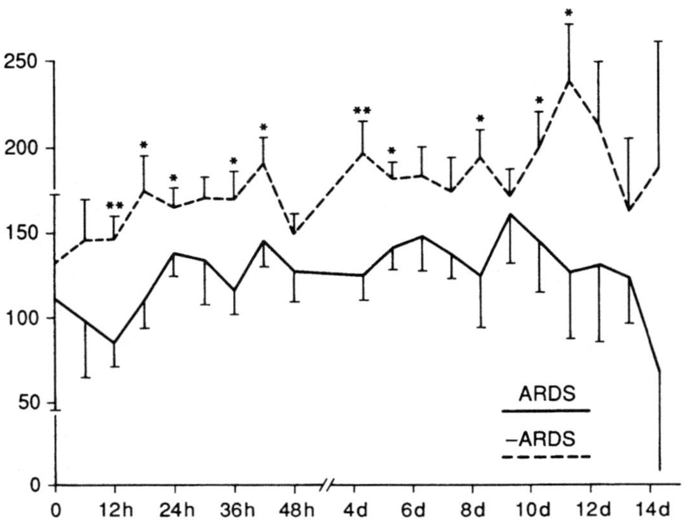

Fig. 7. 14-day course of the endogenous clearance of creatinine (ml/min) in both groups of patients (ARDS/non-ARDS). Level of significance * <0.05 ** <0.01; *d*, day

greater circulation were caused by respiratory therapy (increase in PEEP, reversing the relationship between inspiration and exspiration time) and the administration of vasoactive remedies. The cardiac output and cardiac index were used as control parameters for the treatment and showed no differences for both groups of patients. Body temperature, an important parameter of the peripheral circulation, showed differences between the two groups of patients initially and also up to the 12th h. This can be interpreted as indicating a higher total severity of injury sustained in the ARDS group (Fig. 8).

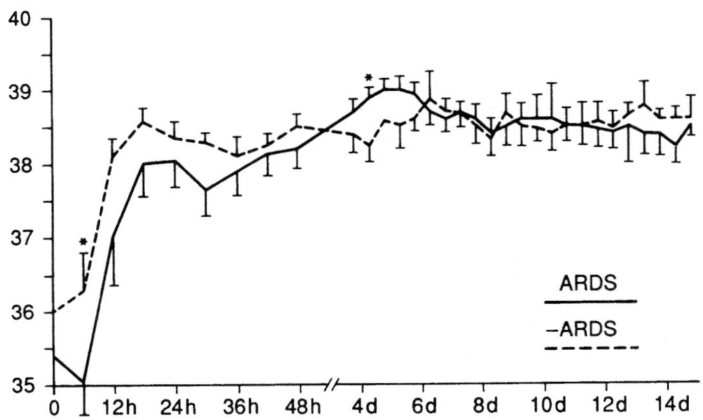

Fig. 8. 14-days course of the highest body temperature in both groups of patients (ARDS/non-ARDS). Level of significance: * <0.05, ** <0.01; *d*, day

Bone Marrow and Blood Cells

The white blood cells in peripheral blood showed no differences between the ARDS and non-ARDS groups over the whole study period, and showed a characteristic posttraumatic course for both groups of patients, with very low variability. A level of 10000 leukocytes/mm^3 up to the 6th day after trauma was followed by leukocytosis of 18000/mm^3 on the 10th–12th day. Monocytes and lymphocytes showed an uncharacteristic course after trauma. Platelets were decreased significantly in the ARDS group over almost the whole study period from the 6th h after trauma. From the 12th h, the platelet count of the ARDS group fell below the threshold of 100000 platelets/mm^3. There was minimal variation in the values between the 12th h and 9th day for the ARDS group. The values for the non-ARDS group showed a significantly higher but parallel course up to the 4th day, and then rapidly increased in platelet count up to normal values of 400000/mm^3, with little variation (Fig. 9).

The hemoglobin levels in the ARDS group initially showed a highly significant difference. This indicated the much more serious injuries. After 12 h, the course of hemoglobin levels in all patients was constant at a level of 11 g/dl with minimal variation (Fig. 10).

Conclusion

Comparison of the Essen and Hannover group showed that the basic morphometric data and the therapeutic interventions did not influence

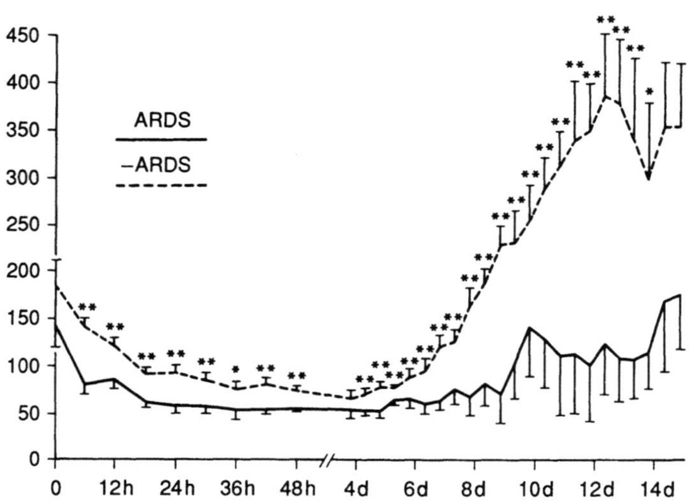

Fig. 9. 14-day course of the platelets in both groups of patients (ARDS/non-ARDS). Level of significance: * <0.05, ** <0.01; *d*, day

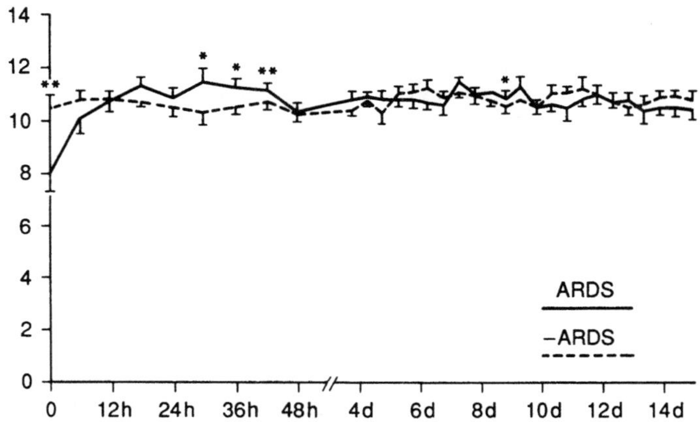

Fig. 10. 14-day course of the hemoglobin (g/dl) in both groups of patients (ARDS/non-ARDS). Level of significance: * <0.05, ** <0.01; *d*, day

prognosis in respect of ARDS and survival. In spite of this there were significant differences in terms of time of death and extent of organ failure. In the patient group in Hannover, the time of death was mainly in the period from the 8th to the 12th day, with progressive pulmonary failure (ARDS) playing a prominent role. In Essen, the patients usually survived this stage, whereas on the 20th day after trauma there were a number of deaths, with MOF as the major cause.

The Hannover Polytrauma Score (PTS) and other parameters which are an expression of the more serious injuries such as hemoglobin level, body temperature, GLDH, γ-GT (Table 2) were indicators of the prognosis and lethality of ARDS. The ARDS and non-ARDS groups of patients could be separated by significant differences in pulmonary functional parameters (compliance, OQ, Q_S/Q_T, PAP_m) and by parameters such as peripheral platelet count and ECC. EVLW (from the 4th day after trauma) and serum bilirubin level (from the 9th day after trauma) were further descriptive parameters.

Table 2. Parameters of prognostic value for the development of ARDS and MOF

ARDS	severity of injury compliance OQ ($PAO_2 - PaO_2/PAO_2$) PAP_m Q_S/Q_T platelets creatinine clearance
Lung/liver organ failure	EVLW bilirubin level

Table 3. Distribution of lethal outcome among all patients in both centers

		Early (<12th day)	Late (>12th day)	
ARDS	Essen	1	4	17
	Hannover	10	2	
Non-ARDS	Essen	1	3	4
	Hannover	0	0	
		12	9	21

If we postulate the multiple reactions after trauma to be manifestations of similar reactions at different organs and organ systems, we see typical posttraumatic changes in the kidney, lung, liver, and bone marrow. In each system we were able to see significant, sometimes early, changes indicative of prognosis. Kidney function, however, was maintained – with significant differences – in both the ARDS and the non-ARDS groups of patients. Pulmonary and hepatic failure were the most frequent causes of posttraumatic death, with a mean time of death from progressive pulmonary failure on the 10th day and from progressive hepatic failure on the 20th day after trauma.

We found a predominance of progressive pulmonary failure in patients at Hannover and a predominance of hepatic failure and MOF in patients at Essen (Table 3). Total lethality and total morbidity from ARDS were almost the same in the both the Essen and Hannover groups.

Progressive Organ Failure

M.L. NERLICH

Introduction

In the past 2 decades progressive failure of several organ systems has accounted for the majority of deaths in intensive care patients. The syndrome of multiple organ failure (MOF) has been described by Baue [1] as a sequence of organ failures initiated by shock, trauma, or sepsis. The definition of MOF is arbitrary, the number and rank of the organ systems involved varying and depending on the individual judgment of the investigators [1, 2, 6, 11]. The methods of measuring changes of "normal," "insufficient," and "failing" organ function vary greatly [1, 3, 6, 7, 11]. Determination of the extent of organ failure therefore is not standardized or schematic.

In an attempt to further describe MOF, scores like the Acute Physiology Chronic Health Evaluation (APACHE II) [9], Sepsis Severity Score (SSS) [15], and Multiple Organ Failure (MOF) Score [8] have been developed to differentiate the degree of organ failure and to summarize larger numbers of parameters indicative of organ function.

In a clinical study on a group of well-defined multiple-injured patients, the extent of organ failure was evaluated prospectively, applying scores to a large number of measured parameters.

Material and Methods

Thirty-eight multiple-injured patients met the study criteria, which were:

1. Severity of injury of more than 30 points on the Polytrauma Score (PTS) [14]
2. Age, 15–65 years
3. Prehospital therapy-free interval less than 60 min

Department of Trauma Surgery, Hannover Medical School, Kanstanty-Gutschow-Str. 8, W-3000 Hannover, 61, FRG

J.A. Sturm (Ed.)
Adult Respiratory Distress Syndrome

4. Accident-admission time less than 120 min
5. Glasgow-Coma Scale (GCS) more than 8 points
6. No steroids, colloids, or protease inhibitors
7. Constant and uniform therapeutic regimen in the intensive care unit.

The Hannover Polytrauma Score (PTS) is an anatomically oriented injury severity score more practicable than the Injury Severity Scale (ISS). Injuries with more than 30 points have a lethality of about 50%.

Cardiocirculatory, pulmonary, renal, hepatic, gastrointestinal, and cerebral organ functions were followed over a 2-week time course by daily measurements, within the first 48 h after accident by 6 h checks.

A retrospective of definition sepsis was used to describe the septic state including the following criteria:

1. Temperature maximum over 39°C
2. Central-peripheral temperature difference more than 8°C
3. Positive fluid balance, +1500 ml/24 h
4. Decrease in oxygenation quotient more than 100/24 h
5. Increase in extravascular lung water (EVLW) more than 3 ml/kg body wt./24 h
6. Platelet count less than 100 000/μl and/or decrease of 30%/24 h
7. Leukocyte count change of 5000 μl/24 h
8. Factor II and/or factor V decrease of 30%/24 h.

If five of these eight criteria were met, the patient was considered to be in a septic state.

Positive bacteriological findings such as positive blood culture or an infectious focus like pus secretion were not necessary for this retrospective definition of sepsis.

For a comparative analysis the study population was divided into patients with and without septic state. To both groups three scores were prospectively applied, the APACHE II [9], the SSS [15], and the MOF score (Goris et al. 1987). In addition to the retrospective definition of sepsis, an index was generated to further quantitatively describe the extent of organ failure and the septic state. In the first step, using a factor analysis, a reduction of 180

Table 1. Morphometric data on the polytrauma study group

	Septic patients n = 18	Nonseptic patients n = 17
Age (years)	39.7	34.2
Rescue time (min)	63.9	59.3
Perhospital volume therapy (ml)	4617	3776
PTS (n)	42.6	42.0
ISS (n)	29.6	28.7
Blood replacement (1/24 h)	10.2	8.8
Crystalloids (1/24 h)	20.2	19.2
Lethal outcome	13	1

measured parameters to 80 variables could be achieved. To further eliminate nonsignificant parameters a comparison of the septic versus the nonseptic patient group (according to the retrospective definition of sepsis) was performed by the Mann-Whitney test (U-test). The resulting these means an equation of discriminant factors was established which differentiated between septic and nonseptic patients.

Results

The comparison of morphometric data between both groups showed no significant differences. Eighteen septic patients were compared with 17 patients being judged as not septic. The lethality in both groups was significantly different. Seventy-two percent of the septic patients died whereas only one of the nonseptic patients (18%) had a lethal outcome (Table 1).

Adult respiratory distress syndrome (ARDS) as a major contributing feature was recorded in 14 out of 18 septic patients, whereas only 1 patient developed ARDS without septic reaction. A number of highly significant hemodynamic differences could be detected between the 4th and 10th day after trauma. Most impressive was the increased pulmonary artery pressure in the septic patients with a significant difference 12 h after the injury (Fig. 1). The cardiac index showed a significant decrease a septic patients around the 4th day (Fig. 2). A hyperdynamic sepsis phase could not be detected.

The largest differences between the septic and the nonseptic group were found in respiratory parameters. Oxygenation as well as ventilation was impaired in the septic-reacting patients. The alveolo-arterial oxygen differ-

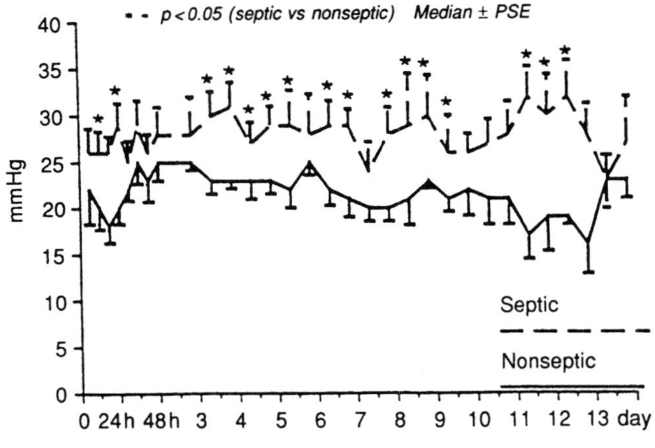

Fig. 1. Pulmonary artery pressure

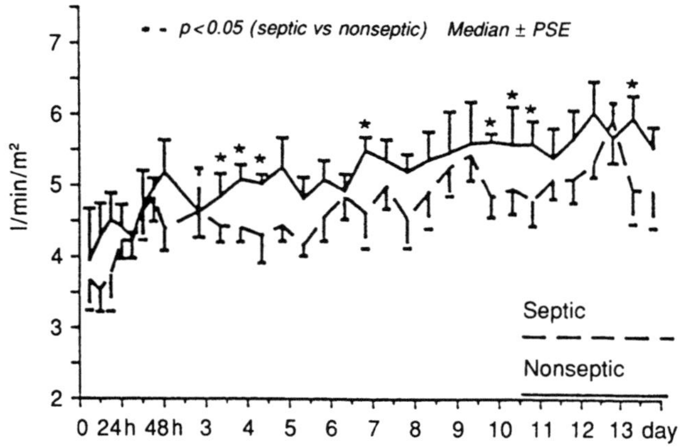

Fig. 2. Cardiac index

ence ($AaDO_2$), a gas exchange index, was significantly reduced in septic patients.

Extravascular lung water was measured according to the method of Lewis et al. [10], using a lung-water computer with the thermal-dye double-indicator dilution technique. EVLW reflects the amount of fluid accumulation in the lung. There was a striking difference between the septic and the nonseptic patients starting the 3rd to 4th day after trauma. The EVLW was used as an indicator for ongoing permeability damage with a consequent interstitial fluid accumulation in the lung (Fig. 3).

The most striking difference in hematological parameters was showed by the platelet count. The recovery of the platelet count after trauma was significantly slowed down in the group of septic-reacting patients (Fig. 4). Significant differences could be shown in the level of urea, with a progressive

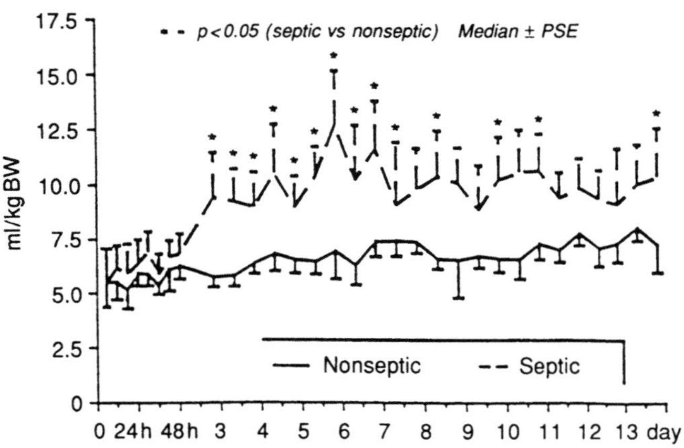

Fig. 3. Extravascular lung water

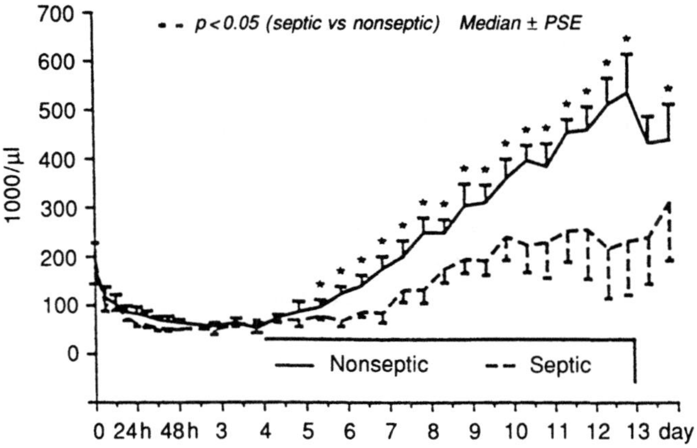

Fig. 4. Platelet count

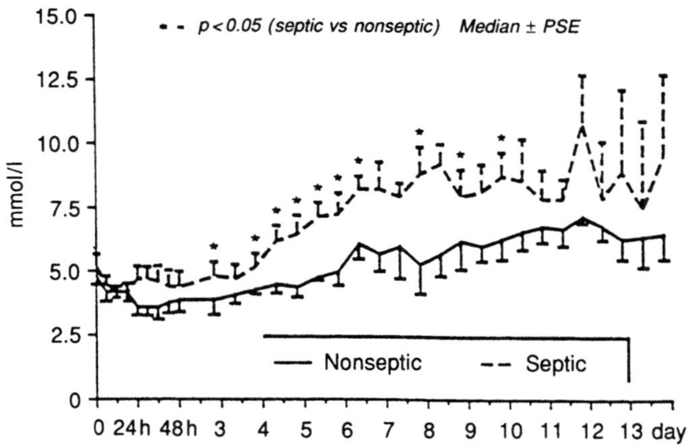

Fig. 5. Serum urea level

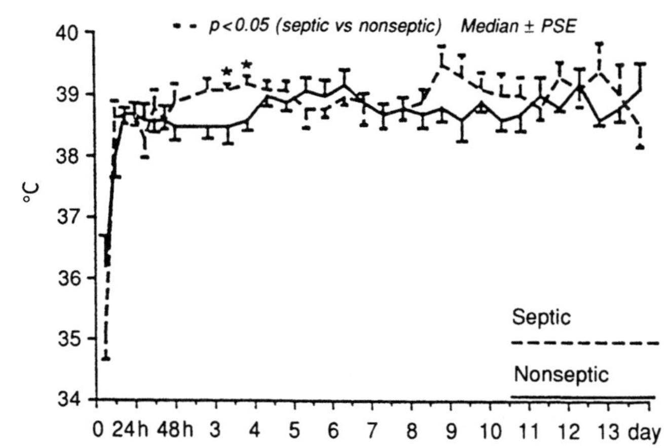

Fig. 6. Maximum body temperature

increase in septic patients starting early after trauma (Fig. 5). The body temperature in both groups was constantly elevated showing fever in both groups. The differences between the groups concerning this classical sepsis parameter were significant around the 4th day after trauma; nevertheless even the nonseptic patients showed constantly elevated temperatures of around 38.5°C (Fig. 6).

All three scores used showed significant differences between both groups (Figs. 7–9). Using the scores, a trauma-related phase of organ insufficiency can be separated from a secondary insult, concomitant with the septic

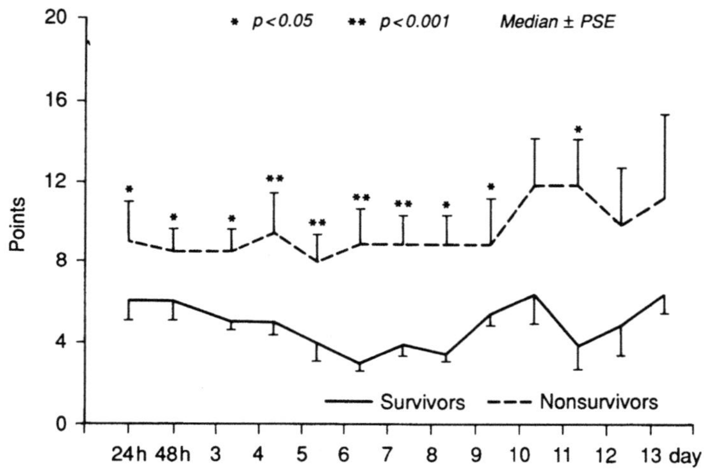

Fig. 7. APACHE II (Knaus)

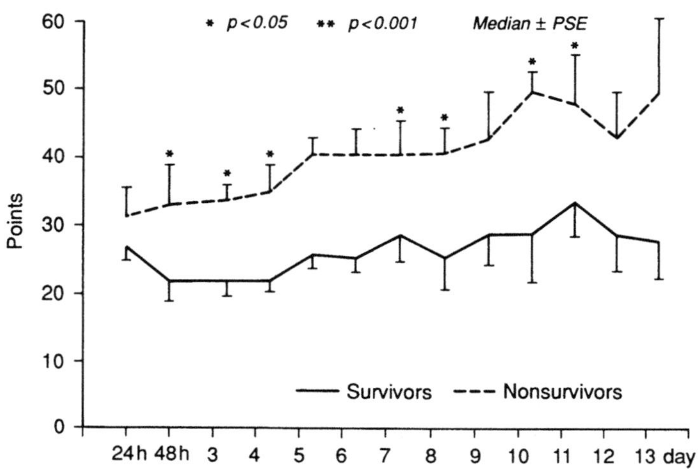

Fig. 8. Sepsis Severity Score (Stevens)

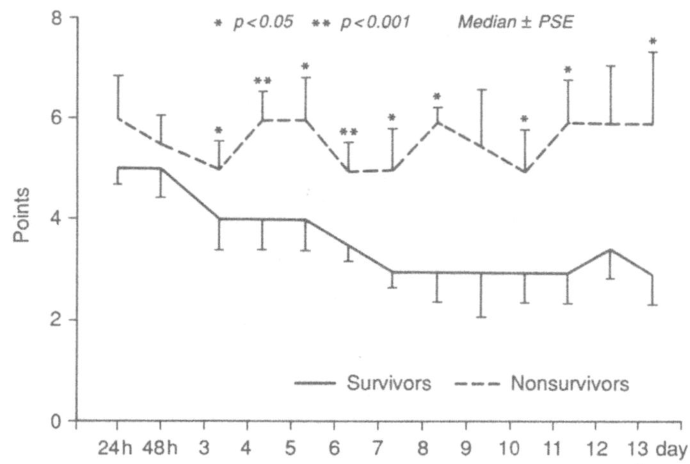

Fig. 9. Multiple Organ Failure Score (Goris)

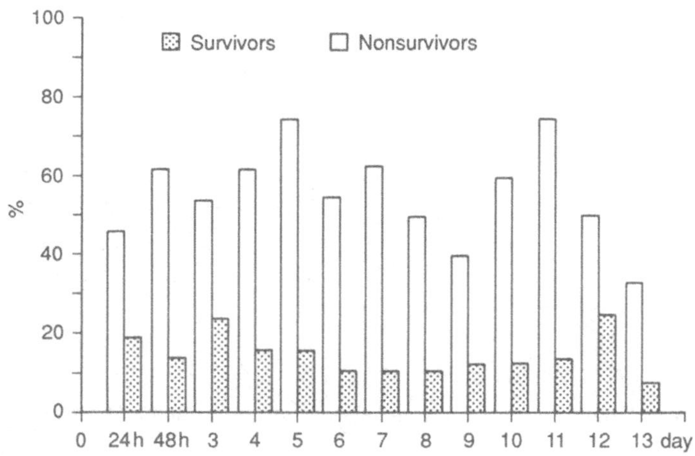

Fig. 10. Cardiac failure (MOF Score, grade II)

reaction starting at the 3rd to 4th day after trauma. The extent of failure of separate organs can be demonstrated with the MOF Score. Besides major differences in the extent of cardiac failure and liver failure, the renal function could be kept in both groups largely normal (Figs 10–12). Differences in hematological reactions, as can be shown by different platelet counts (Fig. 4), reflect major disturbances (Fig. 13).

Comparison of the three scores concerning sensitivity and specificity favored the MOF Score. All three scores satisfactorily showed the differences between both groups and it could be proved that the daily check was useful.

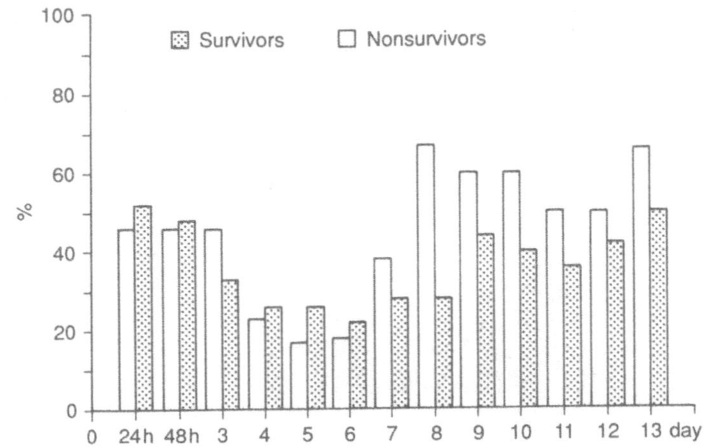

Fig. 11. Hepatic failure (MOF Score, grade II)

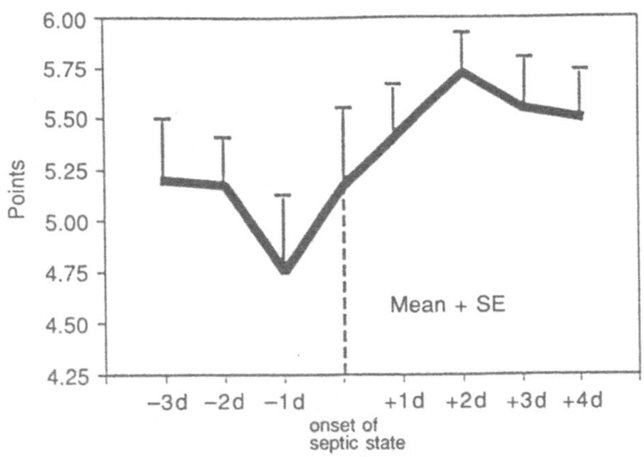

Fig. 12. Multiple Organ Failure Score showing improvement posttrauma and secondary insult

The results of the factor analysis and analysis of discriminance revealed an index consisting of seven parameters which were selected purely by mathematical means. The equation of this index gives the following formula:

$$
\begin{aligned}
&0.54 &&\times \text{ maximum body temperature}\\
&-0.026 &&\times \text{ dynamic compliance}\\
&+0.058 &&\times \text{ nonsegmented granulocytes}\\
&+0.569 &&\times \text{ triclycerides}\\
&+0.119 &&\times \text{ sodium}\\
&+0.0214 &&\times \text{ plasminogen}\\
&+0.00022 &&\times \text{ } N\text{-acetyl-glucosaminidase}\\
&-39.069 &&
\end{aligned}
$$

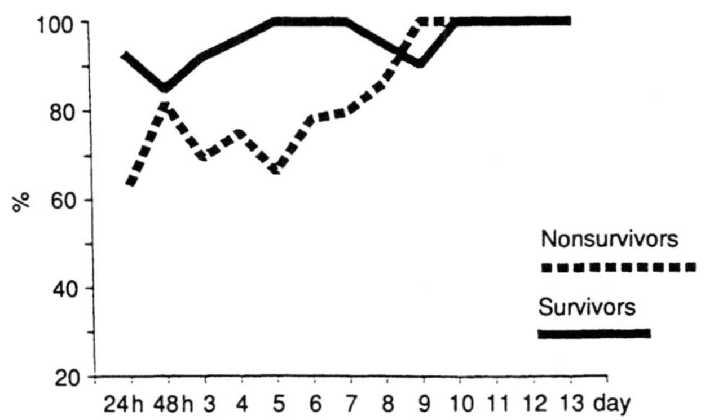

Fig. 13. Hematological function (MOF score)

The results of this formula are shown in Figs. 14 and 15 as comparison of two representative cases and a group comparison. If a patient showed values higher than 0, then he or she developed a septic reaction. The predictive value of this index, with a sensitivity of 80.2% and a specificity of 62.2%, is higher in comparison to the applied scores.

A bacteriological screening with a mean of 21 swabs/patient showed no significant differences between the septic and the nonseptic reacting patients. Of 677 bacterial examinations, 345 (51%) were positive. Of 81 blood cultures, drawn whenever a patient showed a rapid increase in temperature, 38 were drawn from septic patients and 43 from the nonseptic patient group. Three positive blood cultures were detected in the nonseptic reacting patients whereas in the septic patients no blood culture was positive. The bacterial spectrum and the resistance to antibiotics in vitro showed no differences between septic and nonseptic patients.

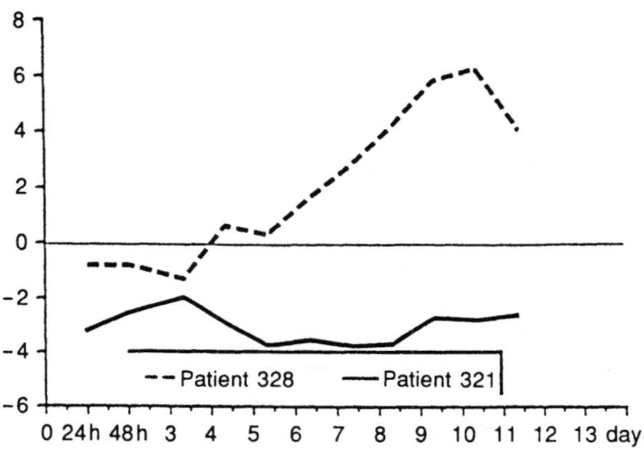

Fig. 14. Discriminant analysis, case comparison

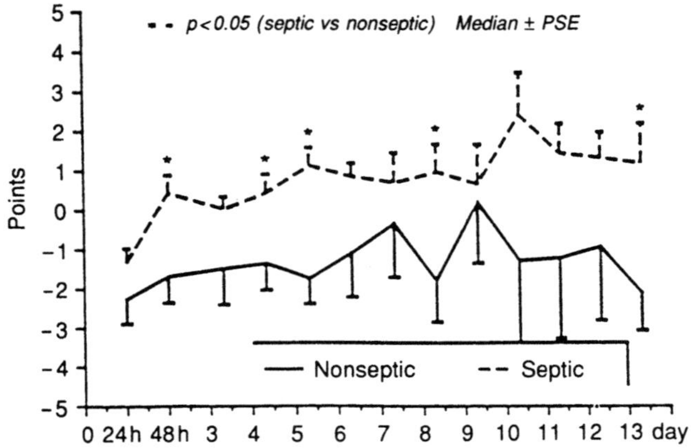

Fig. 15. Discriminant analysis, group comparison

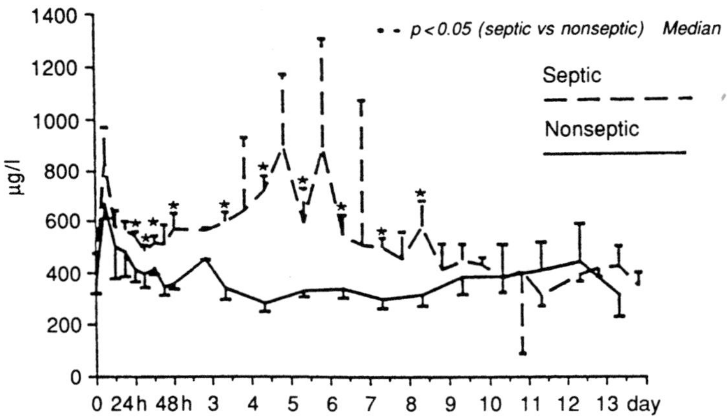

Fig. 16. Elastase-α_1-PI complex. (Courtesy of Dr. Dwenger, Institute for Clinical Biochemistry, University Medical School, Hannover, FRG)

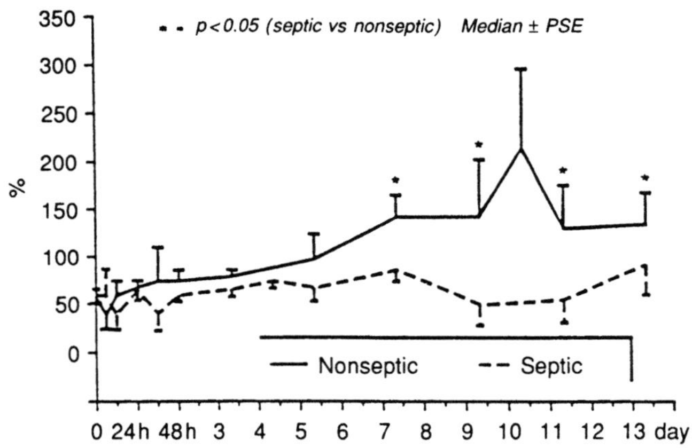

Fig. 17. Granulocyte opsonization capacity. (Courtesy of Dr. Dwenger, Institute for Clinical Biochemistry, University Medical School, Hannover, FRG)

An activation of the nonspecific inflammatory reaction can be inferred from significant increases in the septic patient group concerning the parameter elastase-α_1-PI complex [5]. This proteolytic enzyme seems to be liberated more freely in septic patients from granulocytes (Fig. 16). This is concomitant with a reduced opsonizing capacity of the serum for granulocytes of septic patients (Fig. 17). The significant differences in these parameters show a marked disturbance of granulocyte function. This parallels the development of a generalized permeability damage. The septic reaction seems to be closely related to this permeability damage [12].

Discussion

Quantification of organ failure requires exact definition of the terms "normal," "insufficient," and "failed." As this definition depends on methods of measurements, up to now there has not been a uniform basis for quantification of organ failure [3]. The use of scores improves this situation as scores combine a number of individual parameters otherwise being looked upon as solitary measurements [8]. The application of scores to a highly selected group of severely injured patients and the continuous and close follow-up of these patients for over 2 weeks forms a basis on which the validity of scores can be investigated. In the described study group after trauma a secondary phenomenon leading to a septic state could be detected. There is evidence that this secondary insult is closely correlated to an increase in capillary permeability resulting in interstitial edema formation [12, 13]. This can be detected in the lung by measurements of the EVLW. Parallel to the pulmonary insufficiency and progressive failure other organs as well show pathologic features which can be described satisfactorily by means of the scores.

The pathogenesis of the secondary insult is unclear. Sepsis is regarded as the major contributing factor for multiple organ failure [2, 4, 6, 11]. In our study the pattern of infection in patients with septic reactions showed no difference from patients without septic reaction. These data do not support evidence for a dominant role of sepsis after trauma as the cause of the demonstrated secondary insult. The close correlation of the onset of the septic reaction and the increase of inflammatory signs such as granulocyte protease liberation indicates a massive inflammatory reaction. From the clinical point of view this inflammatory reaction mimics the body's response to a systemic infection [7, 13].

Quantification of organ failure requires exact definitions of basic terms such as "normal" values of parameters. "Normal" in the sense of "necessary," such as a normal versus a necessary cardiac output, has to be clarified and adapted to the individual situation of the patient. The best cardiac output for a patient after severe trauma does not equal the values derived from healthy controls. The quantification of organ failure may help in further differentiation of the causes of the syndrome and help to control, compare, and improve therapeutic regimens.

References

1. Baue AE (1975) Multiple progressive, or sequential systems failure. Arch Surg 110:779–781
2. Bell RC, Coalson JJ, Smith JD, Johanson WG (1983) Multiple organ system failure and infection in adult respiratory distress syndrome. Ann Intern Med 99:283–288
3. Carrico CJ, Meakins JC, Marshall JC, Fry D, Maier R (1986) Multiple-organ-failure syndrome. Arch Surg 121:196–208
4. Crump JM, Duncan DA, Wears R (1988) Analysis of multiple organ system failure in trauma and nontrauma patients. Am Surg 34:702–708
5. Dwenger A, Regel G, Neumann C, Schweitzer G (1986) Pathomechanisms for the adult respiratory distress syndrome (ARDS): elastase contents of polymorphonuclear leukocytes and elastase release during passage across the blood/air barrier. Fresenius Z Anal Chem 324:360–361
6. Fry DE, Pearlstein L, Fulton RL, Polk HC (1980) Multiple system organ failure. The role of uncontrolled infection. Arch Surg 115:136–140
7. Goris RJA, Boekholtz WKF, van Bebber PT, Nuytinck JKS, Schillings PHM (1986) Multiple organ failure and sepsis without bacteria. Arch Surg 121:897–901
8. Goris RJA, Nuytinck HKS, Redl H (1987) Scoring systems and predictors of ARDS and MOF. Prog Clin Biol Res 236:3–15
9. Knaus WA, Draper EA, Wagner DP, Zimmermann JE (1985) APACHE II: a severeity of disease classification system. Crit Care Med 13:818–829
10. Lewis FR, Elings VB, Hill SL, Christensen JM (1982) The measurement of extravascular lung water by thermal green-dye indicator dilution. Ann NY Acad Sci 384:394–410
11. Manship L, McMillin RD, Brown JJ (1984) The influence of sepsis and multisystem and organ failure on mortality in the surgical intensive care unit. Am Surg 50:94–101
12. Nerlich ML (1988) Multiorganversagen und Sepsis nach Trauma: eine klinische und experimentelle Untersuchung zur Pathogenese des pulmonalen Permeabilitätsschadens. *Habilitationsschrift*, University of Hannover
13. Nuytinck HKS, Offermans JMW, Kubat K, Goris RJA (1988) Whole-body inflammation in trauma patients. An autopsy study. Arch Surg 123:1519–1522
14. Oestern HJ, Tscherne H, Sturm JA, Nerlich ML (1985) Klassifizierung der Verletzungsschwere. Unfallchirurg 88:465–472
15. Stevens LE (1983) Gauging the severity of surgical sepsis. Arch Surg 118:1190–1192

II Activation of Humeral Cascade Systems

Adult Respiratory Distress Syndrome and Complement: Significance of C3a in Diagnosis and Prognosis

G. Zilow, U. Rother, and M. Kirschfink

Introduction

The adult respiratory distress syndrome (ARDS) is a well-known complication of traumatic and septic shock. Although other different triggering events cause the development of ARDS, its pathology is surprisingly consistent. It is characterized by intestinal and alveolar edema, hypoxemia due to the intrapulmonary shunting of blood, decreased pulmonary compliance, and increased microvascular permeability in the lungs.

Complement-induced activation of polymorphonuclear leukocytes (PMNs) and pulmonary leukostasis have been considered important pathogenic factors in the development of ARDS. The assumption is based on observations in patients undergoing hemodialysis and cardiopulmonary bypass, where neutropenia and pulmonary leukostasis could be linked to pronounced complement activation [3, 4, 6, 14]. The pathophysiological relevance of complement activation was supported by several animal experiments, where the infusion of zymosan-activated serum [19] or the intratracheal application of the anaphylatoxin C5a [23] induced acute lung injury and respiratory failure similar to human ARDS. Lung damage was shown to depend on complement activation as well as on granulocytes [26], since drug-induced neutropenia prevented the development of pulmonary dysfunction after complement infusion [4] and after endotoxemia [8]. The pathogenic role of complement activation can also be deduced from experiments with C5-deficient mice [27]. Intravenous injection of cobra venom factor produced acute lung injury in normal mice while a marked reduction in the extent of lung injury in C5-deficient mice indicated the need for C5 in the development of lung injury. Addition of a polyclonal antibody to C5a to endotoxin-activated plasma prevented leukocyte aggregation in vitro and septic primates treated with this anti-C5a antibody did not develop an increase in extravascular lung water [25].

Institute of Immunology, University of Heidelberg, Im Neuenheimer Feld 305, W-6900 Heidelberg, FRG

J.A. Sturm (Ed.)
Adult Respiratory Distress Syndrome

From several clinical studies the central role of the complement system in the pathogenesis of ARDS is becoming increasingly evident [12, 21, 24]. The importance of complement activation in the early phase of the disease should be reflected by high plasma levels of split products, thereby providing a possible predictor of the development of ARDS. To find such an indicator was the aim of the work described in this paper.

Materials and Methods

Plasma Samples

Blood was drawn immediately upon admission to the intensive care unit and at intervals of 6 h during the first 48 h. The time interval between injury and admission did not exceed 2 h. From day 4 to day 14 samples were taken once every morning. The samples were centrifuged immediately. Ethylenediaminetetraacetic acid (EDTA) plasma samples as well as serum were frozen and stored in aliquots at −70°C until assayed.

Bronchoalveolar Lavage Samples

Bronchoalveolar lavage (BAL) fluid was recovered by a modification of the method of McGuire et al. [18]. Quantities of 25–30 ml were collected in a sterile graduated plastic container and 1 part of sodium citrate solution was added to 9 parts of fluid to avoid coagulation. The fluid was then filtered through gauze and layered on a modified two-step discontinuous Percoll gradient. After centrifugation at 400 *g* at 22°C for 20 min, the upper layers were pooled and centrifuged to remove remaining cells. EDTA was added to the supernatant and aliquots were frozen at −70°C for later examination.

Detection and Quantitation of Complement Proteins

Diagnostic parameters of the complement system and the methods used to quantitate complement levels in polytrauma patients are given in Table 1. Minimum and maximum levels of normal values are listed for each parameter.

Radial Immunodiffusion. Concentrations of plasma C3, C4, and C1 inactivator (C1Ina) were determined by radial immunodiffusion (Behring Diagnostics, Frankfurt, FRG).

Rocket Immunoelectrophoresis. Concentration of plasma C3d was measured by double-decker electroimmunoassay [2] with anti-C3c (Behring, Frankfurt/

Table 1. Parameters measured and methods used for complement determination

Parameter	Method	Normal Range
CH50	FA	80–120 U/ml
APH50	FA	80–120 % standard
C3	RID	0.8–1.4 mg/ml
C4	RID	0.2–0.5 mg/ml
C5	RID	92–120 % standard
Factor B	RID	0.1–0.4 mg/ml
C1Ina	RID	0.2–0.4 mg/ml
C1Ina	FA	20–35 U/ml
Factor H	RIE	84–108 % standard
Factor I	RIE	73–95 % standard
Carboxypeptidase N	FA	160–330 U/l
C3a	RIA	80–220 ng/ml
C5a	RIA	0–12 ng/ml
C3d	RIE	35–70 mU/l
C1rsC1Ina	ELISA	0–7 U/ml
C3bBbP	ELISA	0–5 U/ml

ELISA, enzyme-linked immunosorbent assay; FA, functional assay; RIA, radioimmunoassay; RID, radial immunodiffusion; RIE, rocket immunoelectrophoresis

Main, FRG) and anti-C3d (Fresenius, Oberursel, FRG) in the gel. C3d values were expressed as units. For standardization, a normal serum pool was aged at 37°C for 5 days. The C3d concentration in this pool was defined to be 1000 mU/1. C3d values in plasma samples were calculated by reference to a standard curve.

Concentration of C5, factor H, and factor I (C3b inactivator) in serum was quantitated with rabbit anti-C5 (Behring, Frankfurt/Main, FRG), rabbit antifactor H (Behring, Frankfurt/Main, FRG), and goat antihuman C3b inactivator (Miles Scientific, ICN Biochemicals, Eschwege, FRG). Concentrations were expressed as percentages of a standard serum.

Radioimmunoassay (RIA). Following the method of Hugli and Chenoweth [11], the concentration of the anaphylatoxins C3a and C5a were determined in plasma and BAL by radioimmunoassay obtained from Upjohn Diagnostics, (Kalamazoo, MI, United States) or Amersham Corporation (Braunschweig, FRG).

Functional Assays. Carboxypeptidase N was measured in a modified continuous spectrophotometric assay [20] utilizing furyl-acryloyl-alanyl-lysine (Sigma, Deisenhofen, FRG) for substrate.

The functional assay of C1 inactivator was a modification of the method described by Levy and Lepow [16]. Functional titration of the hemolytic activity of the classical pathway, CH50 [17], and of the alternative pathway,

APH50 [13], was performed according to described procedures. The APH50 was modified by using chicken instead of rabbit erythrocytes.

Enzyme-Linked Immunosorbent Assay (ELISA). The alternative convertase C3bBbP was measured in a sandwich ELISA system with goat antihuman P (Atlantic antibodies Baxter, Unterschleißheim, FRG) immobilized to polystyrene microtiter plates. After saturation of the plates with 0.01 *M* sodium phosphate, 0.15 *M* NaCl pH 7.4 (buffer A) containing 0.5% bovine serum albumin (BSA) (2 h, room temperature), the patient sample (diluted 1:25 in buffer A containing 0.01 *M* EDTA, 0.25% BSA, 0.05% Tween 20) was added and incubated for 1 h at room temperature. Bound C3bBbP was detected with biotinylated antihuman C3c (Dakopatts, Hamburg, FRG) and streptavidin peroxidase (Amersham, Braunschweig, FRG). *O*-Phenylenediamine (OPD) was used as substrate and the reaction was stopped with 12.5% H_2SO_4. The optical density was measured in an ELISA reader (V_{max} Microplate Reader, Molecular Devices) and values were expressed as units per milliliter calculated by reference to a standard curve obtained with inulin-activated normal human serum.

To determine the C1rsC1 inactivator complex, rabbit antihuman C1 inactivator was immobilized to microtiter plates (Nunc, Roshilde, Denmark). Plates were saturated with buffer A containing 0.5% BSA, and samples diluted 1:50 in buffer A containing 0.01 *M* EDTA, 0.25% BSA, 0.05% Tween 20 were incubated for 1 h at room temperature. Goat antihuman C1s (Atlantic Antibodies, Baxter, Unterschleißheim, FRG) was added, followed by peroxidase-labeled rabbit antigoat IgG. 2, 2'Azinobis (3-ethylbenzthiazolinesulfonic acid) (ABTS) was used as substrate and optical density was measured. Values were expressed as units per milliliter calculated by reference to a standard curve obtained with IgG-activated normal human serum.

Statistical Evaluation

Data are expressed as median ± pseudostandard deviation. The significance of intergroup differences was assessed by the Mann and Whitney *U* test.

Results

C3a Levels in Plasma

Complement activation was demonstrated in all patients by increased C3a levels at more than one time point of the observation period. C3a levels changed considerably during the course of the disease. C3a was elevated in the beginning in all patients. Significantly higher values ($p \leq 0.03$) were, however, measured in ARDS patients at 6 h after admission to the intensive

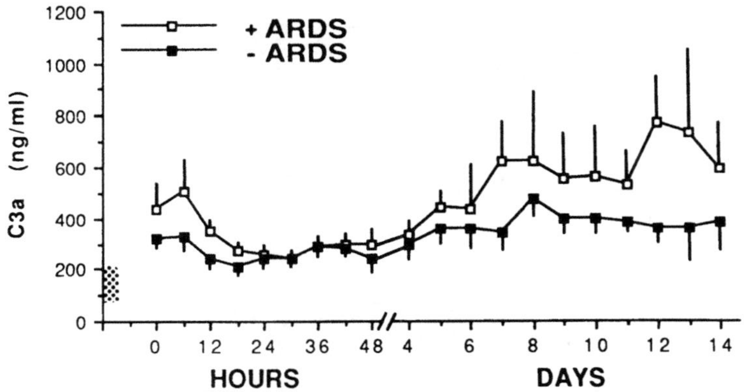

Fig. 1. Elevated C3a plasma concentration (normal range, 80–220 ng/ml) in polytrauma patients with ARDS ($n \leq 25$, *open squares*) and without ARDS ($n \leq 30$, *solid squares*). Data are shown over a period of 14 days as the median ± pseudo-SD. *Bar* indicates normal range

care unit (Fig. 1). While ARDS patients again reached excessively high C3a values 5–6 days after the onset of illness, there was only a minor increase of C3a levels in patients without ARDS ($p \leq 0.07$). Furthermore, C3a levels paralleled the rise in extravascular lung water at days 4–14. If the patients were classified by sepsis and not by severity of the pulmonary dysfunction, a statistically significant difference was noted for C3a values in the late posttrauma phase (data not shown).

C3 and C3a/C3 Levels in Plasma

C3 levels were significantly lower during the first 24 h in patients who developed ARDS (median, 0.56 mg/ml; $p = 0.014$) and also during the course of the disease (median, 0.94 mg/ml; $p = 0.001$) (Table 2). A pronounced increase in C3 levels could be observed later in recovering patients as an expression of an acute phase reaction, whereas the ARDS patients' titers only reached normal values.

The C3a/C3 ratio was determined in all patients. Significantly higher C3a/C3 ratios ($p = 0.04$) were observed in the ARDS patients during the first 24 h with a maximum at 6 h ($p = 0.001$). A second rise of C3a/C3 ratio between days 4–14 could be observed in patients with ARDS but not in patients without ARDS (Fig. 2).

C3a Levels in BAL fluid

In 32 patients of the study group BAL was performed on different days and C3a was measured. The control group consisted of normal volunteers without

Table 2. Complement profile in polytrauma patients with ARDS and without ARDS during an observation period of 14 days

Time after admission	Parameter		With ARDS		Without ARDS		p
			Median (range)	N	Median (range)	N	
0–24 h	CH50	U/ml	70.00 (30.00–107.20)	13	72.40 (32.20–108.00)	17	0.286
	APH50	% standard	31.40 (16.20–170.60)	25	37.60 (15.00– 67.60)	32	0.359
	Factor B	mg/ml	0.11 (0.07– 0.16)	11	0.14 (0.08– 0.18)	11	0.131
	C3	mg/ml	0.56 (0.37– 0.84)	25	0.67 (0.44– 1.02)	32	0.014*
	C4	mg/ml	0.16 (0.11– 0.29)	15	0.21 (0.09– 0.40)	19	0.205
	C5	% standard	54.00 (44.00–135.00)	13	55.60 (48.40–101.00)	17	0.438
30–48 h	CH50	U/ml	73.50 (40.80–117.30)	13	87.50 (63.80–144.00)	17	0.035
	APH50	% standard	57.00 (21.00–128.50)	25	63.30 (24.00–101.50)	30	0.654
	Factor B	mg/ml	0.15 (0.09– 0.24)	11	0.18 (0.18– 0.27)	11	0.212
	C3	mg/ml	0.67 (0.33– 1.06)	25	0.80 (0.34– 1.20)	30	0.009*
	C4	mg/ml	0.18 (0.12– 0.46)	15	0.24 (0.08– 0.50)	19	0.114
	C5	% standard	64.00 (39.00–129.00)	13	70.00 (52.00– 92.00)	15	0.299
4–14 days	CH50	U/ml	119.30 (83.70–226.60)	13	153.30 (105.10–239.30)	17	0.090
	APH50	% standard	75.40 (36.10–194.00)	25	76.00 (20.80–118.50)	32	0.376
	Factor B	mg/ml	0.29 (0.19– 0.39)	11	0.32 (0.13– 0.43)	11	0.168
	C3	mg/ml	0.94 (0.50– 1.50)	25	1.34 (0.66– 1.89)	32	0.001*
	C4	mg/ml	0.27 (0.13– 0.63)	15	0.34 (0.12– 0.75)	19	0.290
	C5	% standard	122.00 (83.80–154.40)	13	121.60 (92.80–157.70)	17	0.544

* significant

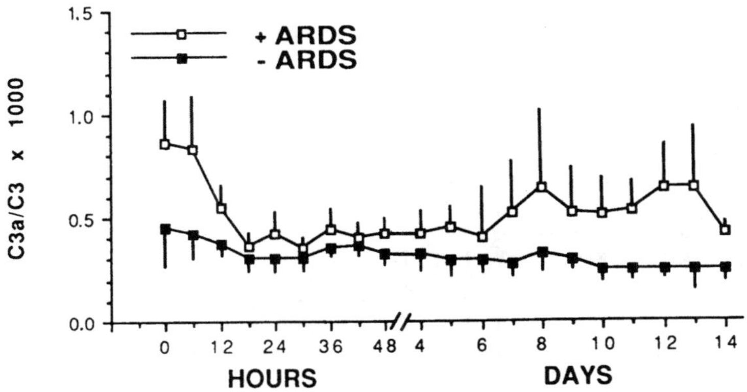

Fig. 2. Ratio of C3a/C3 × 1000 is shown in patients with ($n \leq 25$, *open squares*) and without ARDS ($n \leq 30$, *solid squares*)

pulmonary disease ($n = 10$). In six of ten volunteers C3a concentration in BAL fluid was below the detectable level of 40 ng/ml and it never exceeded 100 ng/ml. BAL is a major technique to evaluate molecular components of the epithelial lining fluid (ELF) of the lower respiratory tract. To quantify the dilution effect caused by saline infusion, urea was used as an endogenous marker and C3a levels were calculated in proportion to the urea concentration. In 12 patients simultaneous plasma and BAL samples were obtained and C3a and urea were determined. During the first 24 h patients who later developed ARDS showed an increase of C3a in the ELF up to about 10 000 ng/ml. BAL samples obtained later on showed low levels of C3a with no difference between the two groups at that time (Fig. 3).

In order to determine the origin of C3a in BAL the ratio of C3a in ELF and in plasma was calculated in 12 patients. In the early posttrauma phase this

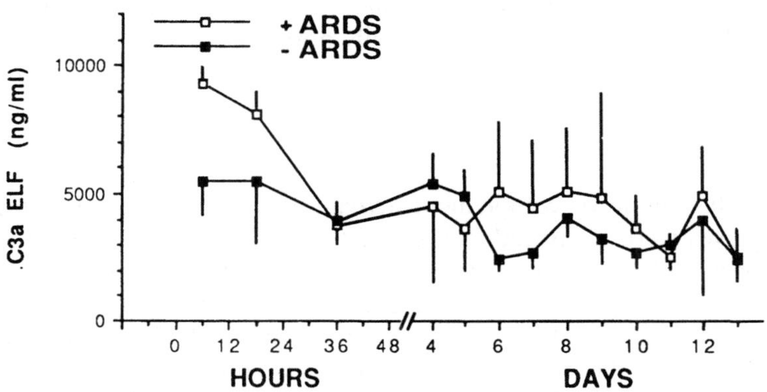

Fig. 3. C3a levels (ng/ml) in epithelial lining fluid (*ELF*). C3a concentration in ELF was calculated based on urea concentration as described. *Open squares* indicate patients with ARDS ($n \leq 6$)

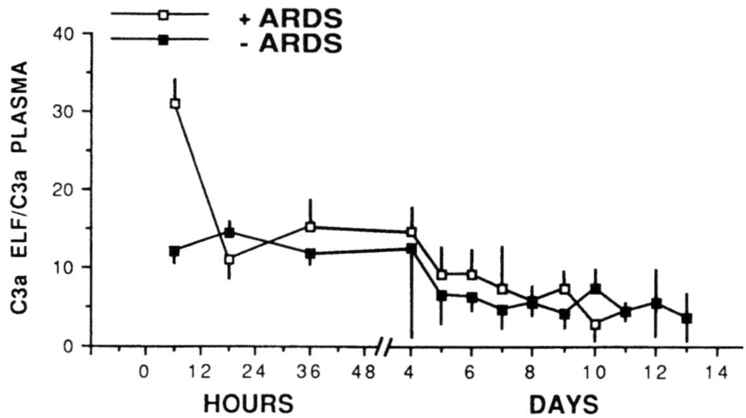

Fig. 4. The ratio C3a in ELF to C3a in plasma obtained at the same time is given of patients with ARDS ($n \leq 6$, *open square*) and without ARDS ($n \leq 6$, *solid squares*)

ratio was extremely high in patients with ARDS (Fig. 4), but even the non-ARDS group had a ratio > 1, indicating a local complement activation in both groups during the course of the illness.

Functional Activity of the Classical and Alternative Pathway

As shown in Table 2 functional activity of the alternative pathway was severely depressed at the beginning (31.4% in ARDS patients and 37.6% in patients without ARDS) and rose after 24 h, reaching nearly normal titers. Although lower titers were consistently observed in ARDS patients, differences between the two groups were not significant. Classical pathway activity (CH50) was slightly depressed from the beginning in all patients. Recovering patients later showed a pronounced acute-phase reaction, whereas the ARDS patients' titers rose to only normal levels.

Activation Products

To investigate the mode of complement activation, two activation-specific protein complexes were measured, the C1rsC1 inactivator complex for the classical pathway and the alternative convertase C3bBbP for the alternative pathway. The two complexes were measured in 12 patients with and 15 patients without ARDS. In the early posttrauma phase, C1rsC1 inactivator levels remained within the normal range. There was, however, an increase from day 4 to day 14 mainly in the ARDS group (Fig. 5). In contrast, activation via the alternative pathway could be demonstrated early in the posttrauma phase with a marked increase at 6 h in the ARDS group

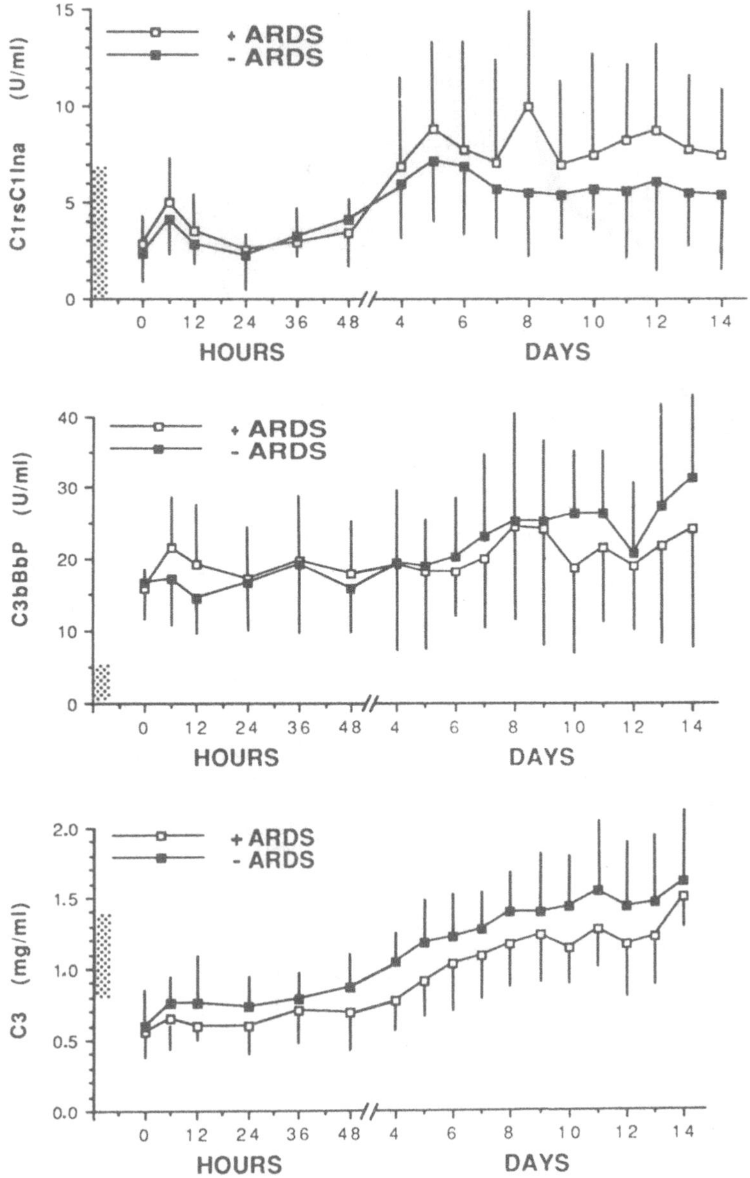

Fig. 5. Activation via the classical (C1rsC1Ina) and alternative (C3bBbP) pathway was measured in some of the polytrauma patients with ARDS ($n \leq 12$, *open squares*) and without ARDS ($n \leq 15$, *solid square*). Data are shown over a period of 14 days as mean ± standard deviation. C3 levels are given of the same patients. *Bars* indicate normal range

Table 3. Inhibitor potential in polytrauma patients with and without ARDS

Time after admission	Parameter		With ARDS		Without ARDS		p
			Median (range)	N	Median (range)	N	
0–24 h	C1Ina	mg/ml	0.25 (0.19– 0.45)	25	0.29 (0.19– 0.41)	32	0.026*
	Factor H	% standard	56.00 (44.40– 86.00)	13	60.40 (36.80– 76.50)	17	0.950
	Factor I	% standard	54.00 (42.00– 81.20)	13	58.80 (37.20– 88.00)	17	0.722
	Carboxypeptidase N	U/l	159.50 (123.00–207.00)	12	175.60 (126.00–245.00)	17	0.232
30–48 h	C1Ina	mg/ml	0.37 (0.29– 0.53)	25	0.41 (0.28– 0.51)	30	0.327
	Factor H	% standard	55.50 (46.50– 97.00)	13	64.00 (46.00– 96.50)	15	0.381
	Factor I	% standard	58.00 (40.50–100.50)	13	62.00 (45.00– 96.50)	15	0.279
	Carboxypeptidase N	U/l	237.00 (171.00–296.00)	12	255.00 (177.00–326.00)	17	0.057
4–14 days	C1Ina	mg/ml	0.54 (0.25– 0.70)	25	0.59 (0.42– 0.79)	32	0.009*
	Factor H	% standard	86.40 (63.50–108.40)	13	90.00 (63.60–129.60)	17	0.249
	Factor I	% standard	89.60 (63.00–123.60)	13	102.50 (56.00–153.80)	17	0.346
	Carboxypeptidase N	U/l	285.10 (190.00–378.00)	13	326.20 (227.00–397.00)	17	0.137

* significant

comparable to the C3a increase at this point. After day 4 a further slight increase developed but there were no longer differences between the two groups. The increase in the C3bBbP complex runs parallel to the increase in the C3 level.

Inhibitor Capacity

Plasma levels of the inhibitors factor H, factor I, carboxypeptidase N, and C1 inactivator (protein and functional activity) were low in all patients in the beginning but reached normal and even elevated levels at a later stage of the disease (Table 3). There was no significant difference between the two groups except for C1 inactivator levels within the first 24 h ($p = 0.026$) and from day 4 to day 14 ($p = 0.009$).

Discussion

Complement-induced aggregation and activation of granulocytes is proposed to be a causative element in ARDS. Quantitation of lung damage is rather difficult in severely traumatized patients. Therefore it would be helpful to find a laboratory parameter which together with clinical parameters could be used to define the severity of pulmonary dysfunction at an early stage. The anaphylatoxins C3a and C5a do not exert a direct toxic effect on lung tissue but they play a key indirect role: they activate neutrophils and stimulate other cells to release their mediators. C5a causes rapid accumulation of neutrophils within the alveolar compartment [9] and is able to induce enzyme release from granules of neutrophils. The release of proteases can lead to an amplification of the response, since neutral proteases stored within the lysosomal granules of neutrophils can cleave C5 and C3 and, thus, in turn yield new chemotactic activity. Finally, C5a has the ability to stimulate neutrophils to produce a series of toxic oxygen products, including H_2O_2, O_2^-, and other oxygen radicals. C3a, while not chemotactic for neutrophils, is able (like C5a) to stimulate the release of lysosomal enzymes from neutrophils and to induce histamine release from mast cells and basophils. Like C5a, it stimulates the metabolism of arachidonic acid [7] and is able to modulate the immune response [29].

In the pathogenesis of ARDS the impact of complement can be described by the following sequence of reactions (Fig. 6): Massive complement activation occurs, e.g., in polytrauma with tissue damage and release of proteases leading to the generation of C3a, C3b, C5a, and C5b-9. These mediators induce aggregation of granulocytes and their accumulation in the lung capillaries. The cells adhere to the vascular endothelium and locally release mediators, e.g., toxic oxygen derivates, enzymes, and prostaglandins

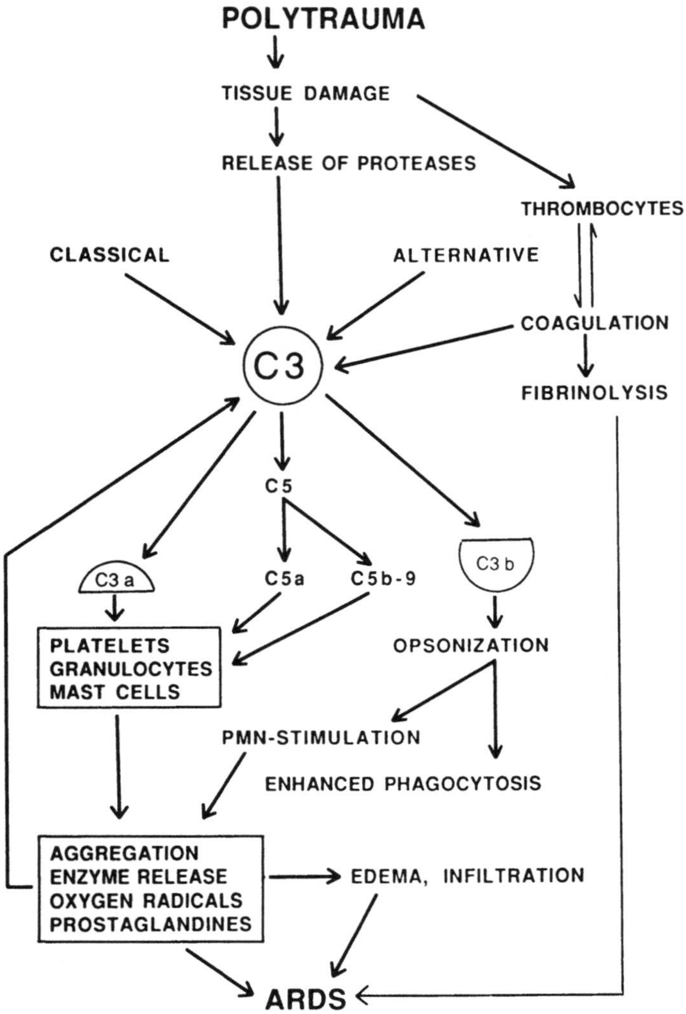

Fig. 6. Factors contributing to the pathogenesis of ARDS

leading to tissue damage. Permeability increase occurs, resulting in frequently fatal edema. This sequence of reactions suggests that complement levels might be used to monitor the development of ARDS. From complement levels measured in this study, a relation between the severity of pulmonary damage and C3a and C3 levels may be assumed. C3a determined during the first 6 h can distinguish between patients later developing ARDS and those who do not. An increased C3a/C3 ratio is associated with the manifestation of ARDS. C3a levels and the ratio of C3a to C3 are therefore of prognostic value in the early phase after severe trauma, identifying those patients who are prone to develop ARDS. Although all patients have evidence of complement activation (the proteins C3, C4, C5 are decreased and the inhibitors factor H, factor I, and carboxypeptidase N show low titers), only high C3a-plasma levels or the calculated C3a/C3 ratios are indicative for the ultimate development of ARDS. Although we found a correlation between the early appearance of the anaphylatoxin C3a and ARDS, C3a should not be considered the most important split product in the pathogenesis of ARDS. More likely it is C5a that causes the fatal complications after polytrauma. C5a, however, could not be detected in the plasma of patients with ARDS, confirming the results of several authors who have shown that C5a cannot be detected in the circulation [21, 24] as it is rapidly bound to its target cells, mainly granulocytes. Differences between our results and those obtained by Hammerschmidt et al. [6] may be due to the test systems applied. PMN aggregation might be more sensitive than an RIA in detecting trace amounts of C5a. It has also been shown, however, that neutrophil aggregation can be induced in the absence of C5a by substances such as leukotriene B_4, platelet-activating factor, and immune complexes [1].

Several other reports in the literature suggest that ARDS is associated with complement activation [10, 12]. On the other hand, there are clinical studies which found no correlation between complement activation and ARDS [22, 31]. C5a-like activity (measured in a leukocyte aggregation assay) was found in the plasma of 81% of ARDS patients (35 of 50 patients developed ARDS).C5a was, however, also present in patients without ARDS and there was no significant difference in mean peak values [5]. In 59 patients with septic shock studied by Schein et al. [22], complement determination of C3, C4, and factor B did not allow prediction of the development of ARDS.

Weinberg et al. [31] found that measurement of C5a desArg and C3a desArg were not useful in predicting the development of respiratory failure, while in a previous report in which the correlation between the extent of complement activation and the severity of abnormal pulmonary function was studied ARDS patients had significantly higher C3a and C5a values [28].

Recent investigations have shown that an influx of PMNs into the lung occurs early in the ARDS [30]. There is evidence that activation of the complement system causes this influx of neutrophils into the lung, where they can damage lung parenchyma by release of proteases and toxic oxygen radicals. Determination of C3a in BAL revealed local complement activation in the early posttrauma phase in ARDS patients and to a lesser degree in patients without ARDS. C5a, however, could only be detected after manifold concentration of the lavage samples. This is in agreement with a recent study where chemotactically active C5a could be measured in ELF of patients with ARDS after 69- to 1200-fold concentration of the BAL [21]. The amount of C5a was correlated to the presence of neutrophils.

The pathway of complement activation has been assessed previously be monitoring protein concentration (C3, C4, factor B) of the alternative and the classical pathway. The measurement of these individual complement components, however, does not accurately reflect complement activation, because the level of these proteins may be influenced by an increased or decreased synthesis. In contrast, the complexes C1rsC1 inactivator and C3bBbP are formed only by activation. After polytrauma, complement is activated via the alternative pathway. This is more pronounced in the ARDS group during the first 6 h, paralleling the C3a increase in this group. There is no activation via the classical pathway at this time. However, in the late posttrauma phase, when most of the ARDS patients develop sepsis, the classical pathway is also affected. We have not been able to confirm the findings that C1rsC1 inactivator concentration and C3bBbP complex concentration preceded ARDS [15].

Conclusion

Our results support the concept that complement activation correlates with the ultimate development of ARDS in patients at risk. In addition to systemic complement activation after polytrauma, which predominantly occurs via the alternative pathway, complement is activated locally in the alveolar space. Anaphylatoxin C3a as well as the calculated C3a/C3 ratio are useful laboratory parameters for assessing and monitoring patients at risk for ARDS.

References

1. Abramson S, Given W, Edelson H, Weismann G (1983) Neutrophil aggregation induced by sera from patients with active systemic lupus erythematosus. Arthritis Rheum 26:630
2. Brandslund J, Siersted HC, Svehag S-E, Teisner B (1981) Double-decker rocket immunoelectrophoresis for direct quantitation of complement C3 split products with C3d specificities in plasma. J Immunol Methods 44:64
3. Craddock PR, Fehr J, Brigham KL, Kronenberg RS, Jacob HS (1977) Complement and leukocyt emediated pulmonary dysfunction in hemodialysis. N Engl J Med 296:769
4. Craddock PR, Fehr J, Dalmasso AP, Brigham KL, Jacob HS (1977) Hemodialysis leukopenia. Pulmonary vascular leukostasis resulting from complement activation by dialyzer cellophane membranes. J Clin Invest 59:879
5. Duchateau L, Haas M, Schreyen H, Radoux L, Sprangers J, Noel FX, Braun M, Lamy M (1984) Complement activation in patients at risk of developing the adult respiratory distress syndrome. Am Rev Respir Dis 130:1058
6. Hammerschmidt DE, Weaver LJ, Hudson LD, Craddock PR, Jacob HS (1980) Association of complement activation and elevated plasma-C5a with adult respiratory distress syndrome. Pathophysiological relevance and possible prognostic value. Lancet 1:947
7. Hartung HP, Bitter-Suermann D, Hadding U (1983) Induction of thromboxane release from macrophages by anaphylatoxic peptide C3a of complement and synthetic hexapeptide C3a 72–77. J Immunol 130:1345

8. Heflin AC Jr, Brigham KL (1981) Prevention by granulocyte depletion of increased vascular permeability of sheep lung following endotoxemia. J Clin Invest 68:1253
9. Henson PM, McCarthy K, Larsen GL, Webster RO, Giclas PC, Dreisin RB, King TE, Shaw JO (1979) Complement fragments, alveolar macrophages and alveolitis. Am J Pathol 97:93
10. Hosea S, Brown E, Hammer C, Frank M (1980) Role of complement activation in a model of adult respiratory distress syndrome. J Clin Invest 66:375
11. Hugli TE, Chenoweth D (1980) Biologically active peptides of complement technique and significance of C3a and C5a measurement. In: Nakamara RM (ed) Future perspectives in clinical laboratory immunoassays. Liss, New York, p443
12. Jacob HS (1980) Complement-induced vascular leukostasis – its role in tissue injury. Arch Pathol Lab Med 104:617
13. Joiner KA, Hawinger A, Gelfand JA (1983) A study of optimal reaction conditions for an assay of the human alternative pathway. Am J Clin Pathol 79:65
14. Kaplow LS, Goffinet JA (1968) Profound neutropenia during the early phase of hemodialysis. JAMA 203:1135
15. Langlois PF, Gawryl MS (1988) Complement activation occurs through both classical and alternative pathway prior to onset and resolution of adult respiratory distress syndrome. Clin Immunol Immunopathol 47:152
16. Levy LR, Lepow DH (1959) Assay and properties of serum inhibitor of C1-esterase. Proc Soc Exp Biol Med 101:608
17. Mayer MM (1961) Complement and complement fixation. In: Kabat EA, Mayer MM (eds) Experimental immunochemistry. Thomas, Springfield
18. McGuire WW, Spragg RG, Cohen AB (1982) Studies on the pathogenesis of the adult respiratory distress syndrome. J Clin Invest 69:543
19. Perkowsky SZ, Havill AM, Flynn JT, Gee MH (1983) Role of intrapulmonary release of eicosanoids and superoxide anion as mediators of pulmonary dysfunction and endothelial injury in sheep with intermittent complement activation. Circ Res 53:574
20. Plummer TH, Hurwitz MY (1978) Human plasma carboxypeptidase N. Isolation and characterization. J Biol Chem 253:3907
21. Robbins RA, Russ WD, Rasmussen JK, Clayton MM (1987) Activation of the complement system in the adult respiratory distress syndrome. Am Rev Respir Dis 135:651
22. Schein RMH, Bergman R, Marcial EH, Schultz D, Duncan RC, Arnold PI, Sprung CL (1987) Complement activation and corticosteroid therapy in the development of the adult respiratory distress syndrome. Chest 91:850
23. Shaw JO, Henson PM, Henson J, Webster RO (1980) Lung inflammation induced by complement derived chemotactic fragments in the alveolus. Lab Invest 42:547
24. Solomkin JS, Cotta LA, Satoh PS, Hurst JM, Nelson RD (1985) Complement activation and clearance in acute illness and injury: evidence for C5a as a cell-directed mediator of the adult respiratory distress syndrome in man. Surgery 97:668
25. Stevens JH, O'Hanley P, Shapiro JM, Mihm FG, Satoh PS, Collins JA, Raffin TA (1986) Effects of anti-C5a antibodies in the adult respiratory distress syndrome in septic primates. J Clin Invest 77:1812
26. Till GO, Johnson KJ, Kunkel R, Ward PA (1982) Intravascular activation of complement and acute lung injury-dependency on neutrophils and toxic oxygen metabolites. J Clin Invest 69:1126
27. Tvedten HW, Till GO, Ward PA (1985) Mediators of lung injury in mice following systemic activation of complement. Am J Pathol 119:92
28. Weigelt JA, Chenoweth DE, Borman KR, Norcross JF (1988) Complement and the severity of pulmonary failure. J Trauma 28:1013
29. Weigle WO, Goodman MG, Morgan EL, Hugli TE (1983) Regulation of immune response by components of the complement cascade and their activated fragments. Springer Semin Immunopathol 6:173

30. Weiland JE, Davis WB, Holter JF, Mohammed JR, Dorinsky PM, Gadek JE (1986) Lung neutrophils in the adult respiratory distress syndrome. Am Rev Respir Dis 133:218
31. Weinberg PF, Matthay MA, Webster RO, Roskos KV, Goldstein JM, Murray JF (1984) Biologically active products of complement and acute lung injury in patients with the sepsis syndrome. Am Rev Respir Dis 130:791

Differences in Activation of Coagulation and Fibrinolysis After Polytrauma with Respect to the Development of Adult Respiratory Distress Syndrome

W. SCHRAMM and M. SPANNAGL

Introduction

It is well-known that soluble fibrin is found in dissminated intravascular coagulation (DIC) and it has often been described in the microcirculation of polytrauma patients. This proves the role of thrombin in this disease. A lot of changes in hemostatic factors and end products can be explained by excessive production of thrombin leading to an increase in intermediate and end products (fibrinopeptide A, fibrin monomers, and protease inhibitor complexes), and to the consumption of clotting factors and inhibitors (fibrinogen and antithrombin III, AT III) [5, 13, 19, 22, 23]. For this reason thrombin inhibition has played an important role in therapy for many years, but until now no significant improvement using low-dose heparin therapy or substitution with AT III could be demonstrated in randomized and prospective studies.

Activation of fibrinolysis is induced by the rapid release of t-PA (tissue plasminogen activator) from endothelial cells and is regulated by t-PA inhibitors. The activation of fibrinolysis by t-PA and its subsequent inhibition by plasminogen activator inhibitor (PAI1) have been demonstrated under conditions such as endotoxin infusion, myocardial infarction, or surgery [8, 15, 20, 21]. After polytrauma, a short-term increase in PAI 1 levels with a rapid reverting pattern has been reported. PAI 1 levels peaked after 12 h and returned to base level during the second day after trauma. Because of the rapidly changing PAI 1 levels in plasma, the importance of frequent sample collecting has been emphasized [4, 9, 10]. With regard to fibrin deposition in the microcirculation and interstitium of the lung, the concept of impaired fibrinolysis is of special interest in patients suffering from adult respiratory distress syndrome (ARDS) [1, 2, 3, 6, 11, 14, 17].

Central Medical Clinic, Ludwig Maximilians University Munich, Ziemssenstr. 1, W-8000 Munich 2, FRG

J.A. Sturm (Ed.)
Adult Respiratory Distress Syndrome

Material and Methods

Blood Samples. Blood obtained by venipuncture was mixed 9:1 with 0.11 *M* Na citrate. To determine fibrinopeptide A, blood was mixed 9:1 with 0.9% NaCI containing 1000 U heparin and 1000 KIU aprotinin/ml. Platelet-poor plasma was prepared by centrifugation for 15 min at 2000 g. Aliquots were stored at −30°C until assayed.

Standard Curve. All the standard curves except those for t-PA and t-PA inhibitor were obtained by serial dilution of a human normal plasma pool. Concentrations were presented as a percentage of normal plasma (reference plasma, Immuno, Vienna, Austria).

Prekallikrein. Prekallikrein was determined in diluted plasma after activation with contact activator (ellagic acid and phospholipid) in the presence of Factor XII, (F XII) and HMW kininogen in excess. Kallikrein generated was measured by chromogenic substrate S2302 (KabiVitrum, Munich, FRG).

Factor XII. F XII activity was determined by a partial thromboplastin time (PTT) clotting method using F XII deficient plasma (Behring Werke, Marburg, FRG).

Fibrinopeptide A. Fibrinopeptide A was determined by a radioimmunoassay using polyclonal antibodies (Byck-Mallinckrodt, Neunkirchen, FRG).

DD Fragment. The fibrin degradation product D-dimer (DD fragment) was determined using an enzyme-linked immunosorbent assay (ELISA) system with monoclonal antibodies (Boehringer, Mannheim, FRG).

Cl Inactivator. C1 inactivator was determined by incubating diluted plasma samples with C1 esterase in excess. Resting activity was measured using substrate C1-1 (Immuno, Vienna, Austria) [16]

Plasminogen. Plasminogen was determined by incubating diluted plasma samples with streptokinase in excess. The so formed streptokinase-plasminogen complex catalyzes the amidolytic cleavage of synthetic chromogenic substrate S 2251. *P*-nitroaniline (pNA) release was followed photometrically at 405 nm.

Antiplasmin. Antiplasmin was determined by adding plasmin in excess to diluted plasma samples. The remaining amount of plasmin catalyzes the splitting of pNA from S 2251. pNA release was followed photometrically at 405 nm.

Antithrombin III. AT III was determined by incubating diluted plasma samples with thrombin in excess. Resting thrombin activity was measured using chromozym TH (Boehringer Mannheim, FRG).

t-PA Inhibitors. 2.5 IU of human melanoma t-PA were added to a 25-μl plasma sample. After incubation the reaction was stopped with acetate buffer (pH 3.9). The residual amount of t-PA was determined by plasminogen and soluble fibrin(ogen) fragments in excess and S 2251. The standard curve was prepared in U/ml according to the manufacturer's instructions using human normal plasma with t-PA added (defined as 0 arbitrary units/ml), and acidified human normal plasma without t-PA added (defined as 100 arbitrary units/ml) (KabiVitrum, Munich, FRG) [12].

t-PA Antigen. t-PA antigen was determined by means of an ELISA system using a solid-phase-bound, monoclonal, murine antibody and a second peroxidase (POD)-conjugated, murine, monoclonal antibody against human t-PA. This system recognizes complexed as well as free t-PA. The standard curve is prepared according to the manufacturer's instructions. The supplied standard material is calibrated in ng/ml (Boehringer Mannheim, FRG) [7].

Statistical Evaluation. Data are presented as median ± standard deviation. The Mann-Whitney test was used to prove a significant ($p < 0.05$) or a highly significant ($p < 0.01$) difference between the two groups. For each time within the first 24 h with a significant difference between the two groups, the positive predictive value ($pV_{pos.}$) and negative predictive value ($pV_{neg.}$) were calculated using the formula:

$$pV_{pos.} = \frac{\text{ARDS correctly predicted}}{\text{all patients with ARDS}};$$

$$pV_{neg.} = \frac{\text{no ARDS correctly predicted}}{\text{all patients without ARDS}}$$

The critical values with a true positive prediction ($pV_{pos.}$) of 75% were calculated. These critical values correctly predict 75% of the patients who will develop ARDS. The false positive prediction (100% $pV_{neg.}$) shows the percentage of patients who are wrongly assumed to develop ARDS.

Results

Prekallikrein and F XII (Fig. 1). The parameters prekallikrein and F XII showed low values over the whole observation period; only 6 h after the patient had been admitted to hospital, normal values of over 60% for prekallikrein and over 80% for F XII were reached. At 24 h after admission, prekallikrein levels declined to values below 30% and F XII to 45%.

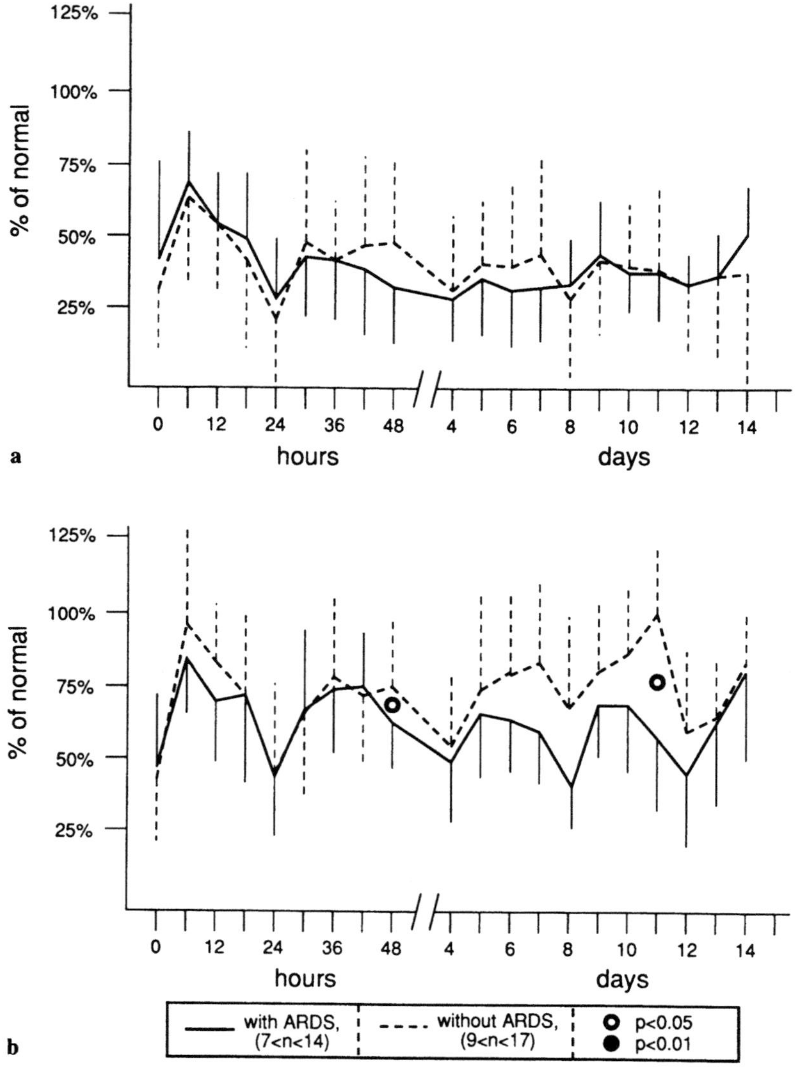

Fig. 1. a Prekallikrein; **b** Factor XII (Hageman factor)

Overall, the values of prekallikrein and F XII did not discriminate between patients with or without ARDS, although there was a significant difference in FXII levels between the two groups at 48 h and 11 days.

Fibrinopeptide A and DD Fragment (Fig. 2). Fibrinopeptide A had very high initial values (40 ng/ml) which went down to a resting level of about 15 ng/ml within 12 h.

In the first 6 days, there were no statistical differences between the levels in the groups with and without ARDS. After 4 days, the fibrinopeptide A

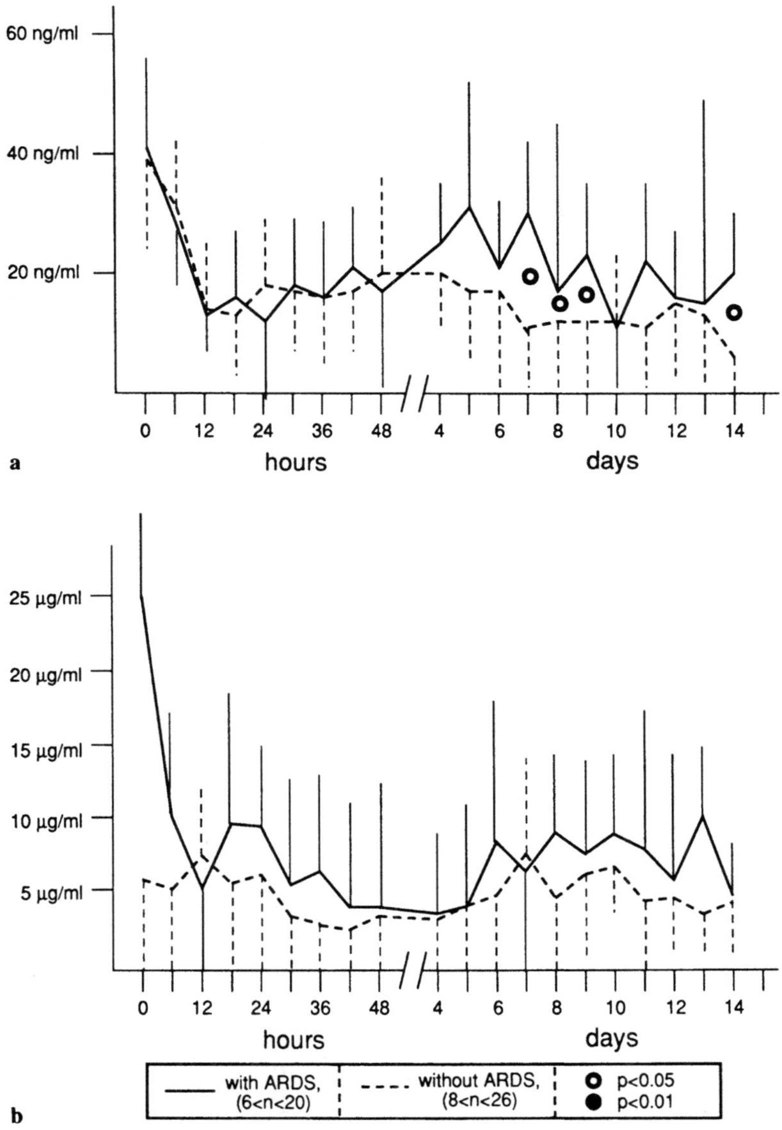

Fig. 2. a Fibrinopeptide A; **b** DD fragment

levels of the ARDS group were higher than those of the group without ARDS. This difference was significant at days 7, 8, 9, and 14.

As with fibrinopeptide A, the DD fragment showed in the ARDS group a very high initial value of 25 µg/ml, which declined to a resting level of about 7 µg/ml within 12 h. The DD fragment showed no statistical differences between the two groups.

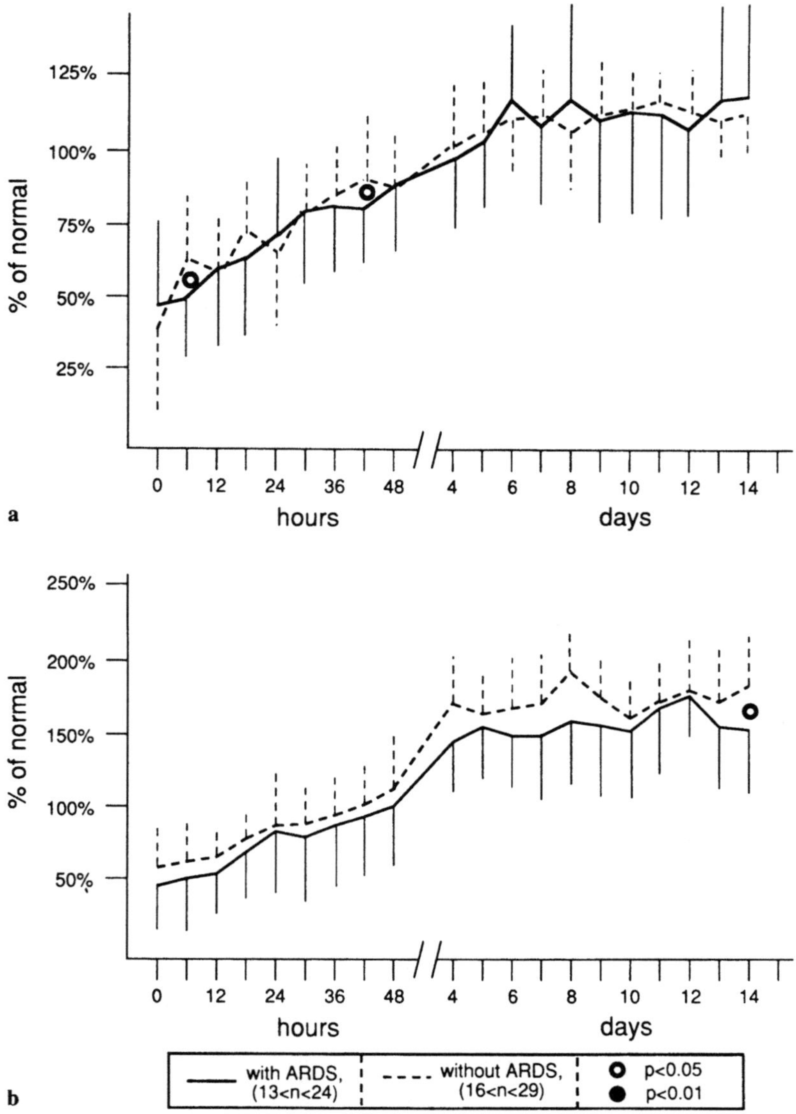

Fig. 3. **a** C1 inactivator activity level; **b** C1 inactivator immunological plasma level

C1 Inactivator (Fig. 3). The activity of the C1 inactivator rose from a initial value of 40% to a plateau of 115% within the first 6 days, while the immunological determination of the C1 inactivator reached a plateau of 170% after 4 days. The ARDS group showed significantly lower 1 inactivator activity at 6 and 40 h and lower antigen levels at 14 days, but on the whole, the two groups were indistingishable both-by the activity and by the immunological measurement.

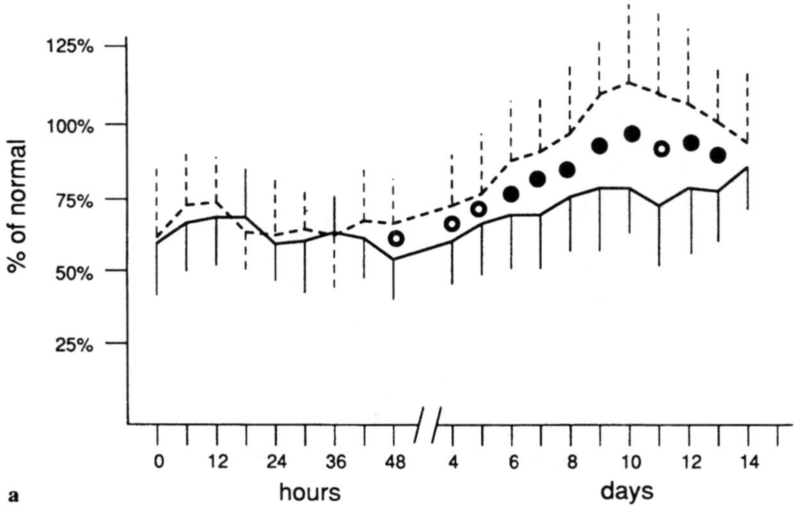

a

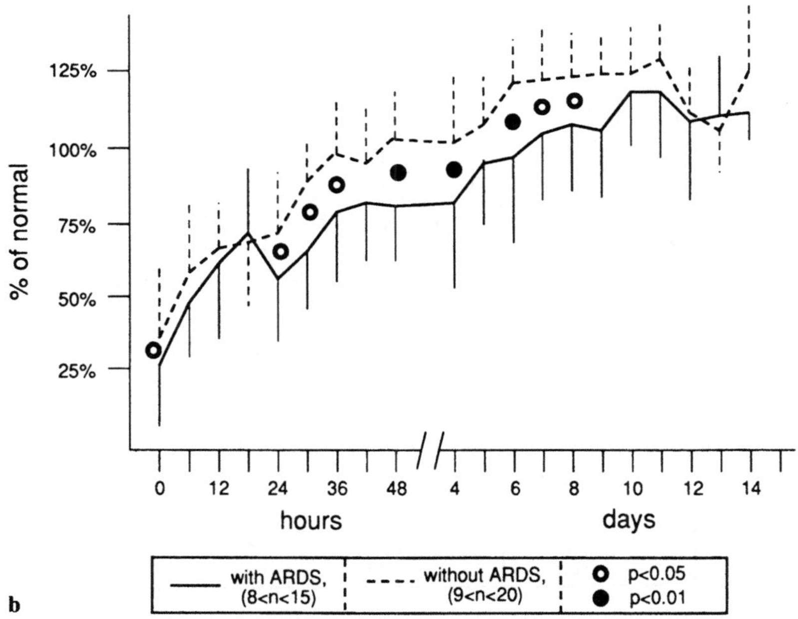

b

Fig. 4. **a** Plasminogen; **b** antiplasmin

Plasminogen and Antiplasmin (Fig. 4). For the first 48 h, plasminogen levels remained stable at about 65% of normal and then rose slowly. At the initial stable phase the two groups showed no significant differences, but after 48 h the rise in plasminogen levels of the group without ARDS was significantly steeper, reaching 114% after 10 days. In the ARDS groups only levels of 79% after 10 days were reached.

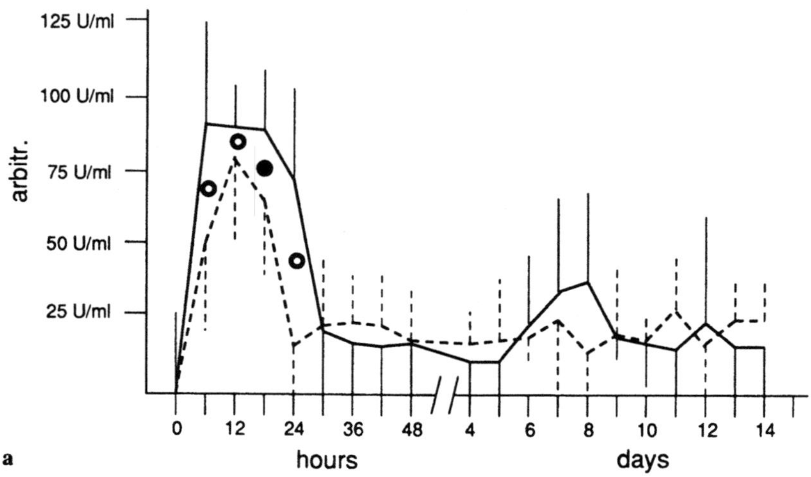

a

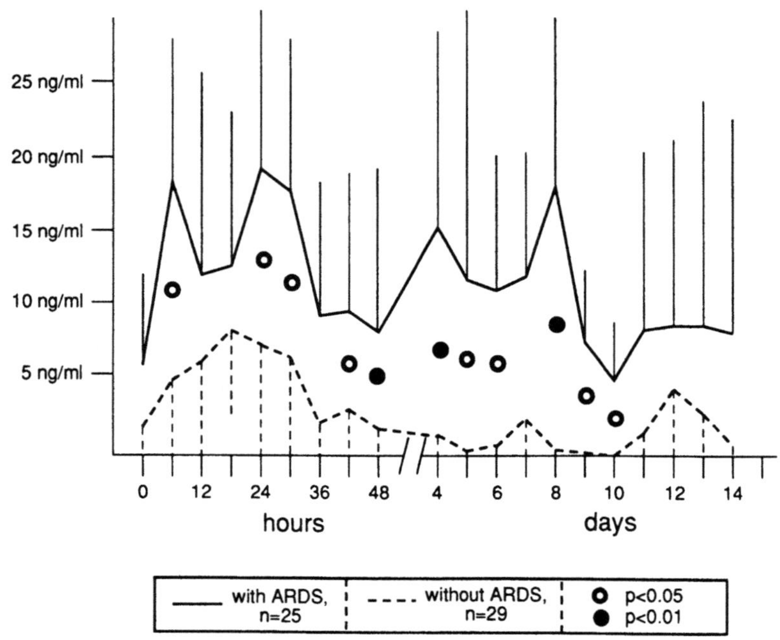

b

Fig. 5. a t-PA inhibitor level; **b** t-PA immunological plasma level

Antiplasmin levels rose from low initial values to a plateau of over 100% after 6 days. The slope of this rise was similar for both group, but the levels of the ARDS group were lower after 24 h and reached a plateau level of 105% compared to 123% in the group without ARDS. These differences were significant at 24, 30, 36, and 48 h and at 4, 6, and 8 days.

t-PA and t-PA Inhibitor (Fig. 5). The t-PA inhibition capacity increased to high concentrations of over 80 U/ml within the first 18 h and declined to a resting level of about 20 U/ml after 30 h. The peak of the ARDS group was significantly higher (up to 91 U/ml) and of longer duration (6–24 h after trauma) than the peak of the group without ARDS (80 U/ml, 12–18 h after trauma). After 30 h, there was no significant difference between the two groups.

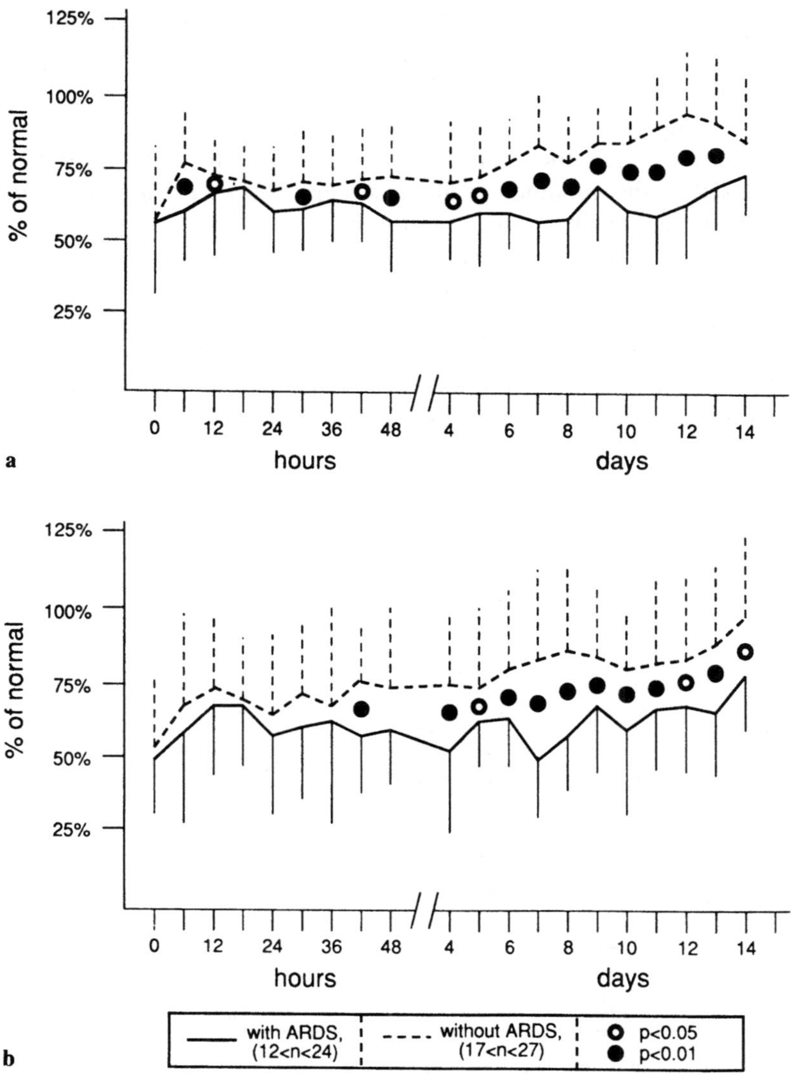

Fig. 6. a Antithrombin III activity level; **b** antithrombin III immunological plasma level

The t-PA antigen levels showed a small peak 6–30 h after polytrauma. While the peak of t-PA inhibition capacity reached base levels 30 h after the patient's admission to hospital, the decrease in t-PA antigen levels was delayed for 6 h, reaching base levels after 36 h. Over the whole experimental period the levels of t-PA concentration in the ARDS groups were higher, with resting levels of about 12 ng/ml, than in the group without ARDS, with resting levels of about 2 ng/ml. These differences were significant at 6, 24, 30, 42, and 48 h and at 4, 5, 6, 8, 9 and 10 days. Moreover ARDS patients showed a slight decrease in concentration at 12 and 18 h after polytrauma, exactly at the time where the t-PA inhibition capacity reached its peak.

Antithrombin III (Fig. 6). The AT III antigen and activity levels were, over the whole observation period, lower in the ARDS group (about 62%) than in the group without ARDS (about 78%). There were significant differences in the AT III activity of the two groups right from the beginning (Fig. 6a). However, due to larger fluctuations and a higher coefficient of variation probably caused by the immunological test system, there were no differences between the antigen levels measured in the two groups within the first 36 h, even though the levels of the ARDS group were persistently lower (Fig. 6b).

Function Versus Immunological Plasma Levels of AT III and C1 Inactivator (Fig. 7). While for AT III, the time course of activity and immunological measurement was equal, the immunological measurement reached a much higher level in the C1 inactivator as an example of an acute-phase protein.

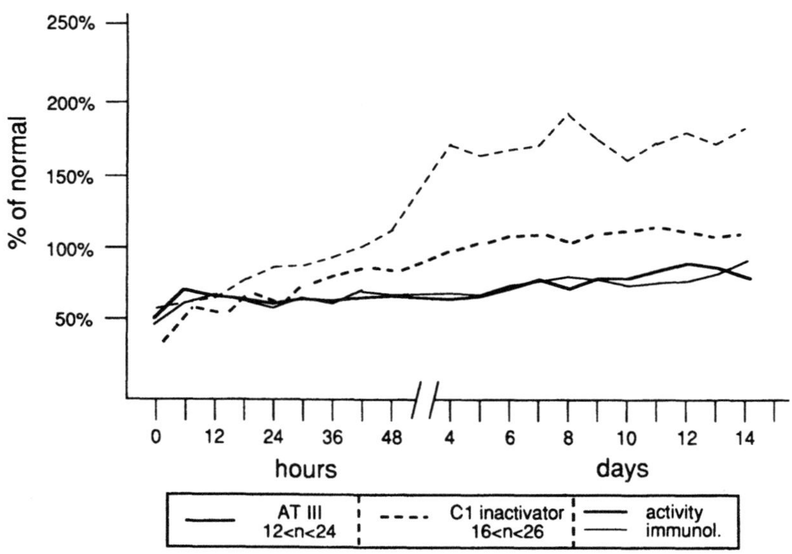

Fig. 7. Comparison of immunological plasma and activity levels measurement of AT III and C1 inactivator

Discussion

As with other factors of the clotting cascade (F VII and F II, Bartels) Prekallikrein and F XII levels were no different in patients with and without ARDS (Fig. 1). Therefore activation of the clotting cascade seems to have been comparable in both groups. The split products of fibrin (DD fragment) and fibrinogen (fibrinopeptide A; Fig. 2) and the main inhibitor of the contact phase (C1 inactivator; Fig.3) are also not involved in the development of ARDS, but are just a secondary phenomenon.

The fibrinolytic system and the inhibition of the clotting cascade seem to be more important for the development of ARDS, because plasminogen, antiplasmin, t-PA, t-PA inhibitor, and AT III levels showed significant differences between the groups with and without ARDS (Figs. 4–6).

The plasminogen levels of the ARDS group stayed low during the whole observation period, while those of the group without ARDS rose after 48 h to normal levels (Fig. 4a). The persistently low plasminogen levels in the ARDS group could be due to dilution as well as lack of synthesis and are therefore probably not a precondition, but a consequence of the development of ARDS. The same might be true for antiplasmin, because the levels of the two groups of patients were indistinguishable from each other between 6–18 h and only later on did the values of the group without ARDS become significantly higher (Fig. 4b).

t-PA antigen, t-PA inhibitor, and AT III showed significant differences between the two groups within the first 24 h (Fig. 5, 6a) and therefore could be in causal context with ARDS. For t-PA and t-PA inhibitor, the values of the ARDS group were higher than for the group without ARDS, and for AT III they were lower. Furthermore, these three parameters could be used as indicators to predict the development of ARDS in an early phase without clinical symptoms.

To predict the development of ARDS using true positive prediction, critical values have to be determined. For t-PA and t-PA inhibitor a large proportion of all patients developing ARDS should lie above these critical values, and for AT III below these values. Since the distribution of the values in both groups overlap, a certain percentage of the patients who would not develop ARDS would be wrongly assigned to the ARDS group (false positive prediction). To allow a reliable prediction of the development of ARDS, the true positive prediction of a certain critical value was set at 75% and the corresponding false positive predictions were calculated (Table 1). They should lie below 35% to obtain to high predictive value for a certain critical value.

The critical values for t-PA inhibitior values at 18 and 24 h, for t-PA antigen at 6 h, and for AT III at 6 h are of high predictive value because less than 35% of the patients would be predicted false positive (Table 1). Therefore, using these critical values, one can predict the patients who will

Table 1. Critical values for a true positive prediction of 75% and the corresponding false positive prediction for t-PA, t-PA inhibitor, and AT III within the first 24 h. The critical values were only calculated if there was a significant difference between the ARDS group and the group without ARDS

		6 h	12 h	18 h	24 h
t-PA inhibitior	critical value [U/ml]	34	77	78	45
	false positive	69%	56%	35%	30%
t-PA antigen	critical value [ng/ml]	8.5	–	–	8.5
	false positive	33%	–	–	42%
AT III activity	critical value [%]	70	76	–	–
	false positive	35%	53%	–	–

develop ARDS and those who will not. The other critical values are of lower predictive value because the percentage of false positive prediction is higher (Table 1).

Only at 6 h did all three parameters show a significant difference between the ARDS group and the group without ARDS (Figs. 5, 6), therefore only at this time was a combinaton of all three parameters possible to improve the predictive value for the development of ARDS. Additionally, it is desirable to predict the development of ARDS as early as possible to start successful treatment.

While at 6 h 83% of the patients of the ARDS group showed t-PA inhibitor levels higher than 34 U/ml, t-PA levels higher than 8.5 ng/ml, and AT III activitly levels lower than 70%, only 27% of the patients of the group without ARDS lay beyond these critical values. If the results of this study are transferable to other collectives, consideration of the combined critical values of t-PA, t-PA inhibitor, and AT III activity 6 h after polytrauma would allow a correct prediction of the development of ARDS in 83% of the cases, while only 27% of the patients who would not develop ARDS would be wrongly assigned to the ARDS group.

References

1. Bachofen M, Weibel EF (1982) Structural alternations of lung parenchyma in the adult repiratory distress syndrome. Clin Chest Med 3:35–56

2. Bone RC, Francis PB, Pierce AK (1976) Intravascular coagulation associated with the adult respiratory distress syndrome. Am J Med 61:585–589
3. Büsing CM, Bleyl U (1977) Plasminogen activatory activity of pulmonary vessels in shock. Thromb Res 11:285–295
4. D'Angelo A, Kluft C, Verheijen JH, Rijken DC, Mozzi E, Mannucci PM (1985) Fibrinolytic shut-down after surgery: impairment of the balance between tissue-type plasminogen activator and its specific inhibitor. Eur J Clin Invest 15:308–312
5. Duswald KH, Jochum M, Schramm W, Fritz H (1985) Released granulocytic elastase: an indicator of pathobiochemical alterations in septicemia after abdominal surgery. Surgery 9815:892–899
6. Eriksson E, Risberg B (1988) Tissue plasminogen activator and its inhibitor following major surgery in relation to ventilatory pattern. Acta Chir Scand 154:57–60
7. Holvoet P, Cleemput H, Collen D (1985) Assay of human tissue-type plasminogen activator (t-PA) with an enzyme-linked immunosorbent assay (ELISA) based on three murine monoclonal antibodies to t-PA. Thromb Haemost 54:684–687
8. Juhan-Vague I, Ailaud MF, De Cock F, Philip-Joet C, Arnaud C, Serradigmin A, Collen D (1985) The fast-acting inhibitor of tissue-type plasminogen activator is an acute phase reactant protein. In: Davidson JF, Donati MB, Cocceri S (eds) Progress in fibrolysis, vol VII. Churchill Livingstone, Edinburgh, pp146–149
9. Kluft C, de Bart ACW, Barthels M, Sturm J, Möller W (1988) Short term extreme increases in plasminogen activator inhibitor I (PAI 1) plasma of polytrauma patients. Fibrinolysis 2:223–226
10. Kluft C, Verheijen JH, Jie AFH, Rijken DC, Preston FE, Sue-Ling HM, Jespersen J, Aasen AO (1985) The postoperative fibrinolytic shutdown: a rapidly reverting acute phase pattern for the fast-acting inhibitor of tissue-typed plasminogen activator after trauma. Scand J Clin Lab Invest 45:605–610
11. McLoughlin GA, Grindlinger GA, Manny J, Valeri CR, Lipinski CR, Mannick JA, Hechtman Hb (1979) Intrapulmonary clotting and fibrinolysis during abdominal aortic aneurysm surgery. Ann Surg 190:623–630
12. Nilsson K, Rosen S, Friberger P (1987) A new kit for the determination of tissue plasminogen activator and its inhibition in blood. Fibrinolysis 1:163–168
13. Ordog GJ, Wasserberger J (1985) Coagulation abnormalities in traumatic shock. Ann Emerg Med 14:650–655
14. Risberg B (1975) Fibrinolysis in the lung. Acta Chir Scand [Suppl] 458
15. Schleef RR, Loskutoff DJ (1988) Fibrinolytic system of vascular endothelial cells: role of plasminogen activator inhibitors. Haemostasis 18:328–341
16. Schramm W (1984) C1-esterase inhibitor. In: Bergmayer HU (ed) Methods of enzymatic analysis, vol 5. VCH, Weinheim, pp 461–466
17. Sitrin RG, Brubaker PG, Fantone J (1987) Tissue fibrin deposition during acute lung injury in rabbits and its relationship to local expression of procoagulants and fibrinolytic activities. Am Rev Respir Dis 126:930–936
18. deleted
19. Spannagl M, Hoffmann H, Siebeck M, Weipert J,Schramm W (1990) A preformed antithrombin III-heparin complex as potent inhibitor of activated clotting factors in endotoxin shock of the pig. Thromb Res (in press)
20. Sprengers ED, Kluft C (1987) Plasminogen activator inhibitors. Blood 69(2):381–387
21. Suffredini AF, Harpel PC, Parrilo JE (1989) Promotion and subsequent inhibition of plasminogen activation after administration of intravenous endotoxin to normal subjects. N Engl J Med 320:1165–1172
22. Watkins J, Wild G (1985) The early diagnosis of impending coagulopathies following surgery and multiple trauma. Klin Wochenschr 63:1019–1027
23. Witte J, Jochum M, Scherer R, Schramm W, Hochstrasser K, Fritz H (1982) Disturbances of selected plasma proteins in hyperdynamic septic shock. Intensive Care Med 8:251–222

III Activation of Cellular Systems

Nonspecific Immune System, Plasma Proteins and Characteristics of the Erythrocyte Insulin Receptor

A. Dwenger[1], G. Regel[2], G. Schweitzer[1], G. Röllig[1], and J. Lindena[1]

Introduction

Several lines of evidence suggest that the imbalance of the humoral-phagocytic immune system conclusively contributes to the development of the adult respiratory distress syndrome (ARDS) [16, 19, 35]. Furthermore, polymorphonuclear leukocytes (PMNLs) are believed to play an essential role in the initiation and amplification of the lung tissue injury processes leading to increased lung permeability and the onset of ARDS. After being stimulated intravascularly, neutrophils adhere to the capillary endothelium, especially of the lung, and then pass across the capillary-interstitial-alveolar space while releasing inflammatory mediators such as arachidonic acid metabolites, oxygen-derived agents, and lysosomal enzymes [26, 29, 33]. These release reactions are coupled to stimulatory response mechanisms in which soluble and/or particulate stimulators cause extracellular release of respiratory burst products and lysosomal enzymes which lead to an increase in photon emission [1].

Therefore, chemiluminescence (CL) probing techniques and modifications thereof can be used to monitor single components of the humoral-granulocytic immune system, as well as the complete system, after trauma.

By the same methods the functional state of neutrophils before (isolated from blood) and after (isolated from bronchoalveolar lavage fluid) passage across the blood/air barrier can be investigated.

Also in vitro stimulation experiments of isolated neutrophils can be used to provide additional information about the functional state of this cell.

Furthermore, three groups of plasma proteins associated with altered pathophysiological reactions occurring after trauma may be investigated: (a) granulocyte-derived enzymes, with the aim of demonstrating their reliability as indicators of posttraumatic neutrophil activation; (b) acute-phase, trans-

[1] Department of Clinical Biochemistry, Hannover Medical School, Konstanty-Gutschow-Str. 8, W-3000 Hannover 61, FRG
[2] Department of Trauma Surgery, Hannover Medical School, Konstanty-Gutschow-Str. 8, W-3000 Hannover 61, FRG

J.A. Sturm (Ed.)
Adult Respiratory Distress Syndrome

port, and opsonic proteins, which may play a critical role in the immediate host defense against bacterial invasion and in the protection of host tissues from autoinjury by the leukocyte-generated mechanisms for bacterial killing and removal of dead tissues [27, 28]; and (c) special marker enzymes to be used as diagnostic or prognostic tools.

In this study, the common destructive influence of neutrophil-secreted lysosomal enzymes on plasma membrane receptors was investigated by means of the insulin receptor-mediated autoregulative process of insulin degradation in erythrocytes catalyzed by glutathione-insulin-transhydrogenase.

Methods

Study Population

Fifty-seven multiply traumatized patients (Injury Severity Score >30 points) were investigated, 26 of them with ARDS and 31 of them without ARDS. Bronchoalveolar lavage fluid (BALF) and citrated venous blood samples were repeatedly obtained from 12 ARDS and 15 non-ARDS patients for up to 14 days after trauma, and once from 12 normals.

Additional blood samples were taken from healthy donors. All parameters were expressed as medians ± pseudo standard error for patients from Hannover (Han), Essen (Es), or both centers (Han + Es), if not stated otherwise. Data were analyzed by means of the Mann-Whitney U test, and differences were assumed to be significant if $p < 0.05$.

Nonspecific Immune System

Chemiluminescence Measurements. By CL probing techniques the following components of the humoral-granulocytic immune system were monitored: (a) the non-opsonized zymosan-induced and luminol-enhanced whole blood CL response, (b) the CL response of isolated PMNL after non-opsonized zymosan and standard plasma stimulation, (c) the patient's plasma opsonic capacity using non-opsonized zymosan and normal PMNL, and (d) the patient plasma CL inhibitory factor to reduce half-maximally the latex-induced CL response of normal PMNL by the use of different dilutions of patient plasma. The experimental procedures have been described previously [6, 9, 12, 18].

Neutrophil Count. After staining with Türk's solution (acetic acid gentian violet solution, Merck, FRG) neutrophils were counted in citrated venous blood samples using a Neubauer hemocytometer.

Adherence. The nylon fiber adherence test according to Dwenger et al. [11] and MacGregor et al. [20] was used with minor modifications. Briefly, replicates of 400 µl MEM (minimal essential medium Dulbecco, Boehringer, Mannheim, FRG) + 100 µl citrated venous blood samples were incubated with (A) and without (B) 5 mg nylon fiber (Leuko-Pak Leukocyte Filter, Code 4 C 2401, Fenwal Division, Travenol Laboratories, Inc., Deerfield, United States) in 3.5-ml polystyrene vials for 20 min at 37°C. After removal of the nylon fiber, neutrophils were counted and adherence was calculated according to:

$$\% \text{ adherence} = \frac{(\text{PMNL/ml}_B - \text{PMNL/ml}_A)}{(\text{PMNL/ml}_B)} \cdot 100$$

Functions and Protein Content of Neutrophils from Blood and BALF

Intra- and Extracellular Elastase and β-N-Acetylglucosaminidase Concentrations/Activities. Elastase (ELA) and β-N-Acetylglucosaminidase (β-NAG) Concentrations and Activities were measured according to previously described methods [5, 6] in plasma, BALF, and PMNL lysate samples (PMNL isolated from blood and BALF, respectively) of eight multiply traumatized patients in comparison with eight blood donors and four normals with the BAL procedure. Briefly, elastase concentration was measured by enzyme immunoassay ("PMN elastase" test, Merck, FRG) with and without the addition of normal plasma, and the activity was determined with pyroGlu-Pro-Val-pNA as substrate (S 2484, KABI Diagnostica, Sweden) at 405 nm and 37°C. β-NAG activity was measured by spectrofflurometric enzyme assay with 4-methyl-umbelliferyl-*N*-acetyl-β-D-glucosaminide as a substrate (Sigma Chemical Co., United States). The epithelial lining fluid (ELF) was determined according to previously described methods [13].

Elastase Receptor System of Human Blood Neutrophils. Competition/inhibition experiments with isolated human PMNL and ^{125}I-labeled and nonlabeled human leukocyte elastase were performed and the receptor characteristics were calculated according to previous descriptions [2, 4, 8].

Chemiluminescence Response of BALF and Blood-Derived Neutrophils. Bronchoalveolar lavage fluid and citrated venous blood samples were simultaneously obtained from nine multiply traumatized patients and this procedure was repeated several times during the posttraumatic course. Isolation and CL measurement of PMNL were performed as previously described [6, 7, 10].

In Vitro Stimulation and Enzyme Release of Isolated Neutrophils

Granulocytes were isolated from citrated venous blood samples on days 0, 1, 4, 8, and 12 after trauma according to Dwenger et al. [8] and resuspended in

MEM to give a final cell concentration of 5–10·10^6/ml. To determine enzyme release, four kinds of reaction mixtures were prepared: (a) 1 ml cell suspension at 37°C without prior incubation + 1 ml digitonin/NP 40 solution [6]; this lysate was used to determine the 100% reference values; (b) 1 ml cell suspension at 37°C without incubation with immediate separation of supernatant by centrifugation (2 min at 12000 g); (c) 1 ml cell suspension at 37°C, 60 min incubation, separation of supernatant by centrifugation; and (d) 1 ml cell suspension at 37°C containing 1mg/ml opsonized zymosan A and $2 \cdot 10^{-6}$ mol/l *N*-formyl-L-methionyl-L-leucyl-L-phenylalanine (Sigma Chemical Co., United States), 60 min incubation, and separation of supernatant by centrifugation. In the lysate (a) as well as in the supernatant samples (b), (c), and (d) the following enzymes were determined: lactate dehydrogenase (LDH, EC 1.1.1.27) with the test combination "LDH optimized UV test" (Boehringer, Mannheim, FRG), elastase (ELA, EC 3.4.21.37) enzymatically as described above, and myeloperoxidase (MPO, EC 1.11.1.7) according to Matheson et al. [22]. β-*N*-Acetylglucosaminidase (β-NAG, EC 3.2.1.30), β-galactosidase (β-GAL, EC 3.2.1.23), β-glucuronidase (β-GLU, EC 3.2.1.31), and acid phosphatase (ACP, EC 3.1.3.2) were measured with fluorogenic substrates using a slightly modified test originally described by Yatziv et al. [34]. Enzyme release was determined as a percentage of cellular content. Four different parameters of each enzyme were calculated and plotted versus time: (a) enzyme units/PMNL, (b) percentage of spontaneous enzyme release after 0 min incubation time, (c) percentage of spontaneous enzyme release after 60 min incubation, and (d) percentage of enzyme release after 60 min stimulation minus the value obtained in (c).

Plasma Proteins

Enzymes Released by Neutrophils. The lysosomal acid hydrolases β-*N*-acetylglucosaminidase, β-galactosidase, β-glucuronidase, and acid phosphatase were measured according to Yatziv et al. [34].

Acute-Phase, Transport, and Opsonic Proteins. Albumin was measured by the bromocresol green method, total protein with the biuret method, transferrin, ceruloplasmin, acid α_1-glycoprotein, C-reactive protein, and fibronectin immunological-nephelometrically using reagent sets, protocols, and instrumentation of Immuno Diagnostika GmbH (FRG) according to previous descriptions [6, 13].

Marker Enzymes. As a capillary endothelial cell enzyme angiotensin-converting enzyme (ACE, kininase II, EC 3.4.15.1) was determined spectrophotometrically according to Hurst and Lovell-Smith [17]. Lactate dehydrogenase was measured as a marker enzyme of general cell damage and cholinesterase (CHE, EC 3.1.1.8) was determined colorimetrically as a marker of liver function (colorimetric method, substrate: butyrylthiocholine, test combination Boehringer Mannheim, FRG).

Plasma Insulin Concentration, Erythrocyte Insulin Receptor Characteristics, and Glutathione-Insulin-Transhydrogenase (GIT) Activity

To judge the integrity of the insulin receptor protein and the function of the signal transfer chain "intracellular GIT activity–receptor efficiency–extracellular insulin concentration," four different parameters were determined on posttraumatic days 0, 1, 4, 8, and 12: (a) the plasma insulin concentration measured by radioimmunoassay [3], (b) the glutathione-insulin-transhydrogenase (GIT, EC 1.8.4.2) activity in erythrocytes according to Varandani and Nafz [31], (c) the insulin receptor concentration, and (d) the insulin receptor affinity according to Dwenger et al. [4].

Results

Nonspecific Immune System

Chemiluminescence Measurements. The whole blood CL response reflects the reactivity of the complete humoral-granulocytic immune system in the posttraumatic course (Fig. la). After a common decline of both patient groups within the first posttraumatic day, a complete recovery followed until the 2nd day. Beginning with days 3 or 4 after trauma, a clear dissociation could be seen, in that non-ARDS patients showed a nearly fivefold increase in the stimulatory response, whereas the reactivity of ARDS patients was generally reduced to just above normal values. This differential behavior was not caused by the cellular component of this system. The stimulatory CL response of isolated neutrophils, which represents their metabolic capacity or oxygenation activity, was higher than normal for both patient groups during the entire posttraumatic course (Fig. 1b). The values of ARDS patients were observed to be still higher than the values of non-ARDS patients, indicating the higher potential of ARDS neutrophils to release inflammatory mediators. The opsonic capacity of the patients' plasma, a reflection of the total mediator effect of all plasma opsonins of zymosan and neutrophils, showed decreased values for both patient groups immediately after trauma (Fig. 1c).

In non-ARDS patients the normal opsonin concentration was reconstituted after 6 days, showing a tendency to increase further, whereas the opsonin concentration of ARDS patients remained far below normal throughout the observation period. This behavior was nearly paralleled by the plasma fibronectin concentration, indicating the important role of fibronectin as a nonspecific opsonin (Fig. 2). It was observed that a substance

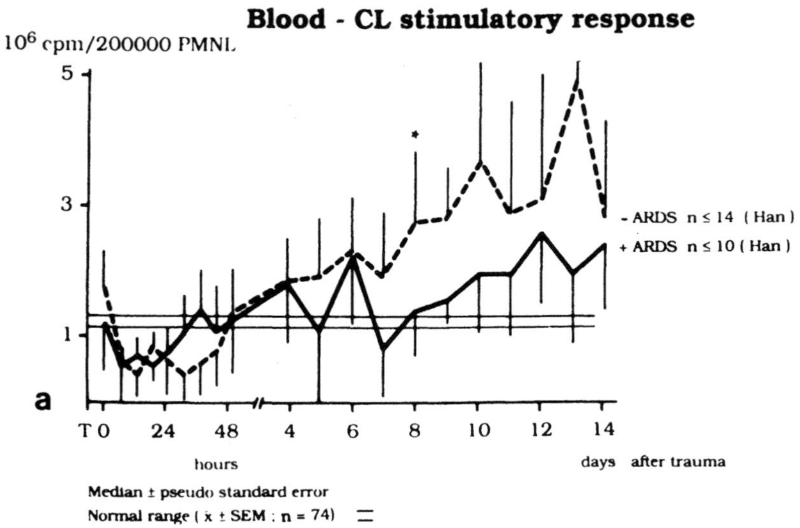

a

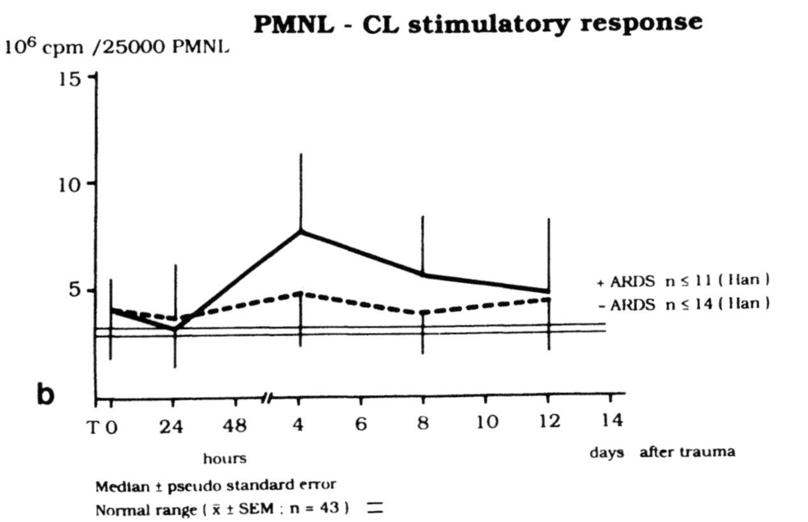

b

Fig. 1a–d. Chemiluminescence measurements: posttraumatic courses of zymosan A induced chemiluminescence response of **a** blood neutrophils, **b** isolated neutrophils and normal plasma, **c** normal neutrophils and patient plasma, and **d** latex-induced chemiluminescence response of normal neutrophils and patient plasma in ARDS and non-ARDS patients. $^{*}p < 0.05$ + ARDS vs − ARDS (U-test); *T*, blood sample obtained at the scene; *O*, blood sample obtained after volume resuscitation

was synthesized immediately after multiple trauma, which suppressed the CL response (Fig. 1d). This was determined by measuring the patients' plasma inhibitory potency to reduce half-maximally the latex-induced CL response of normal neutrophils, which is complement independent and nonspecific. After

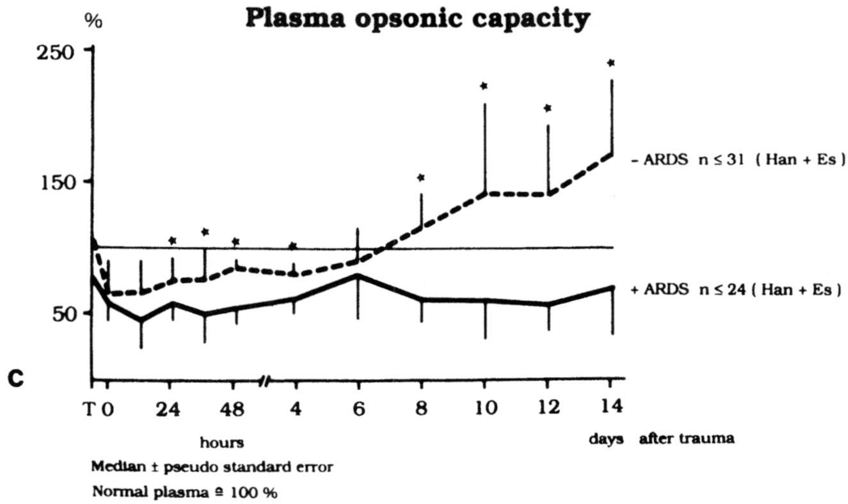

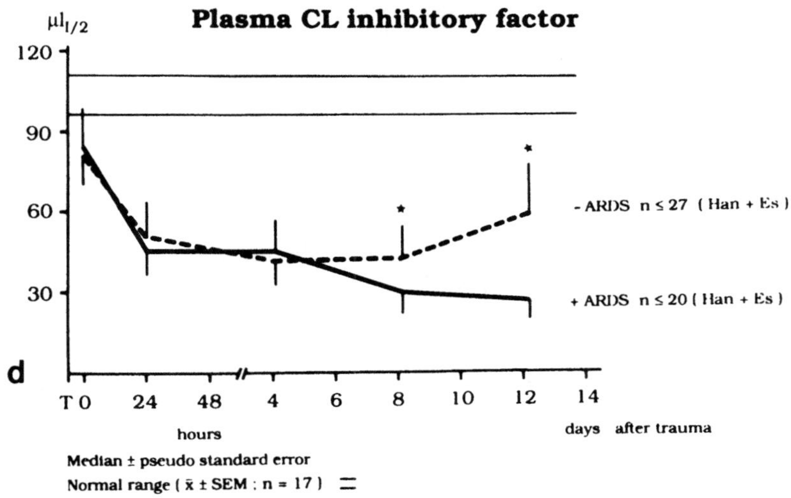

Fig. 1a–d. (Cont.)

an initial rapid increase in this component for both groups, indicated by a rapid decrease of the amount of plasma volume needed to produce the half-maximal CL reduction, this factor was synthesized continuously for up to 14 days in ARDS patients, whereas there was an increased elimination or decreased synthesis in non-ARDS patients beginning at days 6 or 7 after trauma.

Neutrophil Count. After an immediate two fold increase in the blood PMNL count, there was a decrease for up to 12 h after trauma and a further

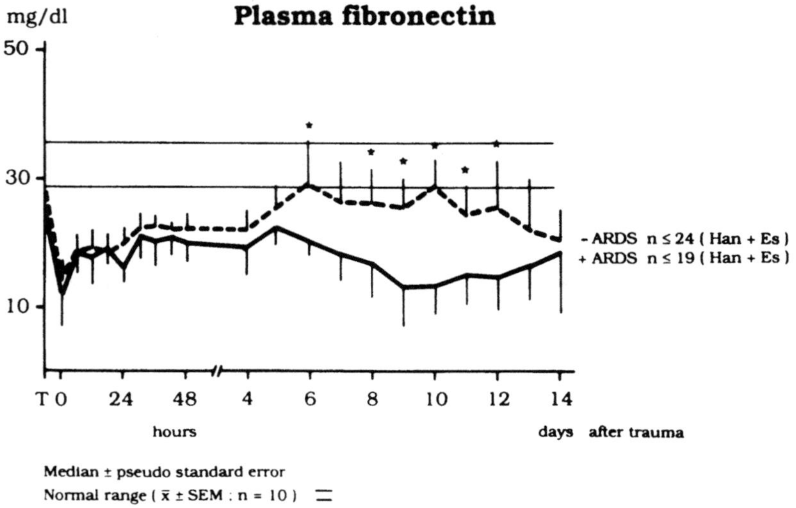

Fig. 2. Posttraumatic course of plasma fibronectin concentrations in ARDS and non-ARDS patients. $^{*}p < 0.05$ + ARDS vs − ARDS (U-test); *T*, blood sample obtained at the scene; *O*, blood sample obtained after volume resuscitation

concomitant increase in both patient groups for up to 8 days (Fig. 3a). From this day on, ARDS patients exhibited a further increase, whereas values for non-ARDS patients declined slightly.

Adherence. Polymorphonuclear leukocyte adherence in whole blood was only measured in the last patients of the study. Due to the small number of patients involved only median values without deviations are shown in Fig. 3b. After an initial decline, a tendency toward steadily increasing adherence could be observed for both patient groups during the complete posttraumatic course.

Functions and Protein Contents of Neutrophils from Blood and BALF

Intra- and Extracellular Elastase and β-N-Acetylglucosaminidase Concentrations/Activities. Both elastase activity and total elastase concentration per 10^9 isolated granulocytes decreased in the order of: blood of normals ($\bar{x}$ = 106 U/9962 µg) > blood of patients ($\bar{x}$ = 67.1 U/6134 µg) > BALF of patients ($\bar{x}$ = 49.6 U/6078 µg); whereas the values for the concentration of complexed elastase increased ($\bar{x} = 1.35 < 3.07 \ll 380$ µg) (Fig. 4a). The plasma elastase concentrations of these patients were found to be elevated ($\bar{x}$ = 424 µg/l) above those of normals ($\bar{x}$ = 84 µg/l). In BALF, complexed and total elastase concentrations ($\bar{x}$ = 423 and 550 µg/l) were increased compared with those of normals ($\bar{x}$ = 11.5 and 8.1 µg/l) (Fig. 4b).

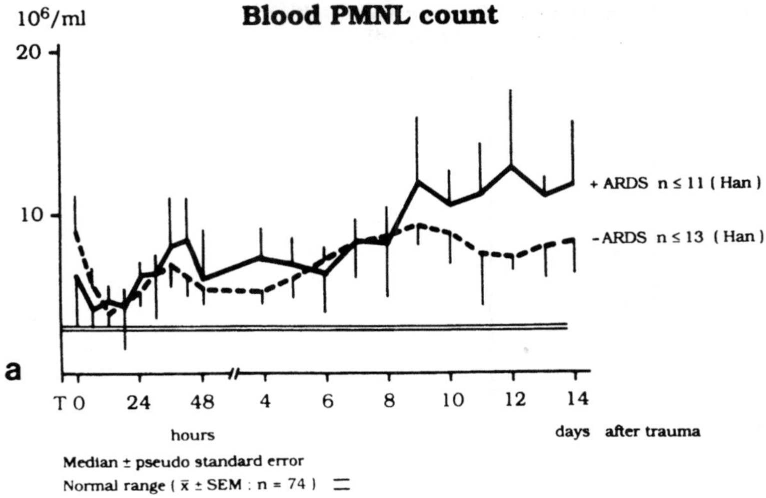

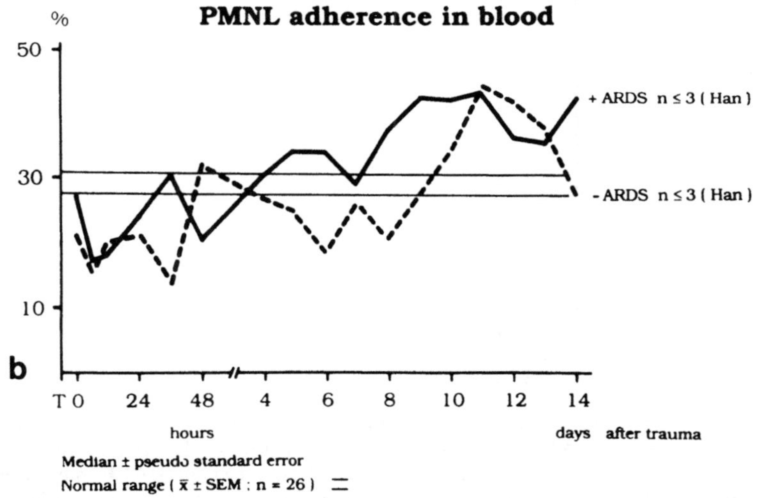

Fig. 3a,b. Posttraumatic courses of blood PMNL count (**a**) and PMNL adherence (**b**) in ARDS and non-ARDS patients. *$p < 0.05$ + ARDS vs − ARDS (U-test); *T*, blood sample obtained at the scene; *O*, blood sample obtained after volume resuscitation

In 3 out of 42 BALF samples, active elastase could be enzymatically detected that was inhibited by α_1-proteinase inhibitor ($\bar{x}$ = 0.049 U/l; n = 42) [5].

In lysates of isolated normal neutrophils, 1.45 mU β-NAG and 9.96 µg elastase were found in 10^6 cells. In epithelial lining fluid (ELF), the mean values were 47.4 U/l β-NAG and 24.3 mg/l elastase-α_1-proteinase inhibitor complex in 12 ARDS patients as well as 68.7 U/l β-NAG and 24.7 mg/l elastase-α_1-proteinase inhibitor complex in 15 non-ARDS patients, indicating

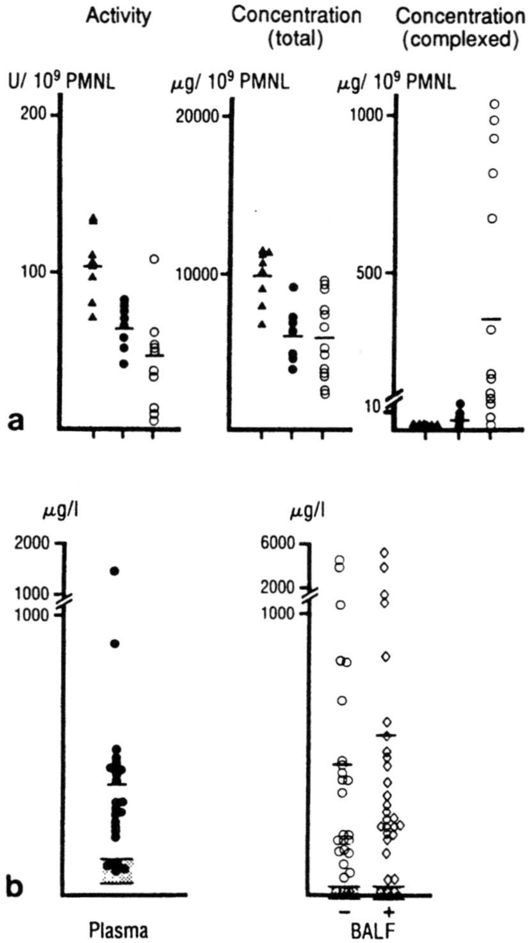

Fig. 4a,b. Elastase activity, total and complexed concentrations (**a**) of neutrophils isolated from the blood of normals (▲) and from the blood (●) and BALF (○) of multiply traumatized patients. Total elastase concentrations (**b**) in plasma (●) and BALF (measured without ○ and with ◊ addition of α_1-proteinase inhibitor) of multiply traumatized patients. *grey* = normal range ($\bar{x} \pm s$); — = means

Table 1. Mean activity of β-*N*-acetylglucosaminidase (β-NAG) and elastase-a_1-proteinase inhibitor complex concentration (ELA) in normal neutrophils ($n = 8$) and in ELF of 12 ARDS and 15 non-ARDS patients; the number of BALF samples is given in parentheses

	10^6PMNL	ELF_{ARDS}	$ELF_{non\text{-}ARDS}$
β-NAG	1.45 mU	47.4 U/l (79)	68.7 U/l (80)
ELA	9.96 µg	24.3 mg/l (75)	24.7 mg/l (66)
β-NAG/ELA	0.14	1.96	2.78
		14-fold	20-fold
		β-NAG increase	

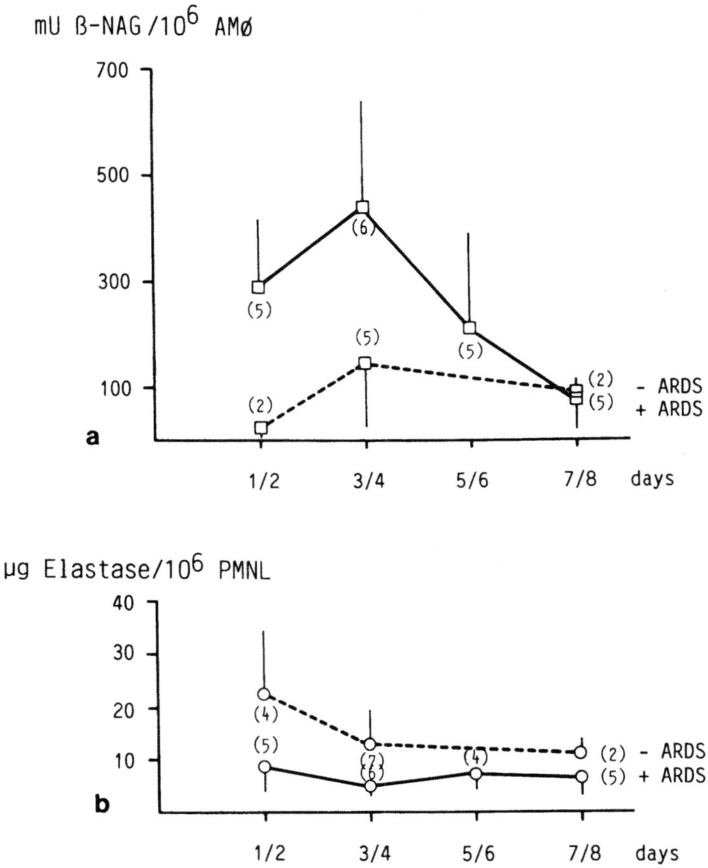

Fig. 5a,b. Posttraumatic courses of β-*N*-acetylglucosaminidase release/10^6 alveolar macrophages (**a**) and elastase release/10^6 neutrophils (**b**) in six ARDS and three non-ARDS patients

a 14-fold and 20-fold β-NAG increase in comparison with the intracellular relationship (Table 1).

Figure 5 depicts the posttraumatic courses of the cell response activities of alveolar macrophages (β-NAG activity/l ELF/alveolar macrophage count/l ELF) and of alveolar neutrophils (elastase concentration/l ELF/PMNL count/l ELF). Total β-NAG activity was corrected for β-NAG activity released by neutrophils.

Elastase Receptor System of Human Blood Neutrophils. A specific elastase receptor system with two independent binding sites was identified on the surface of human granulocytes (Table 2). By simple calculation, the extracellular elastase binding capacity of granulocytes was demonstrated (Table 3).

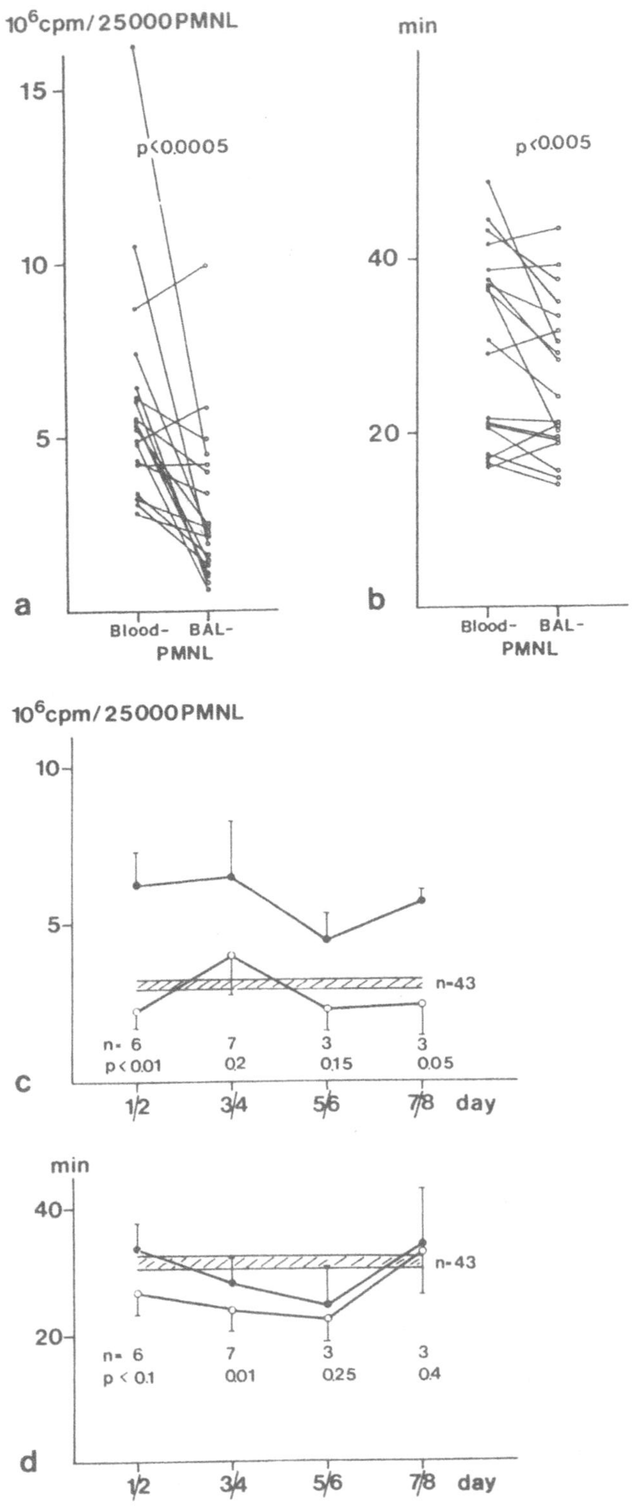

Fig. 6a–d. Zymosan A induced chemiluminescence responses (**a**, peak maximum in cpm/PMNL; **b**, peak maximum time in minutes) of 19 samples of neutrophils isolated from the blood (●) and BALF (○) of nine multiply traumatized patients. Posttraumatic courses (**c**, **d**) of chemiluminescence data of **a** and **b**. *Diagonally striped bars:* normal range ($\bar{x} \pm$ SEM; $n = 43$)

Table 2. Receptor characteristics of neutrophil elastase-binding sites

$K_1 = 2.2 \cdot 10^8$ l/mol	$R_1 = 1.4$ nmol/l $= 0.08 \cdot 10^6$/cell
$K_2 = 5.0 \cdot 10^5$ l/mol	$R_2 = 237$ nmol/l $= 14.0 \cdot 10^6$/cell

K, receptor affinity; *R*, receptor concentration

Table 3. Total receptor-binding capacity for extracellular elastase

Elastase:receptor = 1:1	
Total receptor-binding capacity of $5 \cdot 10^6$ neutrophils/ml ELF	3 μg elastase
Content of $5 \cdot 10^6$ PMNL:50μg	
Release of ~6% (FMLP, LPS)	3 μg elastase
Maximal amounts of noncomplexed elastase/ml ELF measured in ARDS patients	Up to 300 μg elastase

FMLP, *N*-formyl-1-L-methionyl-L-leucyl-L-phenyl-alanine; LPS, lipopolysaccharide

Chemiluminescence Response of BALF and Blood-Derived Neutrophils. Zymosan A stimulation of isolated neutrophils demonstrated a significantly ($p < 0.0005$) reduced CL response of BALF-derived granulocytes in comparison the granulocytes which were isolated from the blood of the same patient (Fig. 6a). Venous blood and BALF were obtained simultaneously. Furthermore, a concomitant and significant ($p < 0.005$) shortening of the time to reach the photon emission maximum was observed for BALF-derived neutrophils (Fig. 6b). The posttraumatic time course of these parameters is shown in Figs. 6c and d.

In Vitro Stimulation and Enzyme Release of Isolated Neutrophils

Lactate dehydrogenase release served as a marker for neutrophil integrity during in vitro incubation. A slight increase in LDH content of isolated neutrophils was observed after 12 days for both patient groups. Spontaneous release after 0 and 60 min, respectively, was normal but showed slightly increased values on day 4, whereas stimulated release was low, constant, and normal for 12 days (Fig. 7). However, for β-NAG (Fig. 8), MPO (Fig. 9), and β-GAL (Fig. 10), stimulated enzyme release peaked above normal values on day 4 whereas there was a nearly identical behavior of their spontaneous release after 0 and 60 min with that of LDH. Significant differences between ARDS and non-ARDS patients were not observed.

Plasma Proteins

Enzymes Released by Neutrophils. In Fig. 11, the time courses of four lysosomal hydrolases are depicted. Significant differences between ARDS

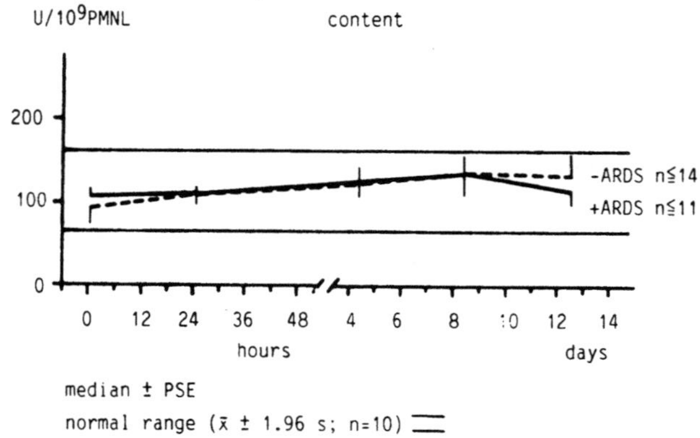

a

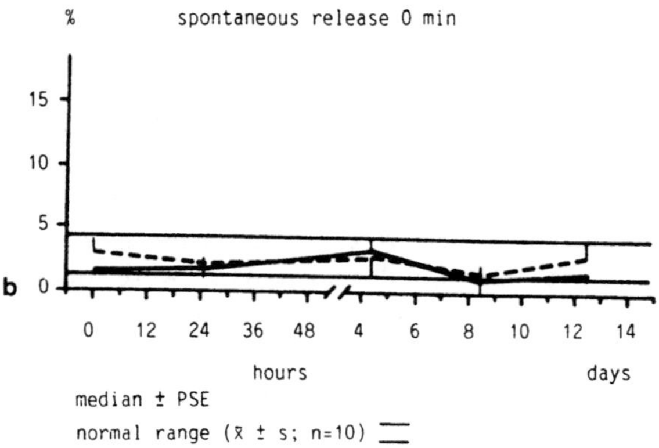

b

Fig. 7a–d. Posttraumatic courses of LDH content (**a**), spontaneous release, immediately (**b**) and after 60 min (**c**), and release after 60 min of stimulation with FMLP/zymosan A (**d**) of neutrophils isolated from the blood of ARDS and non-ARDS patients

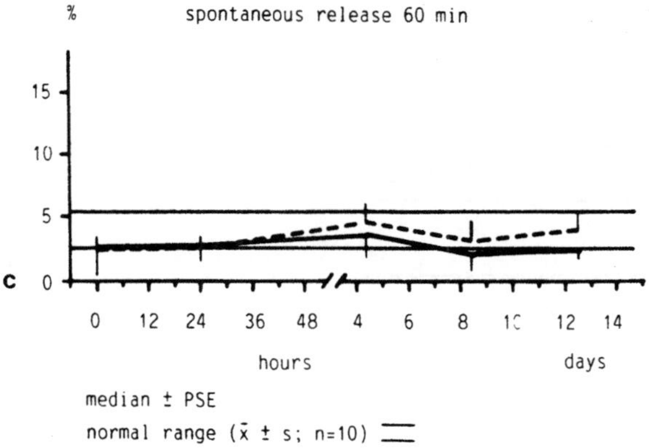
%
spontaneous release 60 min
15
10
5
c
0
0 12 24 36 48 4 6 8 10 12 14
hours
days
median ± PSE
normal range (x̄ ± s; n=10)

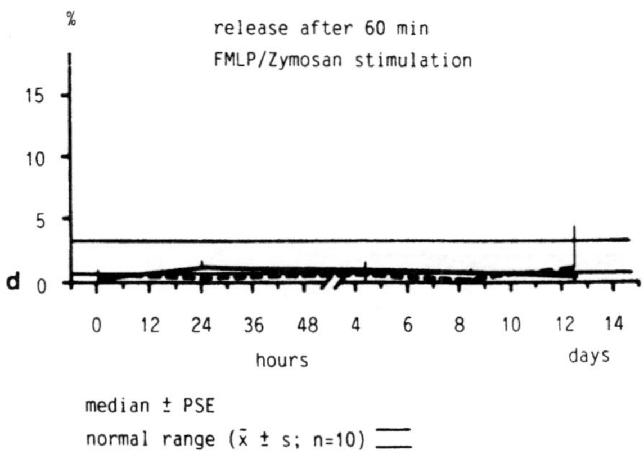
%
release after 60 min
FMLP/Zymosan stimulation
15
10
5
d
0
0 12 24 36 48 4 6 8 10 12 14
hours
days
median ± PSE
normal range (x̄ ± s; n=10)

Fig. 7a–d. (Cont.)

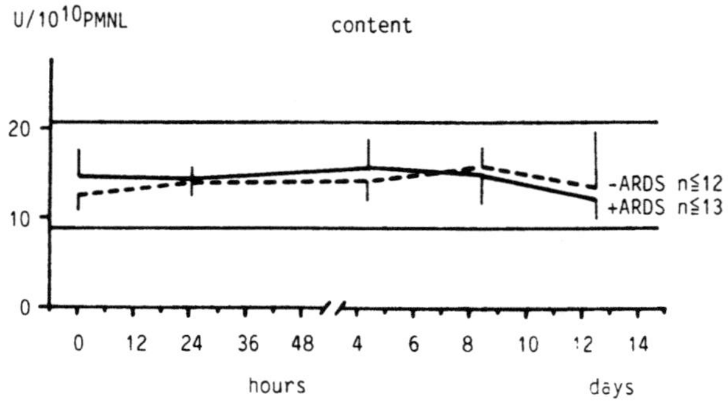

a

median ± PSE
normal range (x̄ ± 1.96 s; n=10)

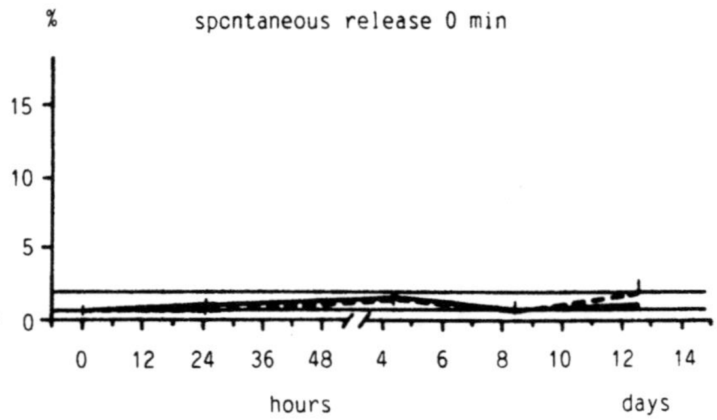

b

median ± PSE
normal range (x̄ ± s; n=10)

Fig. 8a–d. Posttraumatic courses of β-*N*-acetylglucosaminidase content (**a**), spontaneous release, immediately (**b**) and after 60 min (**c**), and release after 60 min of stimulation with FMLP/zymosan A (**d**) of neutrophils isolated from the blood of ARDS and non-ARDS patients

c

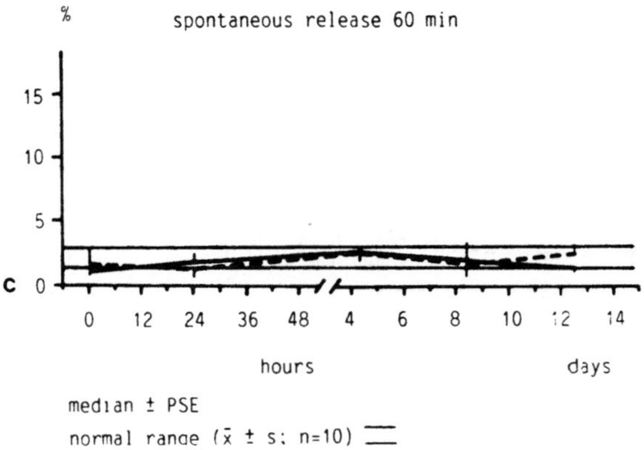

d

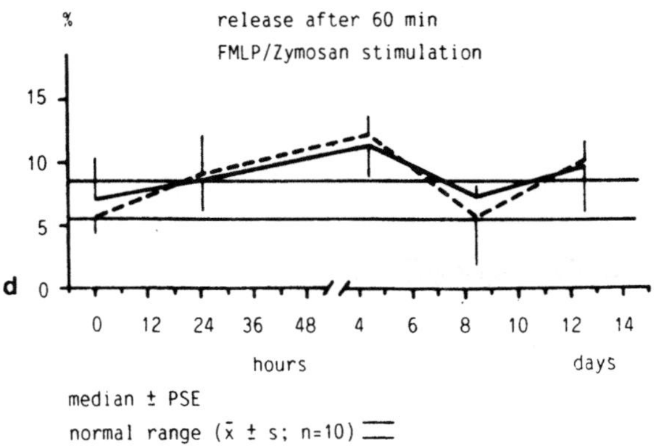

Fig. 8a–d. (Cont.)

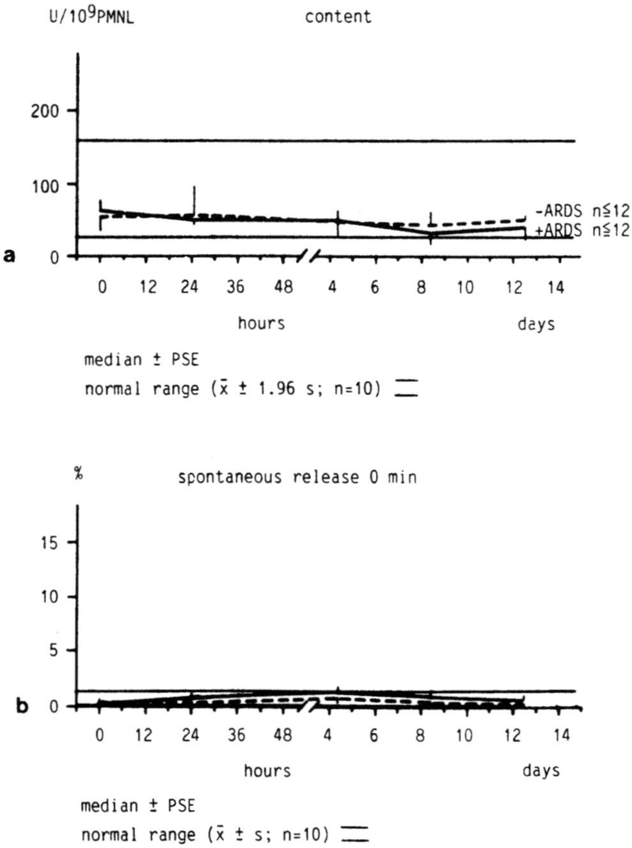

Fig. 9a–d. Posttraumatic courses of myeloperoxidase content (**a**), spontaneous release, immediately (**b**) and after 60 min (**c**), and release after 60 min of stimulation with FMLP/zymosan A (**d**) of neutrophils isolated from the blood of ARDS and non-ARDS patients

c

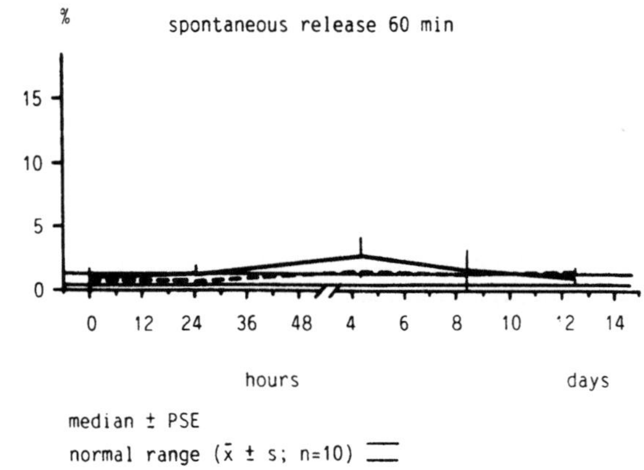

d

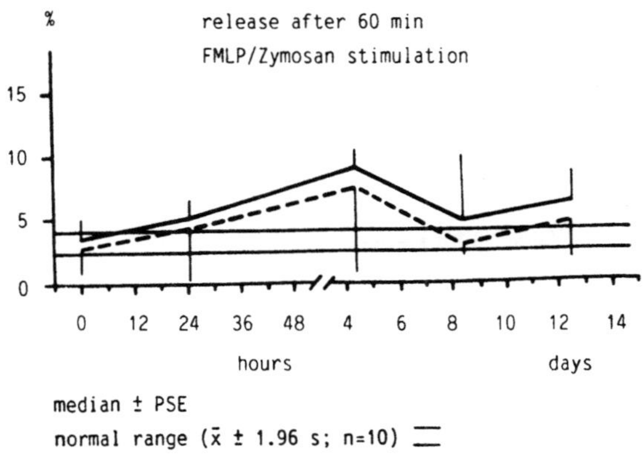

Fig. 9a–d. (Cont.)

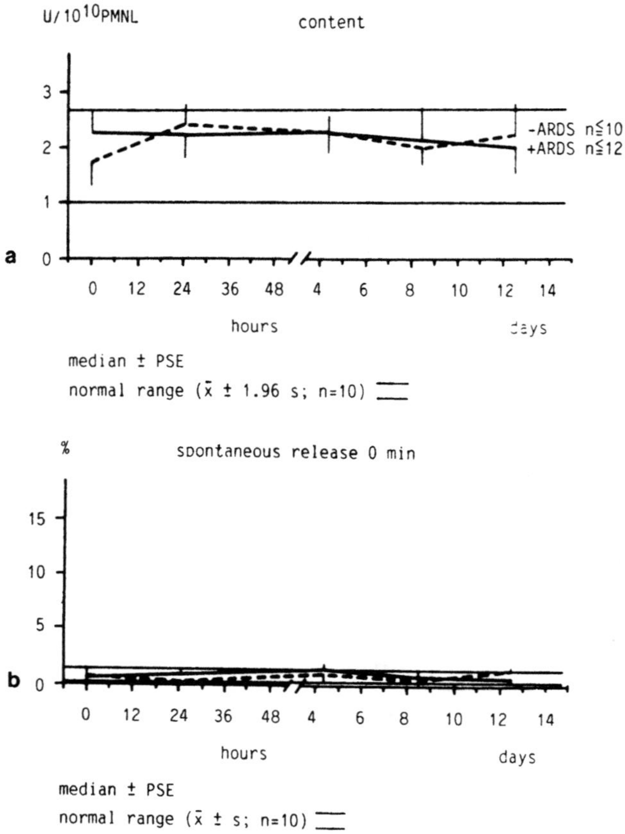

Fig. 10a–d. Posttraumatic courses of β-galactosidase content (**a**), spontaneous release, immediately (**b**) and after 60 min (**c**), and release after 60 min of stimulation with FMLP/zymosan A (**d**) of neutrophils isolated from the blood of ARDS and non-ARDS patients

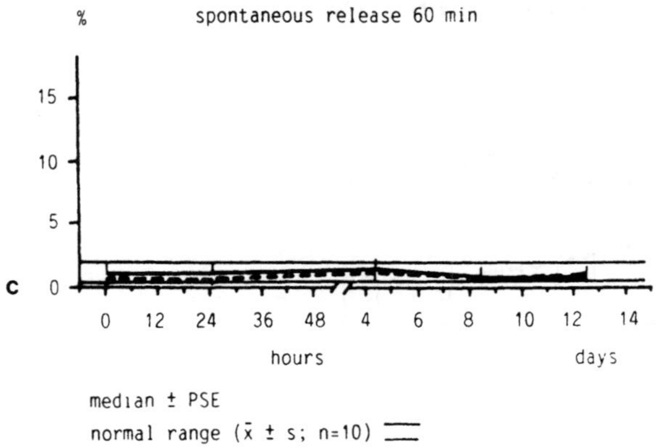

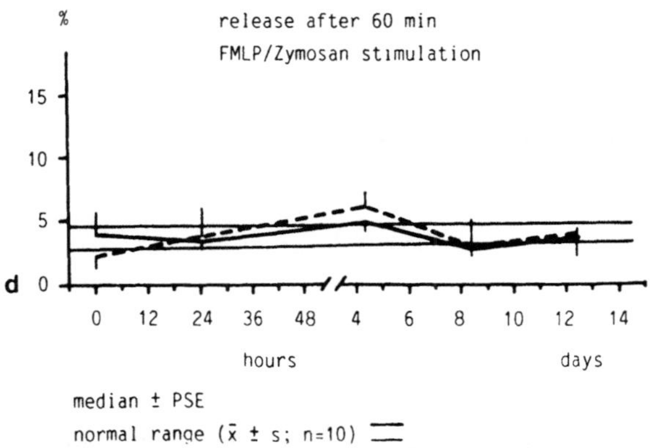

Fig. 10a–d. (Cont.)

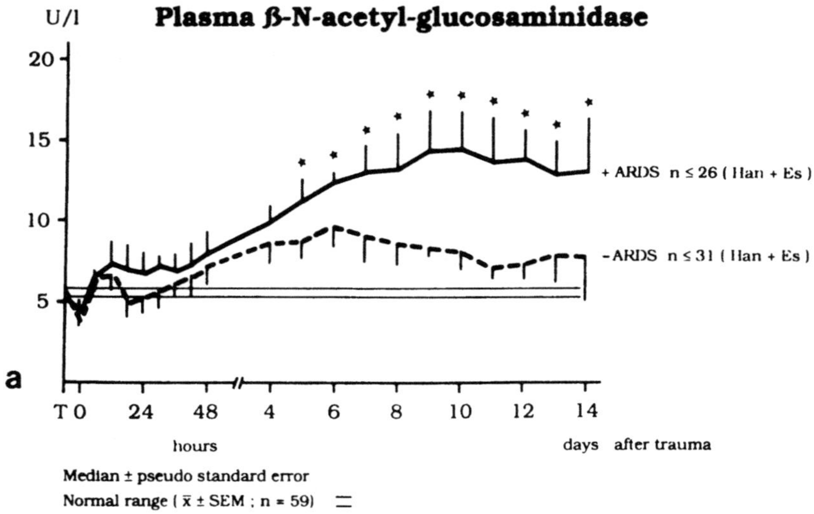

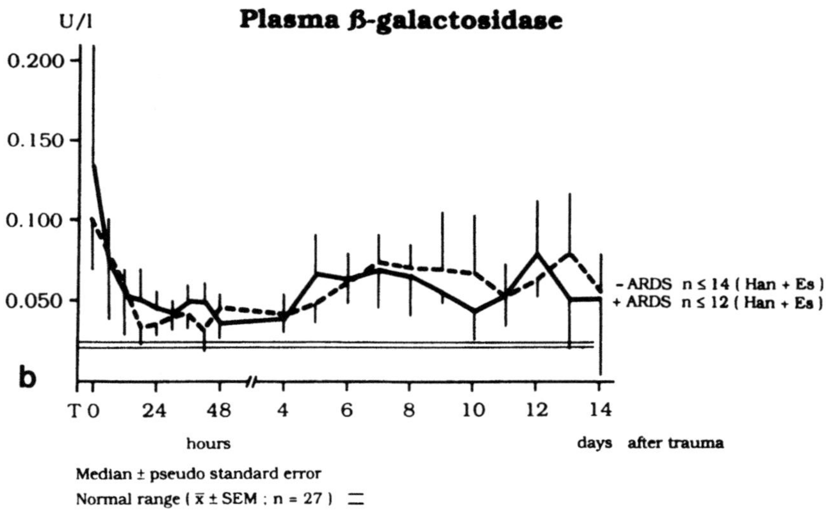

Fig. 11a–d. Posttraumatic courses of plasma β-*N*-acetylglucosaminidase (**a**), β-galactosidase (**b**), acid phosphatase (**c**), and β-glucuronidase (**d**) in ARDS and non-ARDS patients. * $p < 0.05$ + ARDS vs − ARDS (U-test). *T*, blood sample obtained at the scene; *O*, blood sample obtained after volume resuscitation

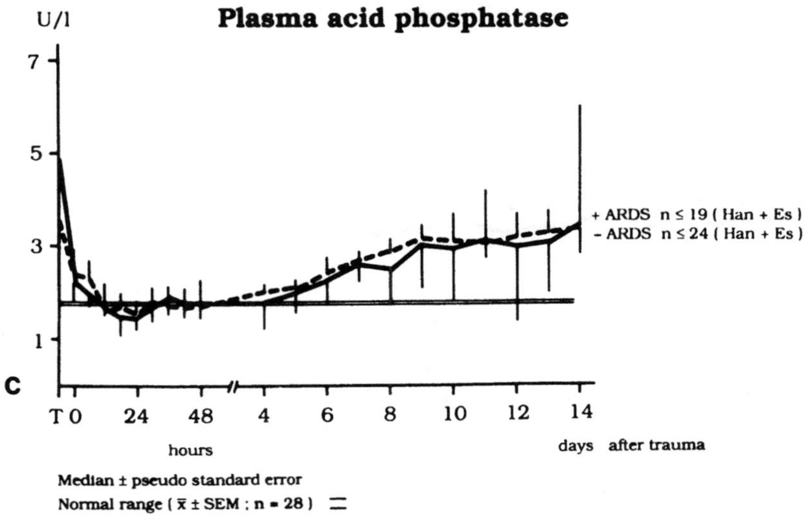

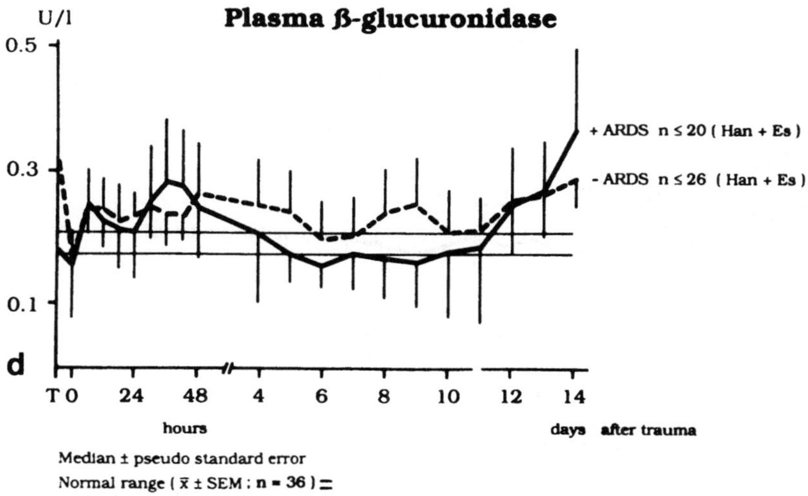

Fig. 11a–d. (Cont.)

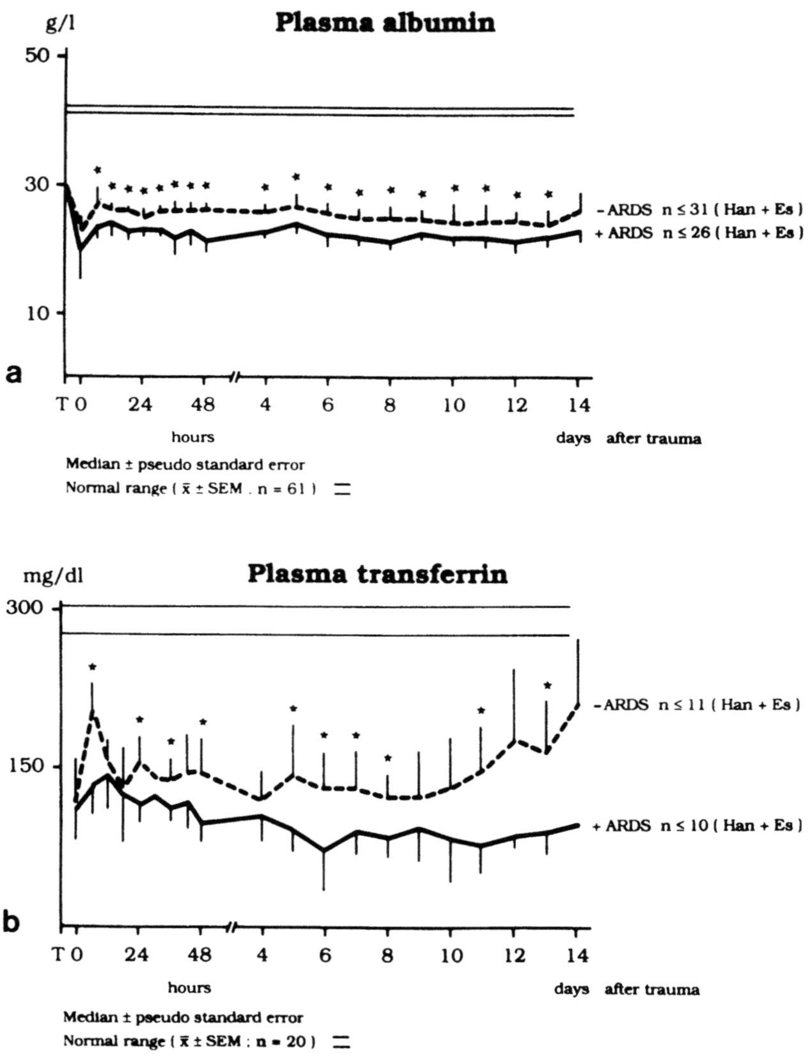

Fig. 12a,b. Posttraumatic courses of plasma albumin (**a**) and transferrin (**b**) in ARDS and non-ARDS patients. *$p < 0.05$ + ARDS vs − ARDS (U-test); *T*, blood sample obtained at the scene; *O*, blood sample obtained after volume resuscitation

and non-ARDS patients could only be observed in β-*N*-acetyl-glucosaminidase.

Acute-Phase, Transport, and Opsonic Proteins. In the posttraumatic course transport protein concentrations (albumin, transferrin) decreased slightly for both patient groups, especially for ARDS patients (Fig. 12), whereas acute-phase proteins (C-reactive protein, α_1-proteinase inhibitor, ceruloplasmin, acid α_1-glycoprotein) showed a rapid and continuous increase which was faster for non-ARDS patients than for ARDS patients during the early course (Fig. 13). After an initial decrease at time point 0, total protein concentrations increased continuously for up to 14 days in both patient groups, non-ARDS patients having significantly higher values than ARDS patients (Fig. 14).

Marker Enzymes. As can be seen in Fig. 14, kininase II showed an initial decrease and followed a constant time course for both patient groups. Also, cholinesterase exhibited an initial decrease and continued to decrease slightly for both patient groups. On the contrary, LDH exhibited above normal values during the entire posttraumatic course with slightly higher values for ARDS patients in comparison to those of non-ARDS patients (Fig. 14).

Plasma Insulin Concentration, Erythrocyte Insulin Receptor Characteristics, and Glutathione-Insulin-Transhydrogenase (GIT) Activity

Between days 4 and 12 after trauma, the intracellular GIT activity of ARDS patients decreased significantly, whereas the plasma insulin concentration remained unchanged (Fig. 15). On the other hand, the erythrocyte receptor affinity and receptor concentration decreased slightly for both patient groups in the posttraumatic course, indicating a slight but progressive insulin receptor defect (Fig. 15). This could be further substantiated by calculating the insulin concentration/GIT activity relationship as well as the receptor concentration × GIT activity product (Fig. 16). In the case of a receptor defect, an increase in the aforementioned ratio (caused by an increase in insulin concentration and decrease in GIT activity) as well as a decrease in the above product (caused by decreases in receptor concentration and GIT activity) should be and was observed.

Discussion

In recent years, the essential role of the PMNL as an initiator and amplifier of the development of ARDS has become more and more clear. Certain results of the present study confirmed previous findings of other authors, and other results have completed our knowledge about the nonspecific granulocyte-humoral immune system and its influence on ARDS development.

In accordance with the results of others [15], we found an identical posttraumatic increase in the course of PMNL levels in the blood but could not predict ARDS development accordingly as postulated by others [30]. At the humoral site, we saw a posttraumatic plasma opsonin deficiency, especially in ARDS patients, as well as a continuous synthesis of a

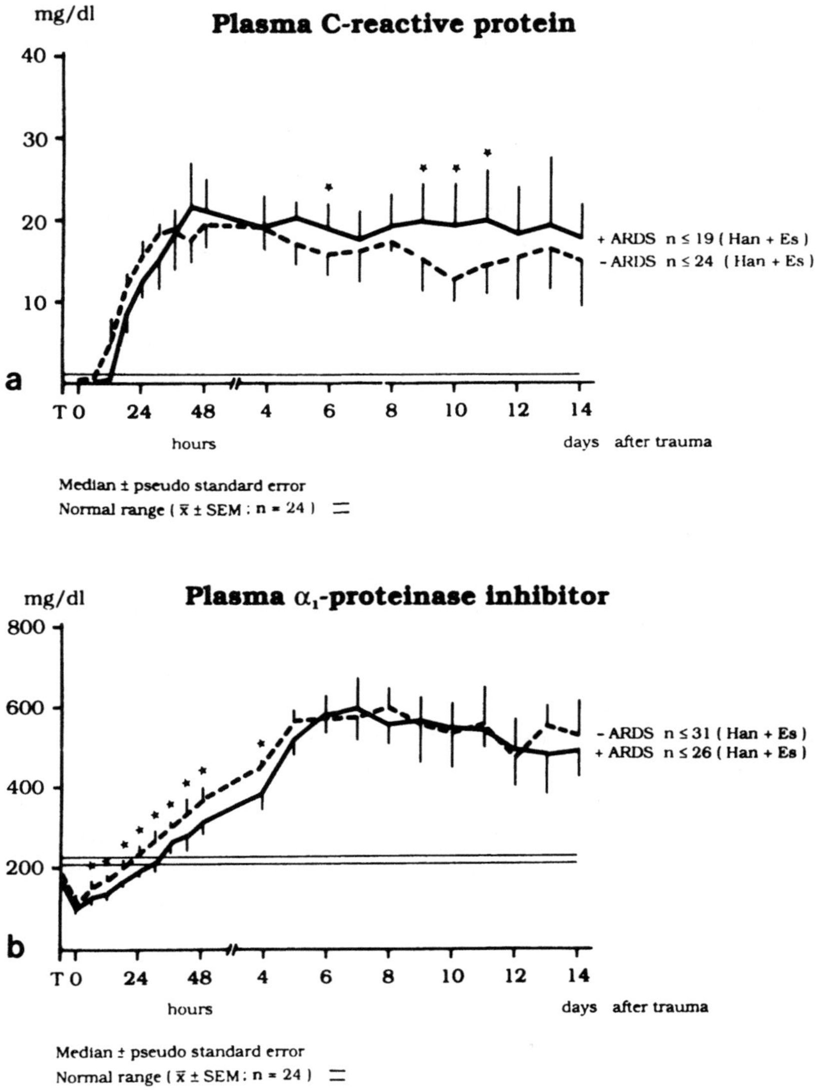

Fig. 13a–d. Posttraumatic courses of plasma C reactive protein (**a**), α_1-proteinase inhibitor (**b**), ceruloplasmin (**c**), and α_1-acid glycoprotein (**d**) in ARDS and non-ARDS patients. $^*p < 0.05$ + ARDS vs − ARDS (U-test); *T*, blood sample obtained at the scene; *O*, blood sample obtained after volume resuscitation

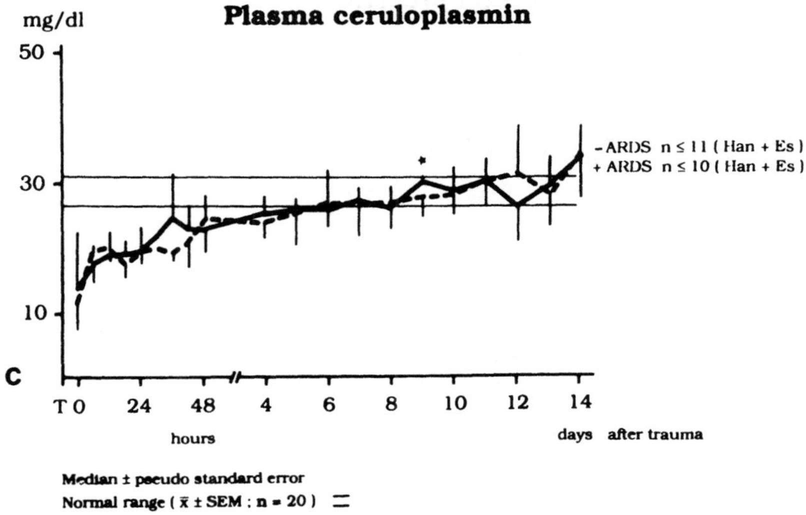

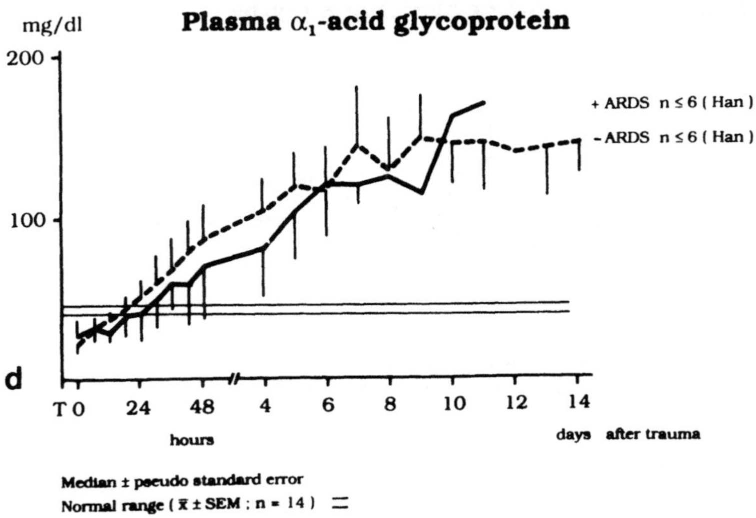

Fig. 13a–d. (Cont.)

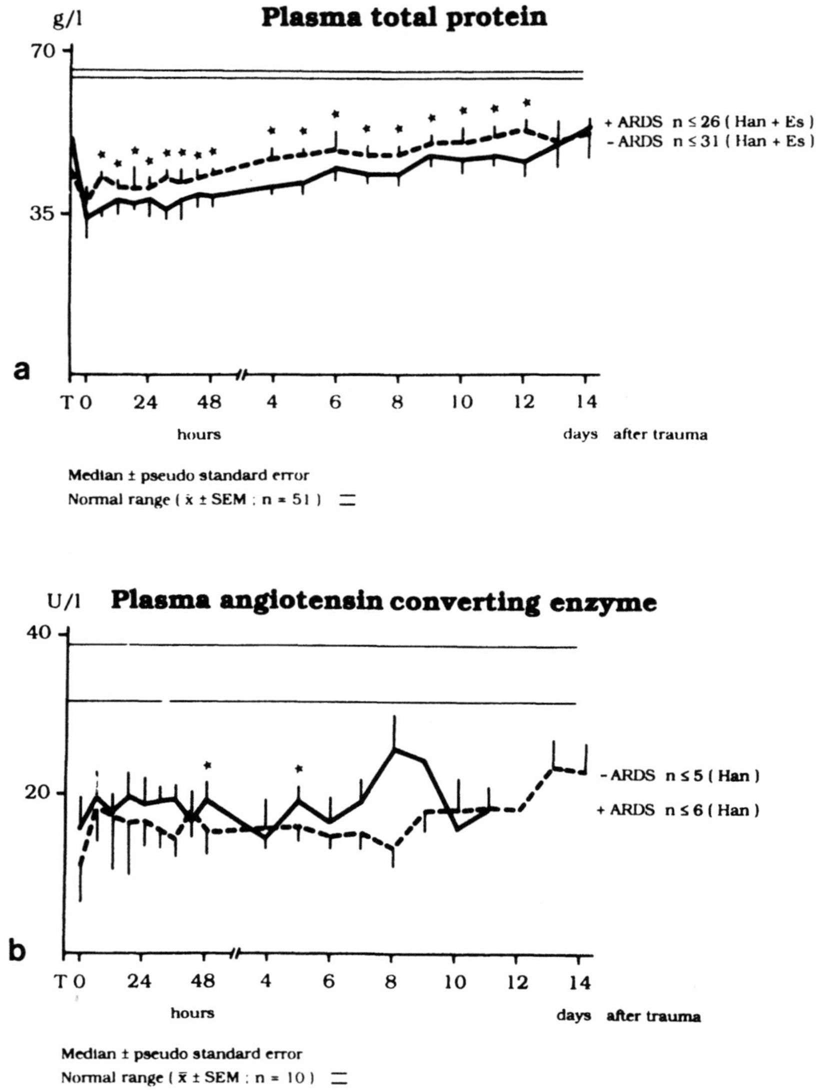

Fig. 14a–d. Posttraumatic courses of plasma total protein (**a**), angiotensin-converting enzyme (**b**), cholinesterase (**c**), and LDH (**d**) in ARDS and non-ARDS patients. $*p < 0.05$ + ARDS vs − ARDS (U-test); *T*, blood sample obtained at the scene; *O*, blood sample obtained after volume resuscitation

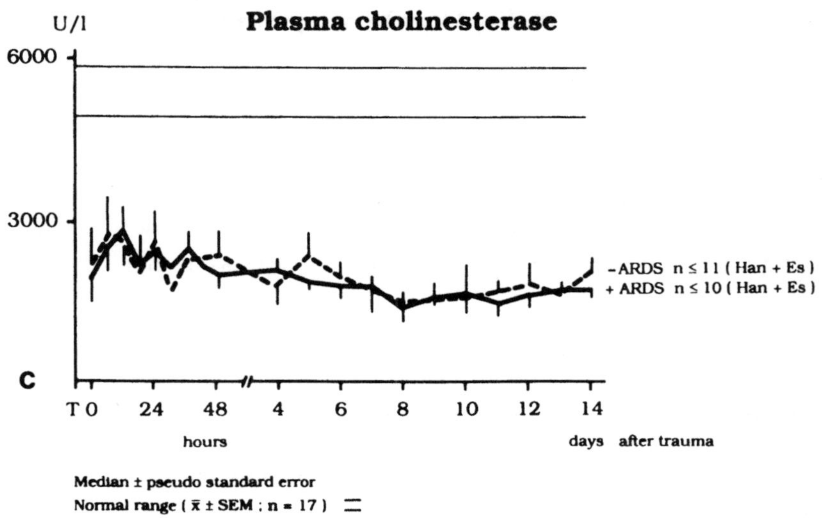

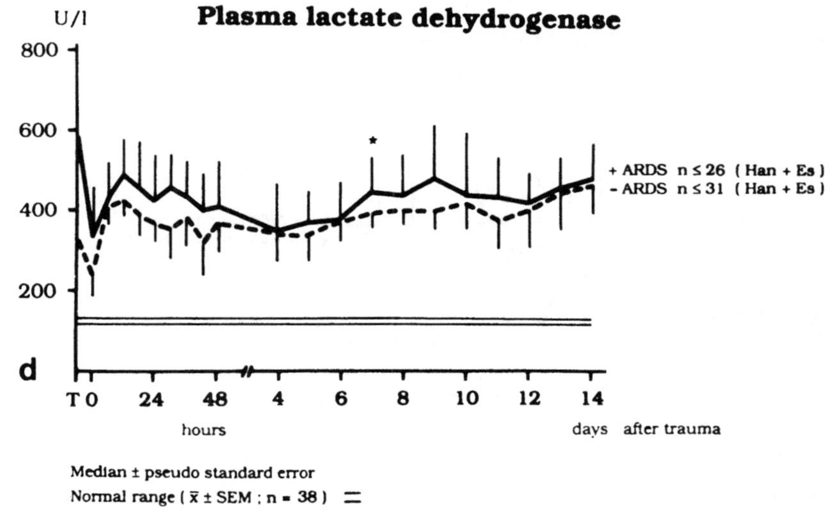

Fig. 14a–d. (Cont.)

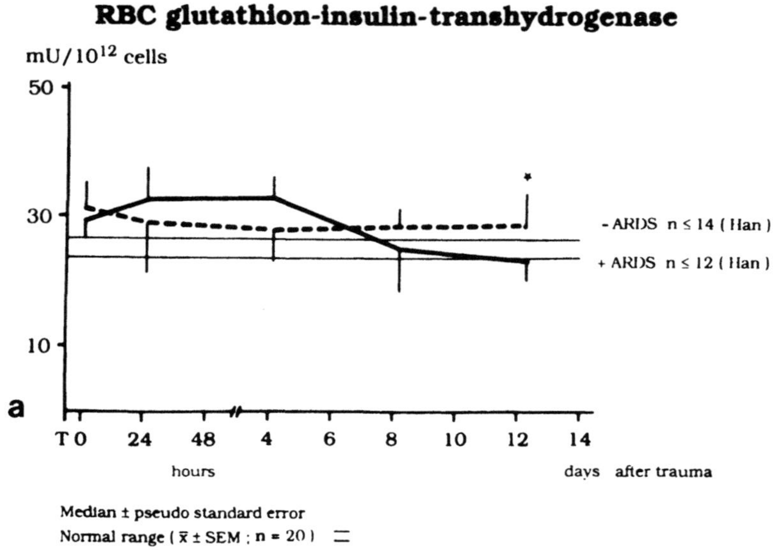

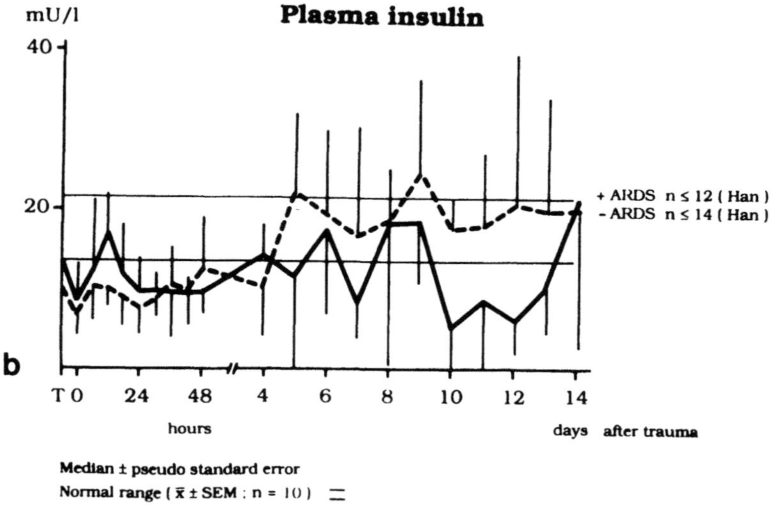

Fig. 15a–d. Posttraumatic courses of red blood cell glutathione-insulin-transhydrogenase (**a**), plasma insulin concentration (**b**), red blood cell insulin receptor concentration (**c**) and affinity (**d**) in ARDS and non-ARDS patients. $^*p < 0.05$ + ARDS vs − ARDS (U-test); *T*, blood sample obtained at the scene; *O*, blood sample obtained after volume resuscitation

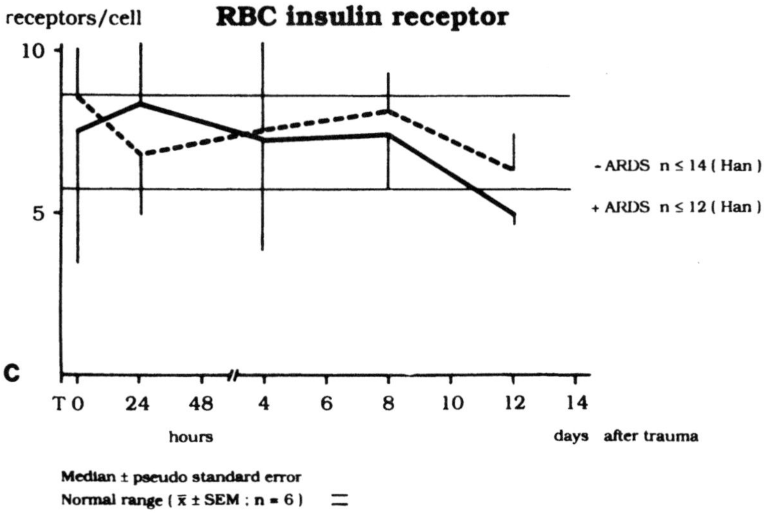

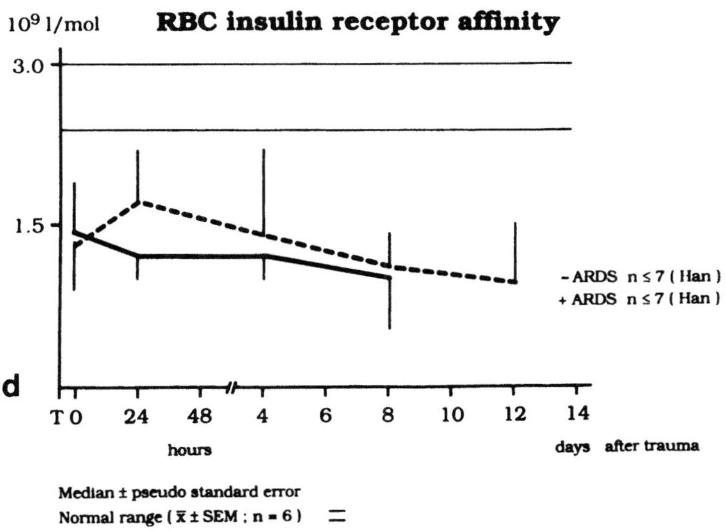

Fig. 15a–d. (Cont.)

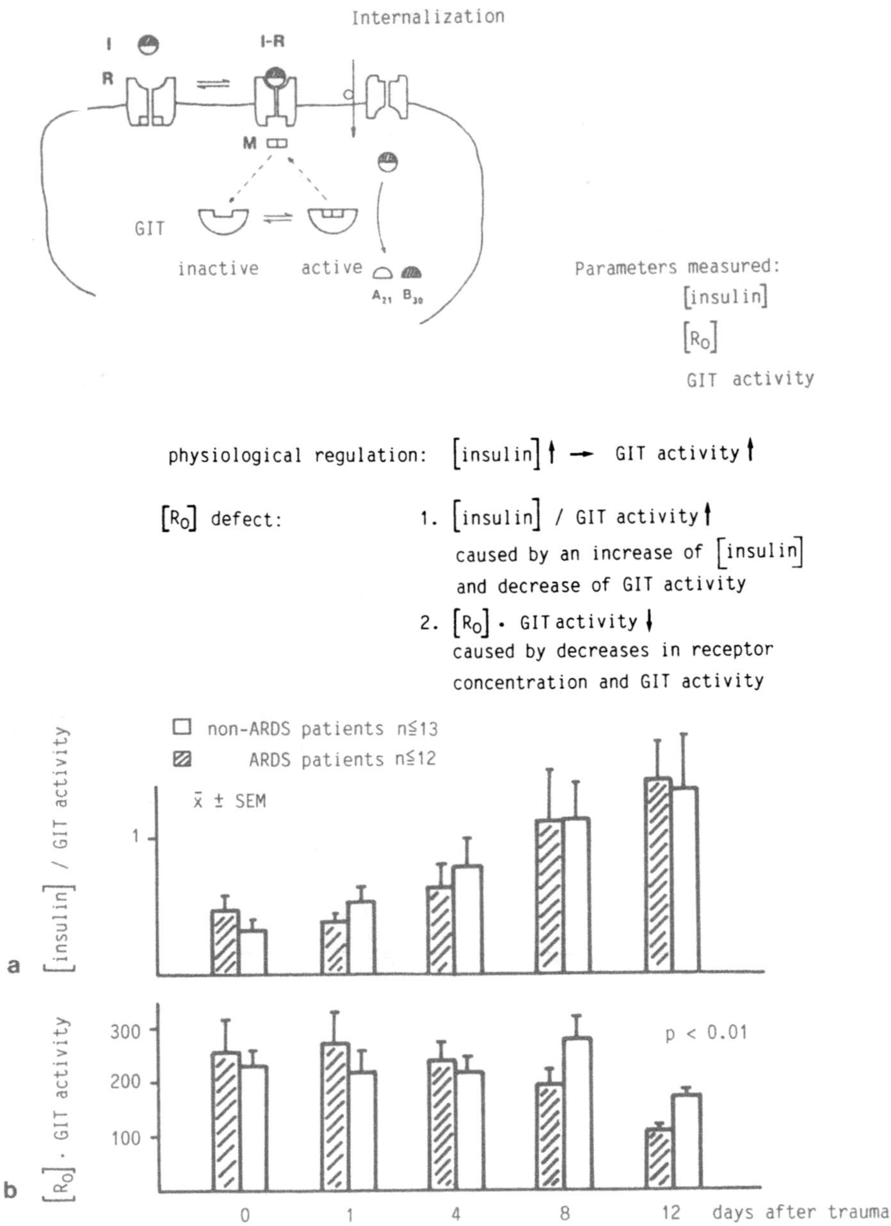

Fig. 16a,b. Regulation of insulin degradation in red blood cells. Posttraumatic courses of insulin concentration/GIT activity ratios (**a**) and receptor concentration × GIT activity products (**b**) in ARDS and non-ARDS patients.

trauma-related plasma factor that suppressed the CL response and presumably also the phagocytosis/killing functions of PMNL in circulating blood [9, 12]. The ARDS patient group seemed to be predisposed to septic complications and sepsis-amplified ARDS development in the later posttraumatic course. Such an inhibition factor has been described in septic patients [19], but our results demonstrated that this factor always seemed to be produced after a traumatic event, irrespective of septicemia. Contrary to others [36], we found a posttraumatic increase in neutrophil adherence and, in accordance with other authors [35], an increased endogenous respiratory burst potential of ARDS neutrophils themselves. This was also confirmed by enzyme release experiments of stimulated neutrophils isolated from patients. As a consequence, this destructive potential of the circulating neutrophils is intravascularly inhibited, although this does not hold true for marginated or adhered cells. The destructive capacity become reactivated upon adhesion and after the neutrophil had left the capillary and entered the interstitial and alveolar spaces. Here, the neutrophils were no longer kept in check by the trauma-related suppression factor, thereby allowing the liberation of the complete set of inflammatory mediators of lung structure damage. This was true for both patient groups, being somewhat more pronounced for ARDS patients, and was also seen by the higher intravascular release of inflammatory mediators and markers such as β-NAG by neutrophils stimulated in vivo. In this context, other lysosomal enzymes cannot be used as such markers because of their respiratory burst-mediated inactivation [32]. The decrease of respiratory burst response and lysosomal enzyme content of neutrophils isolated from BALF in comparison with those derived from blood, as well as the extracellular increase of lysosomal enzyme concentrations, demonstrated the loss of metabolic capacity during passage across the blood/air barrier [5–7, 10, 21, 23–25]. Obviously, the binding capacity of neutrophil receptors for extracellularly located inflammatory mediators did not suffice to prevent tissue damage, as could be demonstrated by elastase binding [2, 6, 8] (Tables 2, 3). Also the α_1-proteinase inhibitor capacity for lysosomal enzymes was totally blocked in some cases in BALF, presumably by α_1-proteinase inhibitor oxidation and inactivation. Therefore, free enzymatically active enzymes, such as elastase, could be found in BALF [5, 26]. Concerning the posttraumatic course of neutrophil alterations, a maximal stimulatory response of blood neutrophils was observed on about the 4th day after trauma in accordance with other biochemical parameters, such as LDH, β-*N*-acetylglucosaminidase, and C-reactive protein plasma concentrations, demonstrating another second event occurring at about this time after trauma, and this resulted in a further differentiation between ARDS and non-ARDS patients. Differences in levels of fibronectin between the patient groups on day 4 after trauma presumably indicate an increasing influence of proteolytic activities only in the ARDS patients (fibronectin serves as a substrate for proteinases), which is also confirmed by the time course of plasma β-*N*-acetylglucosaminidase and elastase- α_1-PI complex concentrations.

Furthermore, this intravascular action of proteinases and hydrolases would also be responsible for the destruction of plasma membrane receptors such as the insulin receptor of erythrocytes and for the inhibition of signal transduction mechanisms. Despite a slight and prolonged continuous impairment of liver function (posttraumatic decrease in cholinesterase levels in both patient groups), hepatocyte protein synthesis of acute-phase reactants increased for C-reactive protein, α_1-proteinase inhibitor, ceruloplasmin, and acid α_1-glycoprotein, whereas there was a decreased production of transport proteins such as albumin and, especially, transferrin. The posttraumatic courses of transferrin demonstrated that this protein behaved as a transport protein rather than as an acute-phase protein, as was expected [28]. In the early posttraumatic course, the acute-phase protein concentrations were found to be higher for non-ARDS patients than for ARDS patients, presumably because of the greater consumption of host defense proteins in ARDS patients. A direct marker for lung endothelial damage was supposed to be the plasma concentration of angiotensin-converting enzyme. However, we found no diagnostic or prognostic value of ACE measurements, which were in accordance with those of others [14]. Assuming a comparable extent of alveolar macrophage and neutrophil damage within the alveoli for ARDS and non-ARDS patients, higher alveolar macrophage activity could be observed in the time course of ARDS development for ARDS patients in comparison to non-ARDS patients, with a maximum occurring at about the 4th day after trauma. On the contrary, the time-dependent response of neutrophils isolated from BALF was lower for ARDS patients, indicating the higher degree of exhaustion during and after their invasion into the alveoli. Accordingly, a role for the alveolar macrophages in the development of ARDS could be proposed, presumably more involved in intercellular reactions rather than as a direct means of destruction.

Conclusion

In conclusion, the results of the present study were integrated into the current pathogenetic concept of ARDS development. A major point was the finding of the depressed intravascular nonspecific immune system after multiple trauma for ARDS patients, which predisposed this patient group to sepsis-amplified ARDS development. Furthermore, blood ARDS neutrophils were found to be in a higher reactive and, therefore, more aggressive state and therefore posed a greater threat to pulmonary endothelial cells.

Another essential finding was the exhaustion of the metabolic capacity of neutrophils during their blood/air passage as assessed by the measurement of functions of neutrophils isolated from both patient blood and BALF obtained simultaneously. The release of inflammatory mediators in the capillary-alveolar area could be demonstrated.

In the posttraumatic course, blood neutrophils seemed to be maximally responsive on about the 4th day after trauma. Beginning on day 4, a distinction in certain biochemical parameters and systems could be seen between ARDS and non-ARDS patients. Some of them are directly affected by neutrophil products liberated extracellularly.

Further investigations will demonstrate whether and how alveolar macrophage stimulation participates in and coincides with the blood neutrophil reactivity, as well as with the response of cells of the specific immune system, in ARDS development.

References

1. Allen RC, Stjernholm RL, Steele RH (1972) Evidence for the generation of an electronic excitation state(s) in human polymorphonuclear leukocytes and its participation in bactericidal activity. Biochem Biophys Res Commun 47:679
2. Dwenger A, Tost P (1986) Elastase-specific receptors on human polymorphonuclear leukocytes. Biol Chem Hoppe Seyler [Suppl] 367:215
3. Dwenger A, Trautschold I (1982) Zum Einfluß von Hämolyse, Harnstoff und Bilirubin auf die Präzision radioimmunologischer Digoxin- und Insulin-Bestimmungen. J Clin Chem Clin Biochem 20:29
4. Dwenger A, Holle W, Tost P, Trautschold I (1983) Zum Einfluß der totalen Hormonkonzentration auf die Ermittlung von Bindungskenngrößen bei der Hormon/Receptor-Wechselwirkung zwischen Erythrocyten und Insulin. J Clin Chem Clin Biochem 21:721
5. Dwenger A, Regel G, Neumann C, Schweitzer G (1986) Pathomechanisms of the adult respiratory distress syndrome (ARDS): elastase contents of polymorphonuclear leukocytes and elastase release during passage across the blood/air barrier. Fresenius Z Anal Chem 324:359
6. Dwenger A, Schweitzer G, Regel G (1986) Bronchoalveolar lavage fluid and plasma proteins, chemiluminescence response and protein contents of polymorphonuclear leukocytes from blood and lavage fluid in traumatized patients. J Clin Chem Clin Biochem 24:73
7. Dwenger A, Regel G, Schweitzer G (1986) Pathomechanisms of the adult respiratory distress syndrome (ARDS): chemiluminescence analysis of polymorphonuclear leukocytes. Fresenius Z Anal Chem 324:360
8. Dwenger A, Tost P, Holle W (1986) Evaluation of elastase and α_1-proteinase inhibitor-elastase uptake by polymorphonuclear leukocytes and evidence of an elastase-specific receptor. J Clin Chem Clin Biochem 24:299
9. Dwenger A, Lindena J, Schweitzer G, Neumann C, Regel G (1987) Opsonophagocytic immune defense mechanisms in multiply traumatized patients with and without the adult respiratory distress syndrome. In: Schölmerich J, Andreesen R, Kapp A, Ernst M, Woods WG (eds) Bioluminescence and chemiluminescence, new perspectives. Wiley, Chichester, pp 41–44
10. Dwenger A, Schweitzer G, Regel G, Neumann C, Funck M (1987) Chemiluminescence response of human polymorphonuclear leukocytes before and after passage of the blood/air barrier. In: Schölmerich J, Andreesen R, Kapp A, Ernst M, Woods WG, (eds) Bioluminescence and chemiluminescence, new perspectives. Wiley, Chichester, pp 45–48
11. Dwenger A, Schweitzer G, Funck M (1988) Lipopolysaccharide-dependent enhancement of adherence- mediated chemiluminescence response of polymorphonuclear leukocytes. J Biolumin Chemilumin 2:35

12. Dwenger A, Schweitzer G, Regel G, Funck M, Sturm JA, Tscherne H (1988) Suppression of neutrophil chemiluminescence response in blood of multiply traumatized patients with and without the adult respiratory distress syndrome (ARDS). Fresenius Z Anal Chem 330:441
13. Dwenger A, Regel G, Joka T, Sturm JA, Tscherne H (1989) Verlust der Molekülgrößen-Selektivität des Alveolarepithels für Plasmaproteine bei Patienten nach Polytrauma. Langenbecks Arch Chir [Suppl] Chirurgisches Forum 1989:109–113
14. Fourrier F, Chopin C, Wallaert B, Wattre P, Mangalaboyi J, Durocher A, Dubois D, Wattel F (1983) Angiotensin-converting enzyme in human adult respiratory distress syndrome. Chest 83:593
15. Hällgren R, Borg T, Venge P, Modig J (1984) Signs of neutrophil and eosinophil activation in adult respiratory distress syndrome. Crit Care Med 12:14
16. Hammerschmidt DE, Weaver, LJ, Hudson LD, Craddock PR, Jacob HS (1980) Association of complement activation and elevated plasma C5A with adult respiratory distress syndrome: pathophysiologic relevance and possible prognostic value. Lancet 1:947
17. Hurst PL, Lovell-Smith CJ (1981) Optimized assay for serum angiotensin-converting enzyme activity. Clin Chem 27:2048
18. Lanser ME, Mao P, Brown G, Coleman B, Siegel JH (1985) Serum-mediated depression of neutrophil chemiluminescence following blunt trauma. Arch Surg 202:111
19. Lanser ME, Brown GE, Mora R, Coleman W, Siegel JH (1986) Trauma serum suppresses superoxide production by normal neutrophils. Arch Surg 121:157
20. MacGregor RR, Spagnuolo PJ, Lentnek AL (1974) Inhibition of granulocyte adherence by ethanol, prednisone, and aspirin, measured with a new assay system. N Engl J Med 291:642
21. Maghsudi M, Sturm JA, Regel G, Oestern H-J, Dwenger A, Schweitzer G (1985) Die Granulozytenfunktion nach schwerem Polytrauma. Langenbecks Arch Chir [Suppl] 99–104
22. Matheson NR, Wong PS, Travis J (1981) Isolation and properties of human neutrophil myeloperoxidase. Biochemistry 20:325
23. Regel G, Dwenger A, Sturm JA, Neumann C, Maghsudi M (1986) Assessment of the functional state of polymorphonuclear leukocytes after multiple trauma. Injury mechanisms in the alveolo-capillary section. Eur Surg Res 18:9
24. Regel G, Dwenger A, Sturm JA, Neumann C, Maghsudi M, Schweitzer G (1986) Eine funktionelle Untersuchung der polymorphkernigen Granulozyten nach Polytrauma-Schädigungsmechanismen im alveolo-kapillären Abschnitt. Langenbecks Arch Chir 369:777
25. Regel G, Dwenger A, Seidel J, Nerlich ML, Sturm JA, Tscherne H (1987) Die Bedeutung des neutrophilen Granulozyten bei der Entstehung des posttraumatischen Lungenversagens. Unfallchirurg 90:99
26. Schraufstatter I, Revak SD, Cochrane CG (1984) Biochemical factors in pulmonary inflammatory disease. Fed Proc 43:2807
27. Sganga G, Siegel JH, Brown G, Coleman B, Wiles CE III, Belzberg H, Wedel S, Placko R (1985) Reprioritization of hepatic plasma protein release in trauma and sepsis. Arch Surg 120:187
28. Stahl WM (1987) Acute phase protein response to tissue injury. Crit Care Med 15:545
29. Tate RM, Repine JE (1983) Neutrophils and the adult respiratory distress syndrome. Am Rev Respir Dis 128:552
30. Thommasen HV, Russell JA, Boyko WJ, Hogg JC (1984) Transient leucopenia associated with adult respiratory distress syndrome. Lancet 1:809
31. Varandani PT, Nafz MA (1976) Insulin degradation. XVIII. On the regulation of glutathione-insulin transhydrogenase in the hyperglycemic obese (*ob/ob*) mouse. Biochim Biophys Acta 451:382
32. Voetman AA, Weening RS, Hamers MN, Meerhof LJ, Bot AAAM, Roos D (1981) Phagocytosing human neutrophils inactivate their own granular enzymes. J Clin Invest 67:1541

33. Worthen GS, Henson PM (1983) Mechanisms of acute lung injury. Clin Lab Med 3:601
34. Yatziv S, Kahane I, Abeliuk P, Cividalli G, Rachmilewitz EA (1979) "Lysosomal" enzyme activities in red blood cells of normal individuals and patients with homozygous β-thalassaemia. Clin Chim Acta 96:67
35. Zimmerman GA, Renzetti AD, Hill HR (1983) Functional and metabolic activity of granulocytes from patients with adult respiratory distress syndrome: evidence for activated neutrophils in the pulmonary circulation. Am Rev Respir Dis 127:290
36. Zimmerman GA, Renzetti AD, Hill HR (1984) Granulocyte adherence in pulmonary and systemic arterial blood samples from patients with adult respiratory distress syndrome. Am Rev Respir Dis 129:798

Morphological and Functional Changes of Alveolar Cells

TH. JOKA[1], U. OBERTACKE[1], J. BRUCH[2], M. REUTER[1], and K.P. SCHMIT-NEUERBURG[1]

Introduction

Inflammatory alveolocapillary membrane disorder is the indicating syndrome and pathophysiological substrate of the acute lung failure in adults known as adult respiratory distress syndrome (ARDS), which essentially involves cascade systems, local and migrated alveolar cell systems, and mediators [1, 3, 8, 15, 17, 18]. The interactions between cells and inflammatory mediators in the alveolar space, and their significance in the development of ARDS remain unclear [4, 12, 13, 16, 17]. By administering bronchoalveolar lavage (BAL) daily in our cohort of patients, it was possible to obtain morphologic data (alveolar cytology). In addition, the appearance and changes in humoral components in the alveolus during the development of ARDS can be directly explained and compared to analogous, potentially occurring changes in the blood [4, 10]. Furthermore, it was possible to obtain and analyze the components and function of the surfactant.

Materials and Methods

The lavage fluid obtained by the described technique [5] was centrifuged in order to separate soluble and cellular components. The cell sediment was used for cytologic studies and functional analysis. The total cell count was determined with the Coulter counter or in a Neubauer hemocytometer. For the differential analysis, hematocrit smears were produced from part of the cell sediment (Cytospin 1, Shandon, Frankfurt, FRG). The smears were dyed using May-Grünwald, Giemsa, and Pappenheim's stains as well as additional special stains (esterase and peroxidase).

[1] Department of Trauma Surgery, University Medical School, Hufelandstr. 55, W-4300 Essen, FRG
[2] Institute for Hygiene and Industrial Medicine, University Medical School, Hufelandstr. 55, W-4300 Essen, FRG

J.A. Sturm (Ed.)
Adult Respiratory Distress Syndrome

The ability of the alveolar phagocytes to liberate oxygen radicals during phagocytic activity was analyzed with the luminol-enhanced chemoluminescence in the LKB luminometer [2]. Each test preparation contained 3.75×10^5 cells in 250 µl phosphate buffered saline (PBS) and 10 µl luminol at 37°C. The peak value (in millivolts) after stimulation with serum-opsonized zymosan (0.4 µg) was used as the parameter for measuring phagocytic activity with liberation of oxygen radicals.

The remaining centrifuged BAL fluids were worked up, frozen at −70°C, and subsequently analyzed at outside laboratories. In particular, the following were determined: complement split products, intracellular enzyme systems (elastase, myeloperoxidase, and lactoferrin), α_1-proteinase inhibitor (α_1-PI), lactate dehydrogenase (LDH), leukotrienes, and selected proteins [7, 10, 16]. All biologically relevant phospholipids of the lung surfactant and the hysteresis area, as an marker of the in vitro function of the surfactant [14], were also determined in the lavage fluid.

Patients with multiple injuries were divided into two different groups (ARDS and non-ARDS) according to a score of lung failure [11]. During the illustration and evaluation of the BAL process, the results of the morphologic investigations were classified into three posttraumatic phases:

First phase	0–48 h
Second phase	days 3–7
Third phase	days 8–14

Results

Morphology of the Alveolar Cells

The total cell count of the alveolus increased within the first phase after trauma. The progress was nearly identical for both group (ARDS and non-ARDS). The relative percentage of alveolar macrophages (AM) distinctively decreased in both groups. The decrease in the ARDS group was significant in relation to the standard value of the alveolar cell distribution. The number of granulocytes (polymorphonuclear neutrophils, PMN) significantly increased in both groups (ARDS and non-ARDS) while the percentage of lymphocytes fell below the normal level after trauma.

For the total number of each cell type averaged over 14 days, a different pattern presented itself. Here, the macrophages showed nearly standard values. It also became apparent that the number of lymphocytes in the ARDS group exceeded twice the number found in the non-ARDS group.

In the presentation of the three posttraumatic phases, our measurements showed the number of macrophages to double in the first phase and then to decrease below the normal level in the third phase. The PMN increased to its tenfold, while the lymphocytes decreased in all three phases (Table 1). Even when tested at different times, the granulocytes ($p = 0.13$) and macrophages ($p = 0.4$) did not show group-specific behavior. In the first 2 days, the ARDS patients exhibited positive correlations between the granulocytes in the alveolus and the pulmonary vascular resistance (PVR) ($r = 0.53$). We did not find any additional correlations to other lung function parameters [$AaDO_2$ (Alveolar arterial difference of O_2^-) protein content].

Table 1. Distribution of alveolar cells (× 10^5/ml) in the BAL of patients with ARDS (n = 9) and patients without ARDS (n = 16) averaged in the three phases

	normal	phase		
		1 –ARDS/ARDS	2 –ARDS/ARDS	3 –ARDS/ARDS
total	126	142/235	149/224	116/105
macrophages	99	123/171	82/130	77/ 34
granulocytes	7	15/ 36	61/ 58	24/ 55
lymphocytes	22	5/ 12	6/ 22	5/ 2

Special Alveolar Cell Compositions

All patients in the ARDS group, exclusively at the moment of marked lung failure, exhibited special alveolar cell compositions. These were identified as lupus erythematosus (LE) cells, hyperplastic type II alveolar cells, PAS-positive neutrophil granulocytes, and immunoblasts. For the LE cells and hyperplastic alveolar cells, we found a good correspondence between the time of their occurrence and the alveolar hypoxia. The presence of PAS-positive cells correlated very well with the onset of the alveolocapillary membrane disorder, which is evidenced by massive movements of proteins into the alveolus.

The morphologic picture of the macrophages also changed in the course of acute lung failure. Initially, small round cells resembling neutrophils in size were found. Later enlarged macrophages appeared. Their big vacuoles indicated increased activity. Finally burst macrophages with cell detritus were observed in the alveolus.

Function of the Alveolar Cells

The functional condition of the alveolar cells after trauma can be represented by the comparative presentation of different humoral and cellular parameters. Alveolarly liberated mediators (C3a, leukotriene, thromboxane) and cellular metabolic products (elastase, oxygen radicals, myeloperoxidase, lactoferrin, and the surfactant) are particularly suited for that purpose.

Complement Split Products. As a marker of general complement activation the complement split product C3a was increasingly evident in the alveolus during the whole course of the disease. In comparison to the non-ARDS group, the alveolar liberation of C3a in the ARDS group increased significantly until the 12th h ($p = 0.05$) and then again from the 6th day ($p = 0.012$). Throughout the whole process, positive correlations to the protein content in the alveolus ($r > 0.5$) and the PVR ($r = 0.5$) were found.

Metabolites of Arachidonic Acid. Leukotriene C_4 (LTC_4) almost exclusively appeared in the BAL of ARDS patients. This correlated with simultaneous evidence of eosinophils in the BAL. In the BAL of patients without complications after multiple trauma, neither LTC_4 nor leukotriene E_4 (LTE_4) was ever found. Thromboxane was detected in the BAL of our patients. In ARDS patients, thromboxane was liberated in distinctly larger quantities.

Chemoluminescence Response. The alveolar phagocytes of patients with multiple injuries liberated greater quantities of oxygen radicals after standardized stimulation. Differences in behavior between the two groups (ARDS/non-ARDS) did not appear. However, the ARDS group showed a slightly greater peak activity. Generally, the chemoluminescence response correlated well with the neutrophil fraction ($r = 0.6$) in the BAL. Similar associations with the macrophages were not detected.

Compared with the usual ability of blood cells, a decreased peak activity generally appeared in the BAL. In some cases of severe lung failure following sepsis, a distinct down-regulation of the PMN was found. The chemoluminescence response was within the normal range of values.

PMN Enzymes. Granulocytic enzymes were detected posttraumatically in greater concentrations in the BAL. Group differences did not exist for the complex elastase, nor for lactoferrin and myeloperoxidase. Throughout the course of the study, the alveolar PMN value and the alveolar concentration of granulocytic enzymes exhibited good correlations ($r > 0.5$).

Proteins. Within the first 48 h, both groups (ARDS/non-ARDS) displayed a distinct leakage of different intra-alveolar proteins. From the 3rd day, the patient groups could be differentiated by the protein leakage in the alveolus. While the protein permeability decreased in the non-ARDS group, high protein concentrations in the alveolus persisted in the ARDS group. Patients with high alveolar protein content were also found to have PAS-positive PMN.

Surfactant. A relation between alveolar protein content and changes in the composition of the surfactant with a deterioration of the surfactant function was discovered in vitro. We found significant correlations between the hysteresis area as the marker of surfactant function and protein content in the alveolus ($r = -0.55$). Overall, distinct changes were evident in the composition of the phospholipids and the apoproteins of the surfactant in the posttraumatic course. The amount of phosphatidylcholine (PC) was distinctly reduced posttraumatically, and significantly lower in the group with ARDS in the second and third phases. The surfactant function was similar as the PC changed. Significant correlations were found between PC and hysteresis area ($r = 0.7$). Morphologically, we found hyperplastic pneumocytes type II cells in the second and third phases of the severe lung failure, a finding which correlates very well with the deterioration in lung function.

Lung Contusion. BAL data from nine patients with lung contusion can be summarized for the early stages up to the 4th day of the trauma. The total cell count and the increase in granulocytes did not change with regard to the known posttraumatic value. The percentage of macrophages was greater than in the ARDS patients. The stimulated activity of phagocytosis in the BAL was within the standard range, in spite of the posttraumatic influx of the granulocytes in the alveolus. At the same time, we detected free elastase even though the physiological inhibitor (α_1-PI) was present. The evidence of free elastase coincided with the liberation of myeloperoxidase and lactoferrin. Both are enzymes of the PMN that take part in the toxic production of oxygen radicals during PMN degranulation.

Discussion

BAL analysis provides important information about the role of the alveolar cells and the humoral factors of the BAL in the pathogenesis of ARDS. In terms of cellular activity, the granulocytes and macrophages are most important initially. Posttraumatically, highly potent granulocytes migrate into the alveolus, resulting in a concentration of ten times their standard value. Especially in the early phase, they correlate well with the PVR. Further correlations with other parameters of lung function, as stated by Weiland [18], could not be detected.

The liberation of oxygen radicals and proteolytic enzymes of the PMN represents a source of the injury to lungs caused by cells [3, 18]. The correlation between PMN and granulocytic enzymes emphasizes the local alveolar significance of the granulocytes. These results confirm the in vitro experiments of Welch [19]. However, the number of alveolar macrophages, which are physiologically the most numerous cells in the alveolus [6], falls distinctly below the standard values in the late stage after trauma. It is possible that this decrease and the simultaneous decrease in lymphocytes in the alveolus cause the weakening of the defense mechanisms of the lung and thus pave the way for infection [9].

Among the humoral factors, the complement split products (i.e., C3a) and the metabolites of arachidonic acid play decisive roles [1]. High concentrations of C3a in the alveolus persist, especially in the ARDS group. Here, we find significant differences in comparison with the group without ARDS. A special inhibitor in the alveolus for this complement split product is not known. The possible consequences include a renewed activation of cell systems in the alveolus, and, therefore, further impairment of the parameters of the lung function [9]. This is also expressed in its correlation to the PVR (pulmonal vascular resistance). The close relation between C3a and the total amount of protein can have only one explanation: we found an higher concentration of C3a in the alveolus than in the blood. This indicates an local liberation of C3a in the alveolus. So the complement split products maintain the protein leakage by repeatedly activating different systems.

Thromboxane is liberated more in the ARDS group. LTC_4, which influences the capillary permeability of the lung, is mainly found in the lavage fluid of the ARDS group. This is possibly an indication of the significance of macrophages and eosinophils within the scope of the pathogenesis of ARDS. The results of early BAL samples in contused pulmonary areas demonstrated a distinctly lowered chemoluminescence response, although more granulocytes were present. At the same time, considerable quantities of free elastase were found in the alveolus. We conclude from this that the granulocytes were activated in the alveolus very early and thus liberated a lot of enzymes and oxygen radicals (respiratory burst). Therefore, it was not possible to stimulate the obtained granulocytes in vitro with zymosan. The liberated oxygen radicals cause a deactivation of the α_1-PI, so that free elastase can take effect in the alveolus. This could explain why lung contusion increases the incidence of ARDS after multiple trauma. Furthermore we found LE cells in this phase, possibly an indication of massive destruction of PMN. Apart from the reaction against nuclear antigens, a reaction against some of the phospholipids of the cell membrane is also possible. The results of these alveolar changes are continuous damage to the alveolocapillary barrier and subsequent protein leakage. Subsequent effects of this alveolar proteinosis are changes in the composition and function of the surfactant. Clinically, the atelectasis produces a deterioration of the parameter of lung function.

Interpreting the changes in the alveolus with respect to the pathogenesis of the ARDS is problematic because local posttraumatic changes in the alveolus are rapidly covered by secondary influences of capillary components due to barrier injury. From our point of view, it should be irrelevant how these damaging factors originated. It is only relevant that these factors appear in the alveolus and remain detectable. There they constitute an adequate stimulus of new injuries to the alveolus.

References

1. Duchateau I, Haas M, Schreyen H, Radoux C, Sprangers I, Noel FX, Braun M, Lamy M (1984) Complement activation in patients at risk of developing the adult respiratory distress syndrome. Am Rev Resp Dis 130:1058
2. Easmon CSF, Cole PJ, Williams AI, Hastings M (1980) The measurement of obsonic and phagocytic function by luminol-dependent chemoiluminescence. Immunology 41:67
3. Fowler AA, Fisher BI, Center RM, Carchmann RA (1984) Development of the adult respiratory distress syndrome: progressive alterations of neutrophil chemotactic and secretory processes. Am J Pathol 116:427
4. Joka Th, Obertacke U, Schönfeld W, Oberste-Beulmann S, Pison U, Kreuzfelder E, Jochum M, Zilow G (1987) Reaction pattern of alveolar cells in the posttraumatic lung failure. In: Schlag G, Redl H (eds) Progress in clinical and biological research, vol 236 A Liss, New York, p 317
5. Joka Th, Obertacke U, Pison U, Neudeck F, Keinecke HO (1985) Die bronchoalveoläre Lavage als Diagnostikum in der Intensivmedizin. Anaesth Intensivther Notfallmed 20:79
6. Joka Th, Nakhosteen J, Obertacke U, Herrmann J, Coenen Th, Brand M, Jochum M, Zilow G, Dwenger A, Kreuzfelder E, (1988) Beeinflußt die BAL das Milieu in der Alveole? Prax Klin Pneumol 42:705
7. Kreuzfelder E, Joka Th, Keinecke HO, Obertacke U, Schmit-Neuerburg KP, Nakhosteen JA, Paar D, Scheiermann N (1988) Adult respiratory distress syndrome as a specific manifestation of a general permeability defect in trauma patients. Am Rev Respir Dis 137:95
8. Lewis RE, Granger HI (1986) Neutrophil dependent mediation of microvascular permeability. Fed Proc 45:109
9. Montgomery AB, Stager MA, Carrico CI, Hudson LD (1985) Causes of mortality in patients with the adult respiratory distress syndrome. Am Rev Respir Dis 132:485
10. Obertacke U, Joka Th, Pison U, Riewendt HD, Stimming W (1987) Normalwerte der Zellverteilung und-Funktion in der menschlichen Alveole. Anaesth Intensivther Notfallmed 22:224
11. Obertacke U, Kalotai J, Coenen Th, Joka Th, Schmit-Neuerburg KP (1988) Ein linearer ARDS-Schweregrad-Score. Intensivmed 25:264
12. Parsons PE, Fowler AA, Hyers TM, Hanson PM (1985) Chemotactic activity in bronchoalveolar fluid from patients with ARDS. Am Rev Respir Dis 132:490
13. Pison U, Brand M, Joka Th, Obertacke U, Bruch J (1988) Distribution and function of alveolar cells in multiple injured patients with trauma induced ARDS. Intensive Care Med 14:602
14. Pison U, Seeger W, Buchhorn R, Joka Th, Brand M, Obertacke U, Neuhof H, Schmit-Neuerburg KP (1989) Surfactant abnormalities in patients with respiratory failure after multiple trauma. Am Rev Resp Dis 140:1033
15. Reid LM (1983) The pulmonary vascular lesions of the adult respiratory distress syndrome. Am J Pathol 112:112
16. Schönfeld W, Knöller J, Brom J, Raulf M, Köller M, Joka Th, König W (1987) Altered arachidonic acid metabolism in granulocytes of polytraumatized patients. Prostaglandins Leukotrienes Med 27:227
17. Tate RM, Repine IE (1983) Neutrophils and the adult respiratory distress syndrome. Am Rev Respir Dis 128:552
18. Weiland IE, Davis WB, Holter JF, Mohammed IR, Dorinsky PM, Gadek IE (1986) Lung neutrophils in the adult respiratory distress syndrome: clinical and pathophysiologic significance. Am Rev Respir Dis 133:218
19. Welch WD, Graham LW, Zaccari I, Thrupp LD (1980) Analysis and comparison of the luminol dependent chemoluminescence responses of alveolar macrophages and neutrophils. J Reticuloendothel Soc 28:275

Functional Changes in Polymorphonuclear Leukocyte Function Following Severe Polytraumatization

J. SEIDEL, J. MIRKHANI, M. BEHRMANN, and W. STANGEL

Introduction

The role of polymorphonuclear leukocytes (PMNL) in the pathogenesis of adult respiratory distress syndrome (ARDS) is widely, although not universely, accepted. ARDS by definition is progressive respiratory distress with hypoxemia following pulmonary dysfunction [1–5]. This situation regularly requires mechanical ventilation. In roentgenograms a so-called white lung is seen based on interstitial edema and fibrosis. Mortality is high and in the range of 80%. This complication is often seen as a consequence of severe polytrauma.

After complement-mediated activation in the circulation, PMNL are believed to be in an increased state of functional activity which causes adherence to the vascular endothelium in the lung. Aggregated PMNL damage the endothelium and underlying tissues by producing oxygen radicals and releasing hydrolytic enzymes [6–12]. This finally leads to pulmonary changes with accumulation of fluid in the interstitium which give rise to the clinically well-known symptoms of ARDS.

Septic complications often also arise which further indicate neutrophilic dysfunction. These septic states may easily lead to multiple organ failure (MOF) which compounds the unfavorable outcome of the disease [13, 14].

To gain more insight into the mechanisms that may precipitate ARDS, in the years 1982–1988 we serially studied some PMNL functions in patients who had suffered severe polytrauma and who were likely to develop ARDS. The PMNL functions we studied were adherence to nylon wool, chemotaxis under agarose, phagocytosis and killing of *Staphylococcus aureus* (*S. aureus*), killing of *Candida* particles, generation of superoxide anion (SA) and hydrogen peroxide (H_2O_2). The intracellular levels of lysozyme (Ly) and myeloperoxidase (MPO) were also determined. Further, patient serum was studied for the presence of chemotactic inhibitors, factors modulating PMNL adherence, and opsonins.

Central Institute for Transfusion Medicine, Eilbektal III, W-2000 Hamburg 76, FRG

J.A. Sturm (Ed.)
Adult Respiratory Distress Syndrome

Patients and Methods

Patients included in this study had suffered severe polytrauma and were admitted to the Department of Traumatology at the Medizinische Hochschule in Hanover. The following criteria had to be met: (a) admittance to the hospital within 2 h at longest after falling victim to polytrauma, (b) no steroids given at rescue, (c) severity of polytrauma scale no lower than 40 points, and (d) no cerebral injury. Blood (20 ml of blood anticoagulated with 10% citrate, 5 ml of whole blood) was drawn immediately after admittance, 24 h later, and at days 4, 8, and 12 after injury. The blood was transferred to the laboratory for separation and to test PMNL functions without any further delay. Blood drawn from healthy blood donors during routine donation at out local blood bank was used for normal controls.

Cell Separation. We carried out cell separation using a modification of Boyum's method [15]. Two parts of blood were mixed with one part of hydroxyethyl starch (Plasmasteril) and left standing for about 30 min in a test-tube. The leukocyte-rich supernatant was then carefully layered on top of 3 ml Ficoll gradient and spun down with 350 *g* at 4°C for 15 min. Contaminating erythrocytes in the pellet were removed by hypotonic lysis. The purified PMNL were then washed twice and the cells suspended in RPMI 1640 to a concentration of 2.5×10^7 cells/ml.

Adherence. We assessed adherence to nylon wool by employing the method detailed by McGregor [16]. The number of PMNL before and after passage through a premoistened and prewarmed (37°C) nylon wool column with defined density (50 mg in an insulin syringe compressed to 1 ml) was determined. PMNL were preincubated in AB serum for 15 min at room temperature before entering the assay. Triple assays were run and the adherence calculated as follows:

$$\%\ \text{adherence} = 100 - \frac{\text{number of PMNL}_{\text{after}} \times 100}{\text{number of PMNL}_{\text{before}}}$$

To study the influence of patient serum on adherence, the behavior of normal PMNL preincubated in AB serum and in patient serum was compared by establishing an index: % $\text{PMNL}_{\text{normal}}$/% $\text{PMNL}_{\text{patient}}$

Spontaneous Migration and Chemotaxis. We performed chemotaxis under agarose as outlined by Chenoweth et al. [17,18]. Agarose (0.7 g/100 ml) and gelatine (0.2 g/100 ml) were boiled in agua bidestillata and then mixed with an equal volume of 2 × minimal essential medium (MEM) which had previously been adjusted to pH 7.4 by adding sodium hydrogen carbonate. Of this solution 2–3 ml were poured into 35-mm tissue culture dishes, which then were left standing to allow hardening of the agarose. With a template, four holes were punched into the agarose in a starlike fashion. Two substances with chemotactic activity were employed, namely, yeast-activated serum (YAS), containing the complement activation product C5a [19], and *N*-formyl-methionyl-leucyl-Phenyl*al*anine (FMLP), a tripeptide with exquisite chemotactic properties [20]. YAS was produced by incubating predried baker's yeast in pooled AB serum (100 mg/1000 ml) for 60min at 37°C in a shaking water bath, after which the mixture was spun down to remove the yeast particles. After a second incubation step at 56°C for 30 min in order to inactivate the carboxypeptidase B, YAS was stored deep frozen at −70°C in 1-ml-portions. FMLP was purchased from Sigma Chemicals and dissolved in MEM (10^{-2} *M*). Starting from this stock solution, the working concentration for the chemotaxis assay (2×10^{-7} *M*) was prepared by further diluting in MEM. The solution was again stored deep frozen at −70°C until further use.

The chemotaxis assay was run as follows: 10 µl FMLP, YAS, or RPMI 1640 were pipetted into the central hole to assess spontaneous migration. Into each of the three outer holes we pipetted 10 µl PMNL suspension (2.5×10^5 PMNL/ml RPMI 1640). Double assays were run each time. The dishes were then covered up and incubated for 3 h at 37°C and at 100% air humidity with 5% CO_2 in an incubator. Afterwards the cells were fixed by pouring 2 ml 10% formaldehyde into the dishes. The agarose was gently removed 24 h later and the cells attached to the bottom stained with Pappenheim's stain. By means of a photographic enlarger the dishes were magnified about tenfold and the distance traveled by the PMNL toward the central hole was measured in millimeters. We calculated the chemotactic difference (CD), i.e., the difference between the distance of chemotactic migration (a) and the migration distance in the opposite direction (b) at the rear of the hole: CD = $a - b$ (mm)

Cell-directed chemotactic inhibitors were studied by preincubating normal PMNL in patient serum and comparing the results of the chemotactic assays (random migration; YAS; FMLP) with those obtained after preincubation of PMNL in normal, pooled AB serum. An index was again calculated as follows:

$$\text{CD PMNL}_{\text{normal}}/\text{CD PMNL}_{\text{patient}}$$

Phagocytosis and Killing of S. aureus. The method employed to study the phagocytosis and killing of *S. aureus* was a modification of the procedure proposed by VanFurth [21]. After phagocytosis, the number of surviving bacteria (a coagulase-positive strain of *S. aureus*) was determined in the supernatant after osmotic disruption of the PMNL. In preliminary experiments it was shown that the strain in use was resistant to serum factors by incubating the bacteria in 10% pooled AB serum. The bacteria were cultured in tryptone soybroth for 24 h yielding a bacterial concentration of about 5×10^8 bacteria/ml. An aliquot of 2 ml was removed and washed twice. The resulting pellet was then diluted 50-fold in RPMI 1640 to a final concentration of about 10^7 bacteria/ml. The exact number of viable bacteria was determined by plating out and colony counting after 24 h incubation.

The PMNL were suspended at a concentration of 10^7/ml RPMI 1640. One milliliter of PMNL suspension and 1 ml of bacterial suspension were mixed in an Erlenmeyer flask and 200 µl of pooled human were AB serum added. This mixture was incubated at 37°C in a shaking water bath. After 90 min, an aliquot of 100 µl was removed and immediately dissolved in 1 ml ice-cold RPMI 1640 to stop any further ingestion and digestion. To determine the total number of viable bacteria (i.e., intra- and extracellular), 100 µl of this suspension were diluted 100-fold in aqua bidestillata. This led to osmotic disruption of PMNL while the osmotically more resistant bacteria survived. The number of viable bacteria was determined by plating out and colony counting. To determine the number of bacteria remaining in the supernatant (phagocytosis), 1 ml of the incubation mixture was again diluted in 1 ml of ice-cold RPMI 1640 and spun down at 4°C for 5 min with 110 *g*. The PMNL were thus pelleted and the number of viable bacteria again determined after appropriate dilution in saline. Each test was run in triple assays. The number of viable bacteria at the beginning of the test (N_o), the total number of bacteria after 90 min of incubation (N_t) and the number of remaining viable bacteria in the supernatant after 90 min of incubating (N_s) were determined. Based on these values the phagocytic index (PI) was calculated as follows:

$$PI = \log No - \log N_s$$

The killing index (KI) as a measure of bactericidal capacity was calculated as follows:

$$KI = \log No - \log N_t$$

To determine serum opsonization the same basic procedure was used. Both AB serum and patient serum were compared in their ability to opsonize bacteria that were then phagocytosed by normal donor PMNL. The opsonic index was established by dividing PI_{pat}/PI_{don}.

Fungicidal Activity. The test germ used to test, fungicidal, activity was *Candida tropicalis* which had previously been shown to be resistant to 10% human AB serum. The yeasts were cultured in tryptone soy broth and after they had been washed twice, brought to a concentration of 10^6 yeasts/ml RPMI 1640. The assessment of fungicidal activity was analogous to the procedure outlined for the determination of bactericidal capacity with the exception that the incubation time was prolonged to 120 min. The candidacidal index was calculated as follows:

$$\text{Candidacidal Index} = \log N_o - \log N_t$$

Generation of SA. Following the procedure proposed by Weening et al. [22] the PMNL were stimulated by preopsonized zymosan and the amount of SA generated determined by reducing cytochrome c. Cytochrome c (100 mg) was dissolved in 30 ml of buffer (0.99 g glucose in 100 ml phosphate buffered solution, PBS) and stored on ice in 1-ml portions until further use. Opsonized zymosan was prepared by incubating 100 mg zymosan in 6 ml pooled AB serum in a shaking water bath at 37°C for 30 min. The suspension was then washed twice, resuspended in 50 ml buffer, and stored deep frozen in 1-ml portions until required. The reaction mixture contained 0.5 ml PMNL suspension (2×10^6 PMNL/ml buffer), 0.5 ml zymosan. 150 µl pooled AB serum, and 250 µl cytochrome c. This mixture was incubated in a shaking water bath at 37°C for 15 min. The vial was then transferred onto ice to stop the reaction. After centrifugation at 4°C for 5 min, the supernatant was measured at 546 nm against a control prepared without zymosan, and the SA concentration calculated as follows (E, extinction):

$$\text{SA nmol}/10^6\ \text{cells/min} = E \times 4.42$$

Generation of Hydrogen Peroxide (H_2O_2). H_2O_2 generation was assessed according to the method described by Pick and Keisari [23]. Horseradish peroxidase (HRPO) catalyzes the oxidation of phenol-red-utilizing H_2O_2 set free by zymosan-stimulated PMNL. Phenol red was dissolved in aqua bidestillata to a concentration of 10 g/l. Horseradish peroxidase type II was purchased from Sigma Chemicals and dissolved in buffer (0.99 g glucose in 100 ml PBS) to yield a concentration of 5 mg/ml. The reaction mixture contained 500 µl PMNL suspension in buffer, 500 µl zymosan suspension, 125 µl pooled AB serum, 12.5 µl HRPO solution, 12.5 µl phenol red solution, and 12.5 µl azid (200 mM) to inhibit cell-standing catalase. This mixture was kept in a shaking water bath at 37°C for 60 min and then spun down for 10 min at 4000 rpm. The supernatant was supplemented with 25 µl NaOH and then photometrically measured at 623 nm. An extinction coefficient had been determined earlier and, based on this finding, the H_2O_2 concentration in the reaction mixture was calculated as follows:

$$\text{nmol } H_2O_2/10^6\ \text{cells/min} = E_{60}\,\text{min} \times 0.883$$

Cellular MPO Content. The oxidative capacity of the myeloperoxidase freed after lysis of PMNL was determined photometrically following the oxidation of dianisidine (3.2 mM in 0.1 M citrate buffer, pH 5.5) [24]. The reaction mixture consisted of 890 µl dianisidine solution, 50 µl 0.2% Triton-X-100, 10 µl 10mM H_2O_2 in aqua destillata, and 50 µl PMNL suspension (2×10^6/ml PBS). The reaction was kept at 25°C in a thermostatically controlled vial and read after 30, 60, and 90 s at 436 nm, and the MPO concentration was calculated as follows:

$$E = (E_{30}\,\text{s}/0.5 + E_{60}\,\text{s}/1 + E_{90}\,\text{s}/1.5)/3 \text{ oxidated dianisidine in nmol}/10^6/\text{min} = E \times 500$$

Cellular Ly Content. After lysis of PMNL, the cellular Ly content was determined using a commerically available test kit (Behring-Werke, Marburg/

Lahn, FRG). PMNL (1×10^7) were suspended in 1 ml 1% Triton-X-100 and left standing for 1 h at room temperature. An aliquot of 25 µl was dissolved in 1.5 ml Ly reactant and immediately read at 546 nm. The Ly concentration was calculated as follows:

$$\text{ly in } \mu g/10^6 \text{ cells} = E \times 220$$

Statistics. Nonparametrical procedures were used for describing and comparing the two patient populations. Medians were established for each time point: testing was done by performing the Mann-Whitney-Wilcoxon U-test.

Results

Of the 38 patients studied, 33 were eligible for evaluation. Fifteen of the patients developed ARDS, 18 of them did not. For each function studied serially, the following results were obtained by comparing the two patient groups with the without ARDS.

Adherence. There was no statistically visible difference between the two groups in the ability of their separated PMNL to adhere to nylon wool (Fig. 1). Studying the influence of patient serum on the adherence of normal PMNL, the serum from non-ARDS patients was seen to enhance the effect by about 20% (Fig. 2).

Random Migration and Chemotaxis. Random migration declined sharply within the first 24 h in both patient groups (Fig. 3). Chemotaxis against a

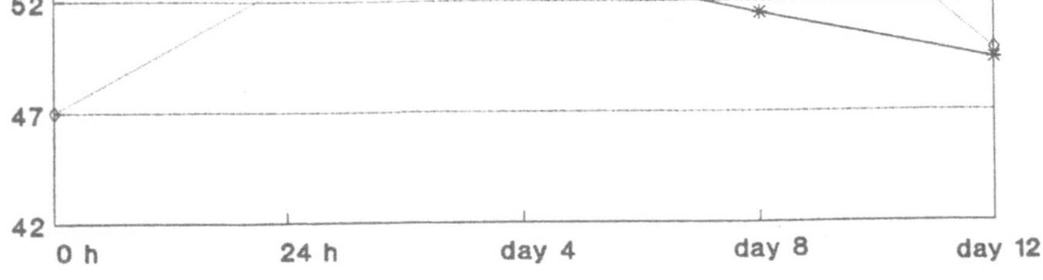

Fig. 1. Percentage of adherence to nylon wool of PMNL from patients with the without ARDS. Data are given as median values. *Asterisk*, patients with ARDS; *rhombus*, patients without ARDS

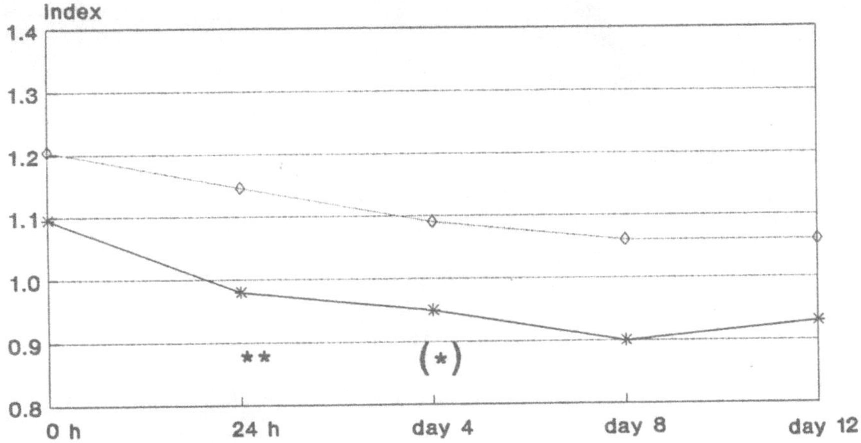

Fig. 2. The influence of patient serum on the adherence to nylon wool of PMNL from patients with and without ARDS. Data are given as median values. *Asterisk*, patients with ARDS; *rhombus*, patients without ARDS; **, $p < 0.05$ (*), not quite significant

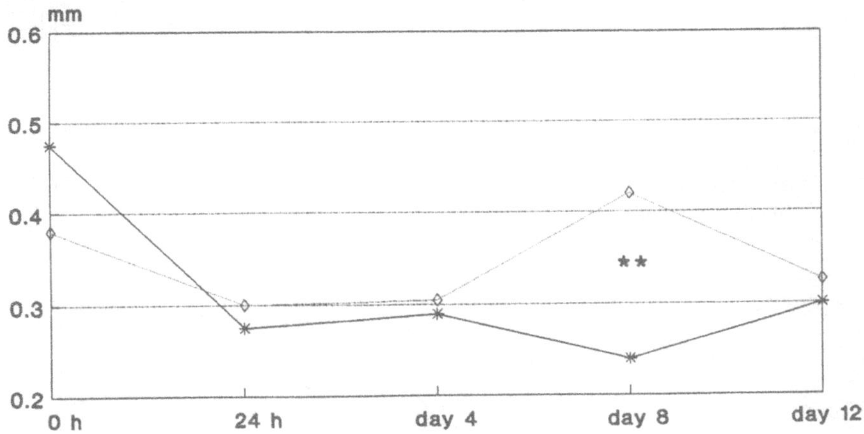

Fig. 3. Random migration of PMNL in patients with and without ARDS. Data are given as median values. *Asterisk*, patients with ARDS; *rhombus*, patients without ARDS; **, $p < 0.05$

gradient of YAS was uniformly impaired in both patient groups within the first 24 h. On day 8 following polytrauma, patients with ARDS were still significantly impaired in their ability to migrate to this chemotaxin whereas patients without ARDS returned to normal (Fig. 4). As far as the ability of patient PMNL to migrate against a gradient of FMLP was concerned, there was a statistically significant reduction in ARDS patients starting with time point O, i.e., shortly after polytrauma. This remained at the same level until day 8 (Fig. 5). Although in absolute figures this impairment was not impressive,

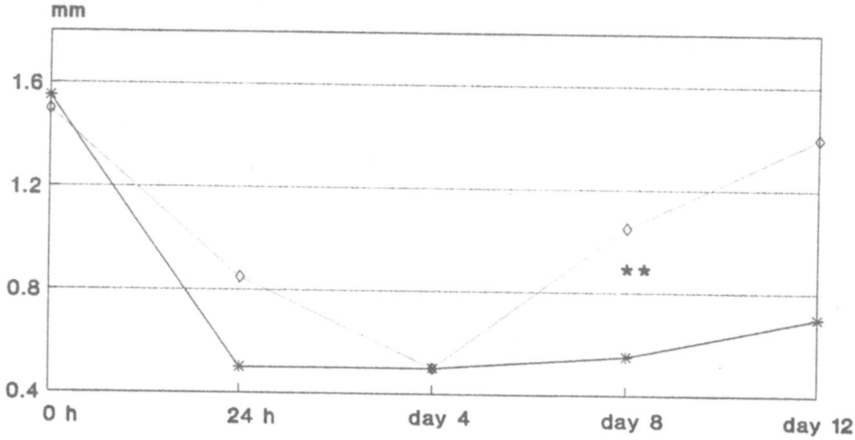

Fig. 4. Chemotaxis of PMNL against a gradient of YAS in patients with and without ARDS. Data are given as medians of chemotactic difference. *Asterisk*, patients with ARDS; *rhombus*, patients without ARDS; **, $p < 0.05$

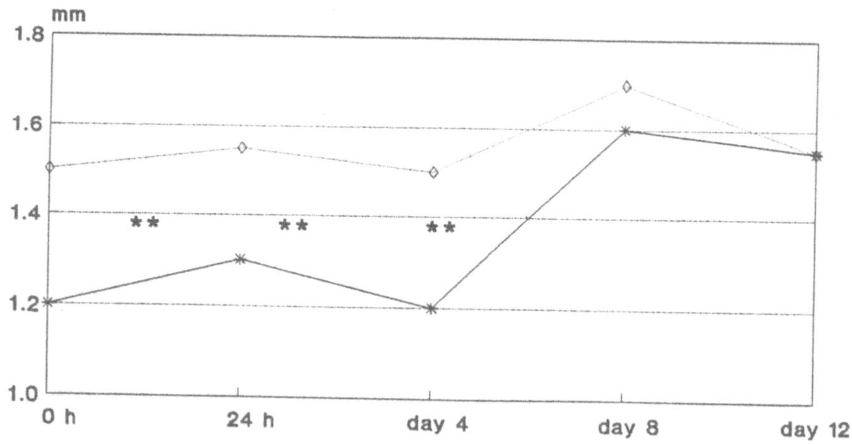

Fig. 5. Chemotaxis of PMNL against a gradient of FMLP in patients with and without ARDS. Data are given as medians of chemotactic difference. *Asterisk*, patients with ARDS; *rhombus*, patients without ARDS; **, $p < 0.05$

the difference between ARDS and non-ARDS patients was striking. Patient serum enhanced both the random migration activity (Fig. 6) and chemotaxis against YAS (Fig. 7) of normal PMNL by about 30%. Enhancement of random migration activity was visible after 24 h, whereas augmentation of YAS chemotaxis was already present shortly after polytrauma. Both these findings are in contrast with the effects of serum on chemotaxis against FMLP; the latter remained unchanged after preincubation of normal PMNL in patient serum (Fig. 8).

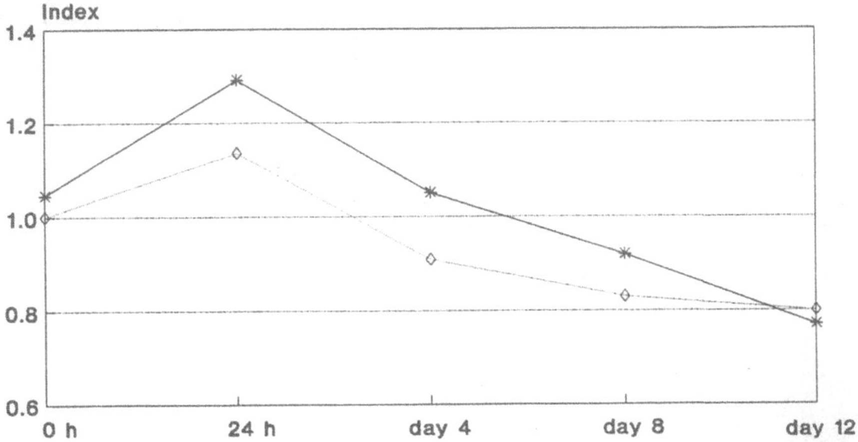

Fig. 6. The influence of patient serum on the random migration of PMNL in patients with and without ARDS. Data are given as median values. *Asterisk*, patients with ARDS; *rhombus*, patients without ARDS

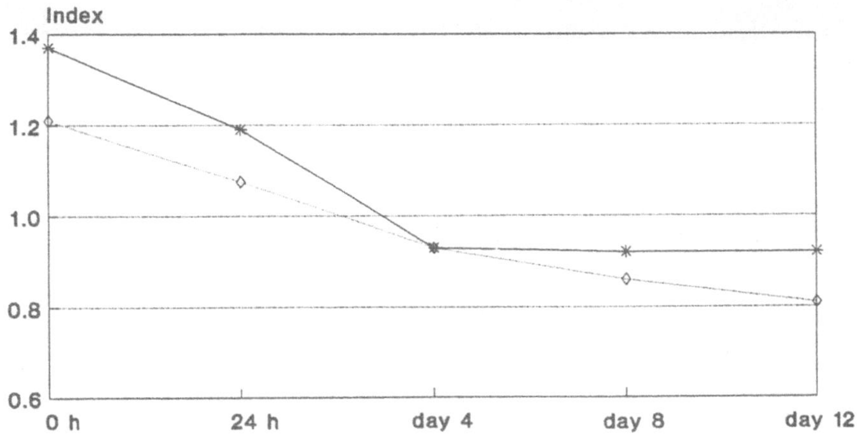

Fig. 7. The influence of patient serum on the chemotaxis of PMNL against a gradient of YAS in patients with and without ARDS. Data are given as medians of chemotactic difference. *Asterisk*, patients with ARDS; *rhombus*, patients without ARDS

Phagocytosis and Killing of S. aureus. Although significant differences between the two patient groups (showing reduction in the capacity of PMNL of ARDS patients to ingest and kill live bacteria) were not seen before day 8, a slight depression in this function in ARDS patients was also suspected earlier (Figs. 9, 10). Looking at the ability of patient serum to opsonize *S. aureus*, there was about 10% impairment in ARDS patient serum to be observed after 24 h (Fig. 11). Impairment in the capacity of patient serum to

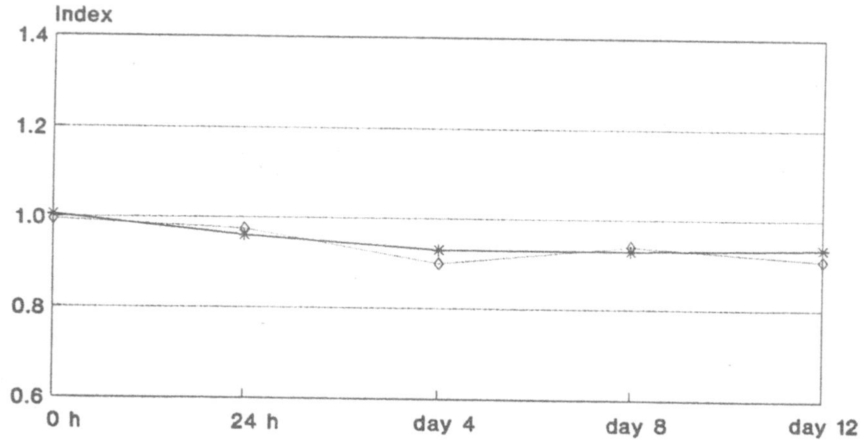

Fig. 8. The influence of patient serum on the chemotaxis of PMNL against a gradient of FMLP in patients with and without ARDS. Data are given as medians of chemotactic difference. *Asterisk*, patients with ARDS; *rhombus*, patients without ARDS

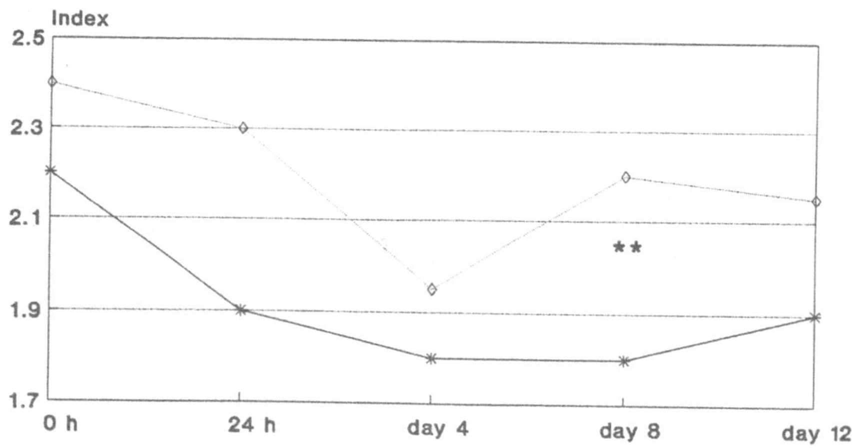

Fig. 9. Capacity of PMNL for phagocytosis of *S. aureus* in patients with and without ARDS. Data are given as median values. *Asterisk*, patients with ARDS; *rhombus*, patients without ARDS

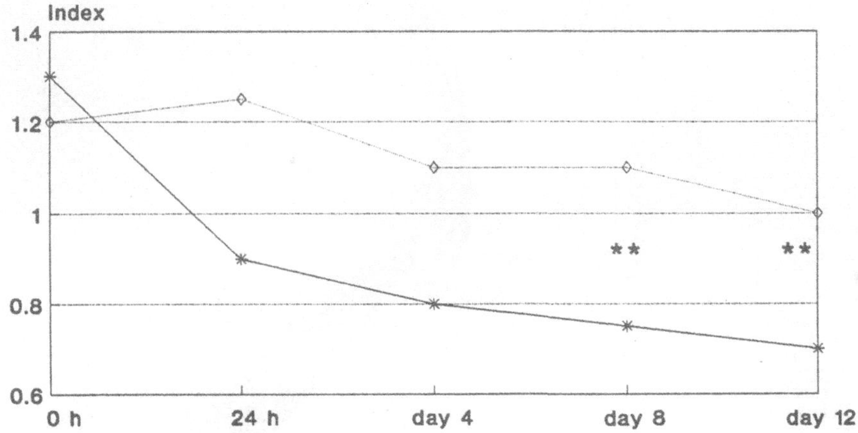

Fig. 10. Capacity of PMNL for killing of *S. aureus* in patients with and without ARDS. Data are given as median values. *Asterisk*, patients with ARDS; *rhombus*, patients without ARDS; **, $p < 0.05$

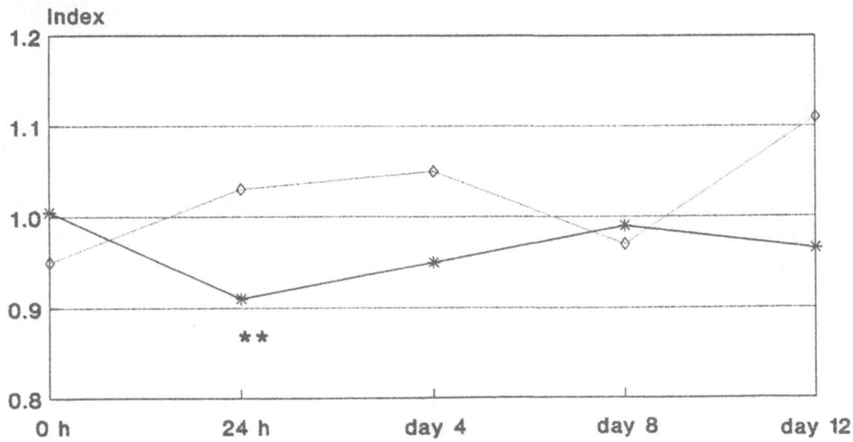

Fig. 11. Ability of patient serum to opsonize *S. aureus* in patients with and without ARDS. Data are given as median values. *Asterisk*, patients with ARDS; *rhombus*, patients without ARDS; **, $p < 0.05$

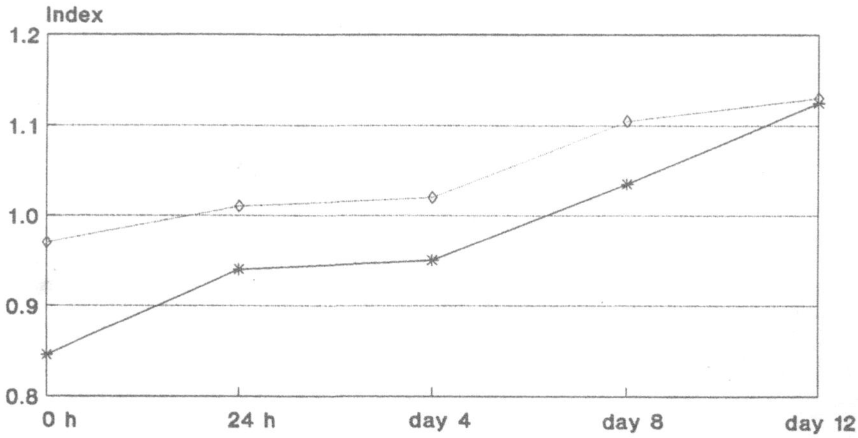

Fig. 12. Ability of patient serum to opsonize *P. aeruginosa* in patients with and without ARDS. Data are given as median values. *Asterisk*, patients with ARDS; *rhombus*, patients without ARDS

opsonize *Pseudomonas aeruginosa* was more pronounced in ARDS patients shortly after polytrauma (Fig. 12).

Fungicidal Activity. At day 4 following polytrauma there was a sharp decline to almost zero in the fungicidal capacity of ARDS patients. At time point O, and 24 h later, there was no difference whatsoever to be noted. This change occurred at the time when the patients developed signs of ARDS, i.e., at day 4. On day 8 there was some recuperation, but the impairment was still visible (Fig. 13).

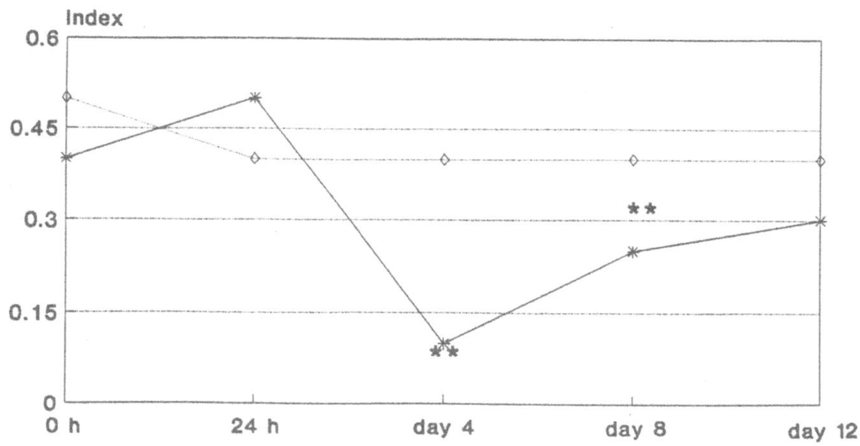

Fig. 13. Fungicidal capacity of PMNL in patients with and without ARDS. Data are given as median values. *Asterisk*, patients with ARDS; *rhombus*, patients without ARDS; **, $p < 0.05$

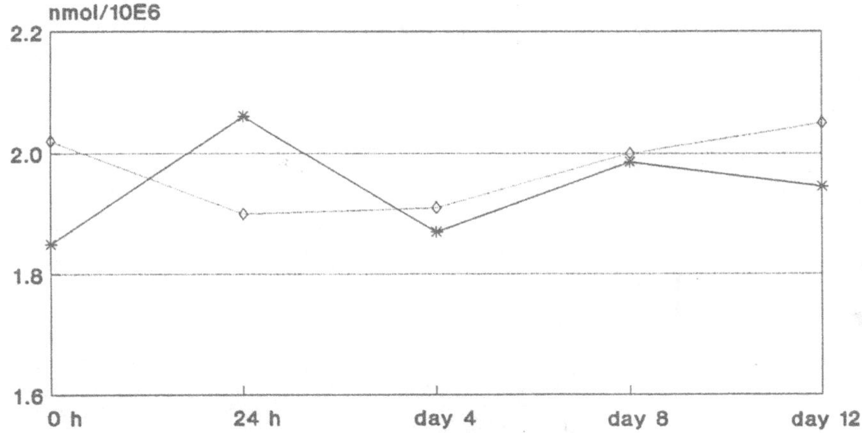

Fig. 14. Superoxide anion (SA) generation in patients with and without ARDS. Data are given as median values. *Asterisk*, patients with ARDS; *rhombus*, patients without ARDS

Generation of SA and H_2O_2. There was no difference between both patient groups, either as far as the generation of H_2O_2 or as the ability to release SA after stimulation with the particulate stimulus of opsonized yeasts were concerned (Figs. 14, 15). It has to be stated, however, that at the time of the patients' admission to the hospital, SA production in patients who eventually develop ARDS was less than in patients with a regular clinical course. This slight reduction was then counterbalanced 24 h later when the level of SA generation in ARDS patients rose above that of the non-ARDS group, although at this point not reaching the level of statistical significance.

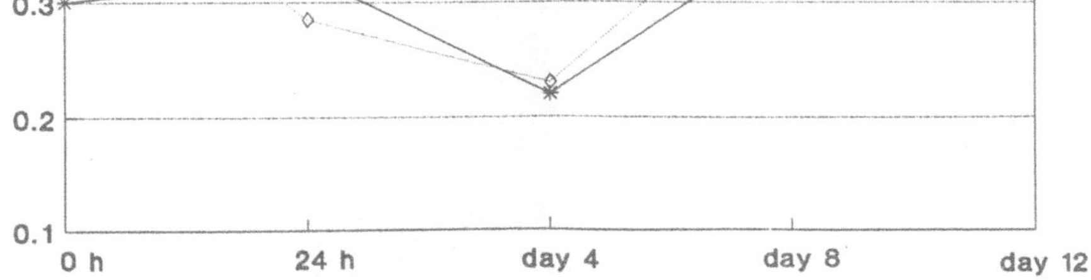

Fig. 15. Hydrogen peroxide (H_2O_2) generation in patients with and without ARDS. Data are given as median values. *Asterisk*, patients with ARDS; *rhombus*, patients without ARDS

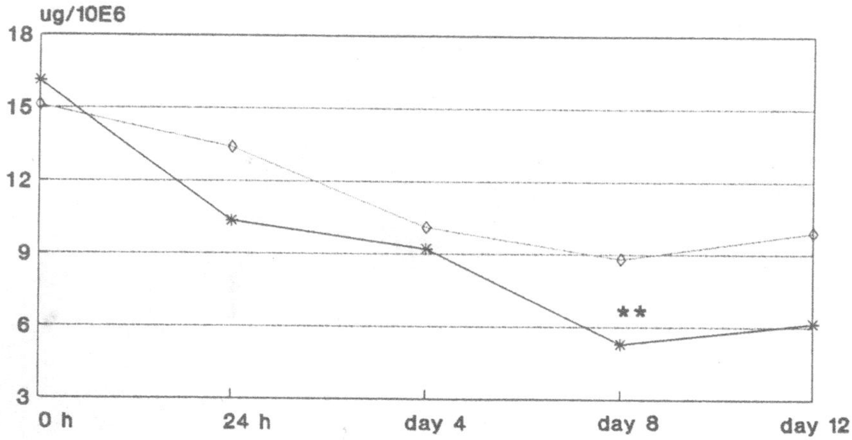

Fig. 16. Cellular lysozyme (Ly) content in patients with and without ARDS. Data are given as median values. *Asterisk*, patients with ARDS; *rhombus*, patients without ARDS; **, $p < 0.05$

Cellular Ly Content. The cellular Ly content decreased during the course of the observation period. On day 8 following polytrauma, patients with ARDS had significantly less cellular Ly in their PMNL than patients without this complication (Fig. 16).

Cellular MPO Content. Although there was a gradual decline in the cellular content of the primary granula constituent MPO, there was no difference between tht two patient groups (Fig. 17).

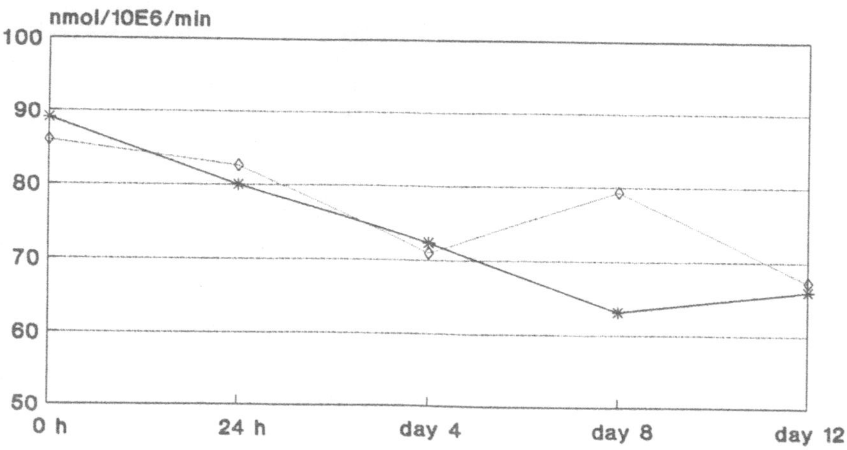

Fig.17. Cellular myeloperoxidase (MPO) content in patients with and without ARDS. Data are given as median values. *Asterisk*, patients with ARDS; *rhombus*, patients without ARDS

Discussion

When we looked for changes that occur early after polytrauma that might predispose for the development of ARDS, the difference in the chemotactic responses to FMLP of both patient groups was striking and statistically significant. Although this impairment of chemotaxis in ARDS patients was not impressive in absolute figures, the different responses have to be attributed to changes in PMNL FMLP-receptor function [25]. Chemotaxis against YAS containing the activated part of complement C5a was only about 50% normal after 24 h in both patient groups. One explanation for this phenomenon may be found in the concept of receptor desensitization. PMNL that have had contact with a chemotaxin become unresponsive to this agent upon second challenge; this is called low-grade desensitization. If this state of chemotactic unresponsiveness is extended to other stimuli as well, this is called high-grade desensitization [26–28].

Assuming that activation of the complement system occurs to a large extent immediately after polytrauma [29–33], PMNL will have had contact with complement-activation products and will become unresponsive to a new challenge with this agent which is present in YAS. Why, in the present study, this phenomenon was not visible at time point O, i.e., immediately following polytrauma, may be explained by the fact that, parallel to the desensitization reaction, there is a chemotaxis-enhancing factor present in the serum that causes enhancement of chemotaxis against a gradient of YAS. This was most pronounced immediately after polytrauma and even more so in patients who eventually developed ARDS (see Fig. 7). After 24 h this effect which augments chemotaxis against YAS was replaced at least to some extent by activity-stimulating random migration. (see Fig. 6). FMLP chemotaxis remained unchanged when patient serum was added (see Fig. 8). Studies investigating receptors for C5a (C5a–R) and FMLP (FMLP-R) have found a decrease in the number of C5a–R. The number of FMLP-R was increased, but the binding capacity of this receptor was depressed [34]. In this situation the release of toxic and thus potentially damaging oxygen radicals was found to be increased after stimulation of FMLP-R [35, 36]. These findings can be imitated in vitro by challenging PMNL first with $C5a/C5a_{desarg.}$ in the form of YAS and secondly with FMLP [37]. The release of oxygen radicals which mediate endothelial cell damage after complement activation of circulating PMNL has already been demonstrated in patients undergoing hemodialysis [38]; this observation eventually led to the engineering of artificial kidneys that did not produce this side effect. In this context it is worth noting that the mechanism of complement-mediated cell alteration also applies to monocyte dysfunction in severe trauma [39] and to burn patients [40, 41]. The untoward effects of oxygen radical release can be greatly reduced, if not abolished, by giving anti-C5a antibodies – a hypothesis that has been successfully tested in primates [42] and by depleting neutrophils from the circulation of test animals [32].

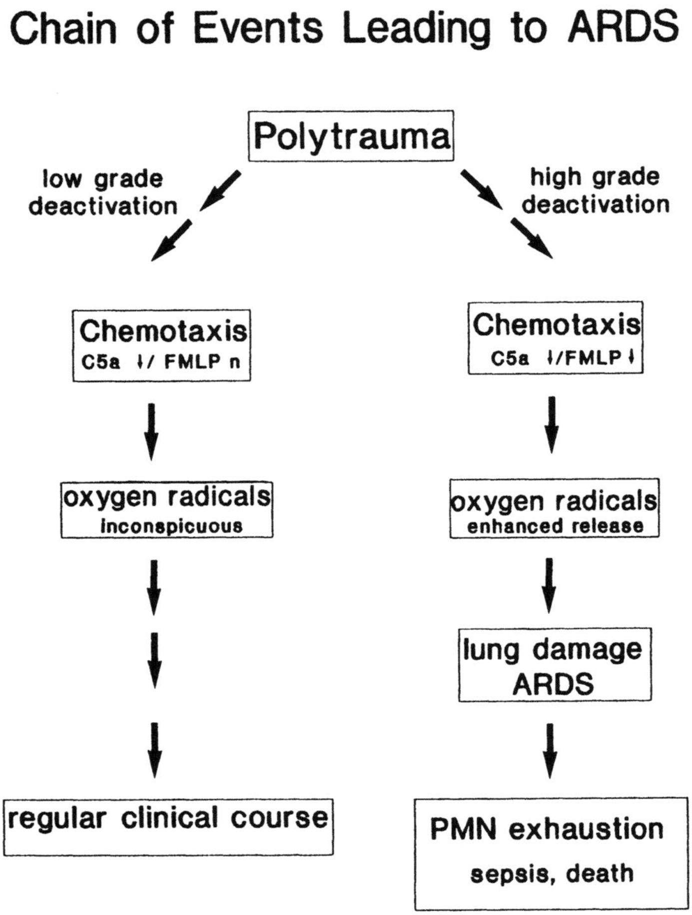

Fig.18. Chain of events leading to ARDS

Interestingly, there is also a type of sterum activity that modulates PMNL adherence. PMNL isolated from patients did not show any differences in our study. When we used patient serum to test PMNL, we noted that adherence seemed to be enhanced shortly after polytrauma in a magnitude of about 10%–20% (see Fig. 1). Serum from patients who did not succumb to ARDS was more active in that respect and remained so, whereas serum from ARDS patients was not so active. There findings are corroborated somewhat by Venezio's observation; when studying adherence to nylon wool in septic patients using whole blood, he observed an increase in adherence of about 30% and also a positive effect mediated by patient serum [43].

Differences in phagocytosis and killing of *S. aureus* and *Candida* particles do not reach levels of statistical significance within the first 4 days although a tendency for less activity can be seen in the group of patients that later develops ARDS. Following day 4 the differences in microorganism-digesting performance become significant between the two groups. Patients with ARDS show a significant reduction in phagocytosis and killing of *Staphylococci* and yeast particles (see Figs. 9–11). This may contribute to the susceptibility of developing septic complications seen in ARDS patients. In this state, PMNL seem to be "exhausted" and no longer able to respond adequately to invading organisms. A similar situation is seen in the lymphocyte stimulatory response in burn patients [44]. Depressed phagocytic activity is not uncommon in surgical patients [45–48]. A slight depression in serum opsonic activity specific for *S. aureus* is manifested in ARDS patients as early as 24 h after polytrauma (see Fig. 11). Opsonization of *P. aeruginosa* is clearly depressed in ARDS patients within the first 24 h (see Fig. 12). For opsonization to function properly, an intact complement system is necessary. This holds true especially for *P. aeruginosa*. The impairment of opsonic capacity seen in ARDS patients early after polytrauma may be an indicator of massive complement activation, that is more pronounced in patients suffering from ARDS.

The release of toxic oxygen products such as SA and H_2O_2 did not differ in the two patient groups – at least not in the way it was tested in the present study using a particulate stimulus in the form of preopsonized zymosan. A stronger generation of SA could be observed in a few patients after challenge with FMLP – a soluble stimulus directly affecting FMLP-R (results not shown).

Looking at our results of PMNL function early after polytrauma and considering evidence presented by other authors, we feel that a possible – but not necessarily the only – pathomechanism for developing ARDS resides with deactivation and the associated toxic oxygen release of circulating PMNL (Fig. 18). Polytrauma patients may either experience low-grade deactivation or high-grade deactivation of PMNL depending on the amount and/or composition of the deactivating substances appearing in the circulation. One factor identified is surely $C5a/C5a_{desarg.}$ It is either the greater amount of $C5a/C5a_{desarg.}$ generated in ARDS-prone patients or else some additional factor that leads to high-grade deactivation – demonstrated by impairment of FMLP chemotaxis – and thus greatly enhanced release of toxic and damaging oxygen radicals. This study clearly demonstrates that PMNL chemotaxis against a gradient of FMLP shows deactivation at time point O less than 2 h after trauma. At this time some determination of the patient's clinical outcome has already taken place. Besides the role of $C5a/C5a_{desarg.}$ mediating deactivation responses in vivo there may be some other factors acting in the same direction. Possible factors are bacterial endotoxins or similar products [49, 50] which may act either directly on PMNL or else via monocyte stimulation. Evidence is mounting that endotoxemia may grossly facilitate the release of toxic oxygen radicals by PMNL and the development of ARDS [49, 51–54]. Monocytes and macrophages are primed to release among other things interleukin-1 or tumor necrosis factor (TNF) which among other actions extert modulatory effects on PMNL function [55–58]. Alveolar macrophages may cause PMNL to secrete azurophilic granule enzymes via a peptide [59]. Bacterial translocation – a possible source of endotoxins – has been shown to occur in traumatic and shock situations [46, 60].

The agents leading to high-grade deactivation have not yet been identified and many details have still to be uncovered. It seems, however, that this factor already exerts its effects in the initial period following severe trauma.

References

1. Rocker GM, Wiseman MS, Pearson D, Shale DJ (1989) Diagnostic criteria for adult respiratory distress syndrome: time for reappraisal. Lancet 1:120–123
2. Norwood SH, Civetta JM (1985) The adult respiratory syndrome. Surg Gynecol Obstet 161:497–508
3. Hyers TH, Fowler AA (1986) Adult respiratory distress syndrome: causes, morbidity, and mortality. Federation Proc 1986; 45:25–29
4. Balk R, Bone RC (1983) The adult respiratory distress syndrome. Med Clin North Am 67:551–556
5. Derderian SS (1980) Adult respiratory distress syndrome. J Am Osteopath Assoc 79:402–406
6. Craddock PR (1984) Complement, granulocytes, and shock lung. Am J Emerg Med 2:78–81
7. Hammerschmidt DE, Weaver LJ, Hudson LD, Craddock PR, Jacob HS (1980) Association of complement activation and elevated plasma-C5a with adult respiratory distress syndrome. Pathophysiological relevance and possible prognostic value. Lancet 1:947–949
8. Sacks T, Moldow CF, Craddock PR, Bowers TK, Jacob HS (1978) Endothelial damage provoked by toxic oxygen radicals released from complement-triggered granulocytes. Prog Clin Biol Res 21:719–726
9. Cochrane CG, Spragg RG, Revak SD, Cohen AB, McGuire WW (1983) The presence of neutrophil elastase and evidence of oxidation activity in bronchoalveolar lavage fluid of patients with adult respiratory distress syndrome. Am Rev Respir Dis 127:25–27
10. Zimmerman GA, Renzetti AD, Hill HR (1983) Functional and metabolic activity of granulocytes from patients with adult respiratory distress syndrome. Evidence for activated neutrophils in the pulmonary circulation. Am Rev Respir Dis 127:290–300
11. Parsons PE, Fowler AA, Hyers TM, Henson PM (1985) Chemotactic activity in bronchoalveolar lavage fluid from patients with adult respiratory distress syndrome. Am Rev Respir Dis 132:490–493
12. Varani J, Fligiel SEG, Till GO, Kunkel RG, Ryan US, Ward PA (1985) Pulmonary endothelial cell killing by human neutrophils: Possible involvement of hydroxyl radical. Lab Invest 53:656–663
13. Grob PJ, Holch M, Brunner W (1987) Posttraumatisches/postoperatives Immundefektsyndrom (Post-traumatic/postoperative immune deficiency syndrome). Schweiz Med Wochenschr 117:471–480
14. Munster AM (1984) Immunologic response of trauma and burns. An overview. Am J Med 76:142–145
15. Boyum A (1968) Separation of leukocytes from blood and bone marrow. Scand J Clin Lab Invest [Suppl. 97] 21:77–82

16. MacGregor RR, Macarak EJ, Kefalides NA (1978) Comparative adherence of granulocytes to endothelial monolayers and nylon fiber. J Clin Invest 61:697–702
17. Chenoweth DE, Rowe JG, Hugli T (1979) A modified method for chemotaxis under agarose. J Immunol Meth 25:337–353
18. Nelso RD, Quie PG, Simmons RL (1975) Chemotaxis under agarose: A new and simple method for measuring chemotaxis and sponateous migration of human polymorphonuclear leukocytes and monocytes. J Immunol 115:1650–1656
19. Repo H, Kosunen TU (1977) Leukocyte migration agarose test for the assessment of human neutrophil chemotaxis. Scand J Immunol 6:211–218
20. Showell HJ, Freers RJ, Zigmond SH, Schiffmann E, Aswanikumar S, Corcoran B, Becker EL (1976) The structure-activity relations of synthetic peptides as chemotactic factors and inducers of lysosomal enzyme secretion for neutrophils. J Exp Med 143:1154–1169
21. VanFurth R, VanZweet TL (1973) In vitro determination of phagocytosis and intracellular killing by polymorphonuclear and mononuclear leukocytes. In: Weir DM, ed. Handbook of Experimental Immunology. Blackwell, Oxford pp 36.1–36.24
22. Weening RS, Wever R, Roos D (1975) Quantitative aspects of the production of superoxide radicals by phagocytizing human granulocytes. J Lab Clin Med 85:245–252
23. Pick E, Keisari Y (1980) A simple colorimetric method for the measurement of hydrogen peroxide produced by cells in culture. J Immunol Meth 38:161–170
24. Kitahara M, Eyre HJ, Simonian Y, Atkin CL, Hasstedt SJ (1981) Hereditary myeloperoxidase deficiency. Blood 57:888–893
25. Snyderman R, Pike Mc (1984) Chemoattractant receptors on phagocytic cells. Ann Rev Immunol 2:257–281
26. Solomkin JS, Cotta LA, Satoh PS, Hurst JM, Nelson RD (1985) Complement activation and clearance in acute illness and injury: evidence for C5a as a cell-directed mediator of the adult respiratory distress syndrome in man. Surgery 97:668–678
27. Solomkin JS, Jenkins MK, Nelson RD, Chenoweth D, Simmons RL (1981) Neutrophil dysfunction in sepsis: II. Evidence for the role of complement activation products in cellular deactivation. Surgery 90:319–327
28. Solomkin JS, Cotta LA, Brodt JK, Hurst JW, Ogle CK (1984) Neutrophil dysfunction in sepsis: III Degranulation as a mechanism for nonspecific deactivation. J Surg Res 36:407–412
29. Robbins RA, Russ WD, Rasmussen JK, Clayton MM (1987) Activation of the complement system in the adult respiratory distress syndrome. Am Rev Respir Dis 135:651–658
30. Olson LM, Moss GS, Baukus O, Das Gupta TK (1985) The role of C5 in septic lung injury. Ann Surg 202:771–776
31. Worthen GS, Henson PM (1983) Mechanisms of acute lung injury. Clin Lab Med 3:601–617
32. Till GO, Johnson KJ, Kunkel R, Ward PA (1982) Intravascular activation of complement and acute lung injury: dependency on neutrophils and toxic oxygen metabolites. J Clin Invest 69:1126–1135
33. Tennenberg SD, Jacobs MP, Solomkin JS (1987) Complement-mediated neutrophil activation in sepsis- and trauma-related adult respiratory distress syndrome. Clarification with radioaerosol lung scans. Arch Surg 122:26–32
34. Solomkin JS, Cotta LA, Ogle JD, Brodt JK, Ogle CK, Satoh PS, Hurst JM, Alexander JW (1984) Complement-induced expression of cryptic receptors on the neutrophil surface: a mechanism for regulation of acute inflammation in trauma. Surgery 96:336–341
35. van Epps DE, Garcia ML (1980) Enhancement of neutrophil function as a result of prior exposure to chemotactic factor. J Clin Invest 66:167–175
36. Bendeer JG, McPhail LC, van Epps DE (1983) Exposure of human neutrophils to chemotactic factors potentiates activation of the respiratory burst enzyme. J Immunol 130:2316–2323

37. Tennenberg SD, Solomkin JS (1987) Surface receptor mobilization in complement-mediated neutrophil activation: characterization and effects of methylprednisolone. J Surg Res 43:143–148
38. Sacks T, Moldow CF, Craddock PR, Bowers TK (1978) Oxygen radicals mediate endothelial cell damage by complement-stimulated granulocytes. An in vitro model of immune vascular damage. J Clin Invest 1161–1167
39. Antrum RM, Solomkin JS (1986) Monocyte dysfunction in severe trauma: evidence for the role of C5a in deactivation. Surgery 100:29–37
40. Nelson RD, Hasslen SR, Ahrenholz DH, Solem LD (1987) Mechanisms of loss of human neutrophil chemotaxis following thermal injury. J Burn Care Rehabil 8:496–502
41. Moore FD, Davis C, Rodrick M, Mannick JA, Fearon DT (1986) Neutrophil activation in thermal injury as assessed by increased expression of complement receptors. N Engl J Med 314:948–953
42. Stevens JH, O'Hanley P, Shapiro JM, Mihm FG, Satoh PS, Collins JA, Raffin TA (1986) Effects of anti-C5a antibodies on the adult respiratory disdress syndrome in septic primates. J Clin Invest 77:1812–1816
43. Venezio FR, Westenfelder GO, Phair JP (1982) The adherence of polymorphonuclear leukocytes in patients with sepsis. J Infect Dis 145:351–357
44. Deitch EA, Landry KN, McDonald JC (1985) Postburn impaired cell-mediated immunity may not be due to lazy lymphocytes but to overwork. Ann Surg 201:793–802
45. Alexander JW, Wixson D (1970) Neutrophil dysfunction and sepsis in burn injury. Surg Gynecol Obstet 3:431–438
46. Deitch EA, Berg R (1987) Bacterial translocation from the gut: a mechanism of infection. J Burn Care Rehabil 8:475–482
47. Alexander JW, Stinnett JD, Ogle CK, Ogle JD, Morris MJ (1979) A comparison of immunologic profiles and their influence on bacteremia in surgical patients with a high risk of infection. Surgery 86:94–104
48. Alexander W. Wixson D (1970) Neutrophil dysfunction and sepsis in burn injury. Surg Gynecol Obstet 431–438
49. Simons RK, Maier RV, Lennard ES (1987) Neutrophil function in a rat model of endotoxin-induced lung injury. Arch Surg 122:197–203
50. Worthen GS, Haslett C, Smedly LA, Rees AJ, Gumbay RS, Henson JE, Henson PM (1986) Lung vascular injury induced by chemotactic factors: enhancement by bacterial endotoxins. Federation Proc 45:7–12
51. Holman RG, Maier RV (1988) Superoxide production by neutrophils in a model of adult respiratory distress syndrome. Arch Surg 123:1491–1495
52. Giomarelli PP, Chiara O, Borrelli E, Betti S, Volterrani L, Lorenzini L, Grossi A (1988) Early diagnosis of adult respiratory distress syndrome: an experimental model of complement-mediated pulmonary injury. J Thorac Imaging 3:15–20
53. Bloom RJ, Simon LM, Benitz WE (1988) Endotoxin and pulmonary cell injury. Surg Gynecol Obstet 167:92–98
54. Griswold J, Maier RV (1988) Neutrophil phagocytosis during endotoxin-induced lung injury. J Surg Res 44:417–424
55. Berger M, Wetzler EM, Wallis RS (1988) Tumor necrosis factor is the major monocyte product that increases complement receptor expression on mature human neutrophils. Blood 71:151–158
56. Baker CC, Yamada AH, Faist E, Kupper TS (1987) Interleukin-1 and T cell function following injury. J Burn Care Rehabil 8:503–508
57. Tracey KJ, Lowry SF, Cerami A (1988) Cachetin/TNF-alpha in septic shock and septic adult respiratory distress syndrome. Am Rev Respir Dis 138:1377–1379
58. Stephens KE, Ishizaka A, Larrick JW, Raffin TA (1988) Tumor necrosis factor causes increased pulmonary permeability and edema Comparison to septic acute lung injury. Am Rev Respir Dis 137:1364–1370
59. Cohen AB, MacArthur C, Idell S, Maunder R, Martin T, Dinarello CA, Griffith D, McLarty J (1988) A peptide from alveolar macrophages that releases neutrophil

enzymes into the lungs in patients with the adult respiratory distress syndrome. Am Rev Respir Dis 137:1151–1158
60. Deitch EA, Winterton J, Berg R (1986) Thermal injury promotes bacterial translocation from the gastrointestinal tract in mice with impaired T-cell-mediated immunity. Arch Surg 121:97–101

Changes in Reticuloendothelial Capacity Associated with Liver Dysfunction in Multiple Trauma*

G. Regel[1], K.F Gratz[2], T. Pohlemann[1], J.A. Sturm[1], and H. Tscherne[1]

Severe trauma is often complicated by the development of multiple organ system failure. In this context mainly dysfunction syndromes of lung and kidney have been described. Distinct disturbances of hepatic function have frequently been noticed. In some cases, however, severe liver failure is seen mostly in association with posttraumatic sepsis [7]. The pathomechanisms relating disturbances of hepatic blood flow, liver cell integrity, and the function of the reticuloendothelial system (RES) in the liver have so far not been clarified [1, 4, 10].

Whether the onset of posttraumatic sepsis is possibly related to one of these mentioned liver functions is still unknown. To elucidate these interactions we investigated perfusion, bile excretion, protein synthesis, and RES clearance of the liver during a prospective follow-up in multiple trauma victims. Our specific questions were:

1. Are alterations of liver perfusion present immediately after trauma and do they differ in patients with additional blunt liver trauma?
2. Are there changes in RES clearance? Are these changes perfusion dependent and are they enhanced in the group of multiple trauma patients with direct liver injury?
3. Does the onset of sepsis correlate with the alterations seen of liver perfusion and RES function?

Patients and Methods

From 1985 to 1987 ten patients suffering from multiple trauma (Injury Severity Score >30) were included in this study, all of whom were primar-

* Supported by the DFG (Deutsche Forschungsgemeinschaft) project nr. TS 14/3–3 and 4

[1] Department of Trauma Surgery, Hannover Medical School, Konstanty-Gutschow-Str. 8, W-3000 Hannover 61, FRG
[2] Department of Nuclear Medicine and Biophysics, Hannover Medical School, Konstanty-Gutschow-Str. 8, W-3000 Hannover 61, FRG

J.A. Sturm (Ed.)
Adult Respiratory Distress Syndrome

Table 1. Analysis of blood

Serum Enzymes
Serum glutamate pyruvate transaminase (SGPT) (u/l)
Serum glutamate oxalacetate transaminase (SGOT) (u/l)
Serum glutamate dehydrogenase (GLDH) (u/l)
γ-Glutamyl transpeptidase (γ-GT) (u/l)
Alkaline phosphatase (AP) (u/l)
Bilirubin
Total serum bilirubin (μmol/l)
Clotting factors
Antithrombin III (AT III) (%)
Choline esterase (CHE) (Ku/l)
Fibrogen (FIB) (g/l)

ily admitted to the trauma center of the Hannover Medical School and transferred to the surgical intensive care unit after initial resuscitation and operation. To monitor liver function, blood was sampled daily, and bilirubin, serum enzymes, and clotting factors were analyzed (Table 1).

Arterial and Venous Blood Flow

In addition we measured the arterial and venous fractions of total hepatic blood flow after injection of a 500-mbq Tc99m DTpA bolus. The activity was measured in 0.2-s increments for up to 50 s. After selection of representative regions such as the lower abdominal aorta, right kidney, spleen, and right hepatic lobe (without the kidney region), separate time activity curves were produced [2]. Three points on the curve were identified:

1. The time the arterial liver perfusion started (first increase of the liver curve: point A in Fig. 1)
2. The time the portal venous perfusion started (second increase of the liver curve, about 7 ± 2 s later: point B in Fig. 1)
3. The beginning of recirculation effects at the end of the first portal passage (point C in Fig. 1).

Integrals were calculated for the time AB (arterial-related flow) and for the additional activity in the time BC. The arterial portion of liver perfusion is given by the formula:

$$\text{Arterial perfusion} = \frac{\text{activity}_{AB} \times 100}{\text{activity}_{AB} + \text{activity}_{BC}} \ (\%)$$

Figure 1 shows a normal curve at the top and a pathologic increase of the arterial fraction in the bottom curve.

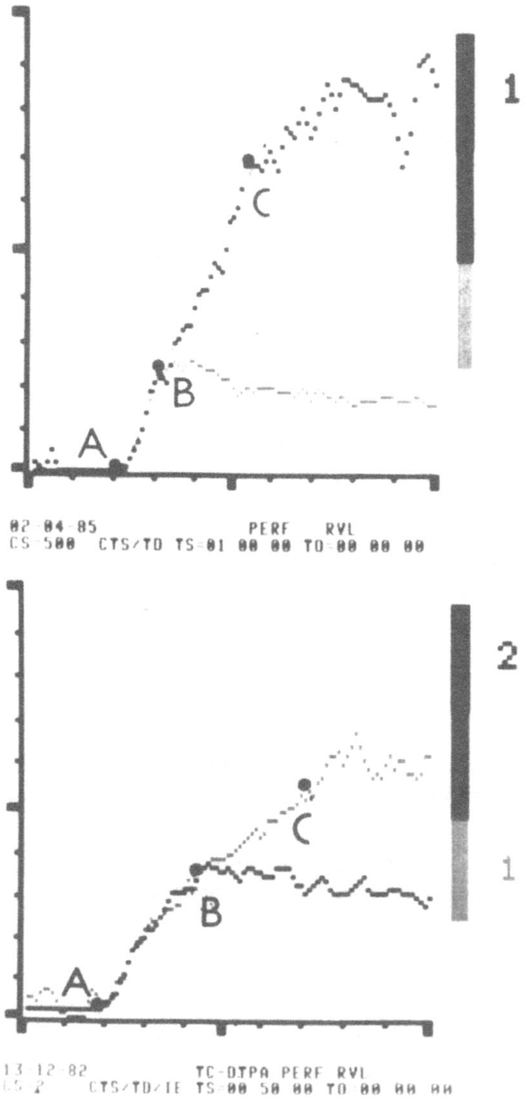

Fig. 1. Determination of the arterial blood flow of the liver after generation of a time-activity curve (500 mBq Tc 99 m DTpA): *A* at the beginning of arterial organ uptake; *B* at the beginning of the portal phase; *C* at the beginning of recirculation

Reticuloendothelial System Clearance

The uptake measurement of labeled millimicrosphere (MMS) into the liver enables the regional in vivo assessment of phagocytic properties of the hepatic RES to be carried out [2]. For this purpose the patients were positioned under a gamma camera, linked to a dedicated computer. After i.v. injection of technetium-99m-labeled human serum albumin MMS (37 MBq), accumulation in the liver was recorded for 18 min in 15-s increments. Time activity

Table 2. Sepsis criteria

1.	Temperature maximum > 39°C
2.	Rectal − peripheral temperature difference > 8°C
3.	Positive fluid balance > +1500 ml/24 h
4.	Decrease in Horovitz quotient paO_2/FIO_2 > 100/24 h
5.	Increase in extravascular lung water > 3 ml/kg body wt./24 h
6.	Decrease in platelets of 30%/24 h
7.	Change in leukocyte count of 5000/μl per 24 h
8.	Decrease in clotting factor II and/or V of 30%/24 h

Five of the eight criteria must be fulfilled to meet the definition of sepsis

curves were generated for the entire liver. A monoexponential fit was performed to calculate the colloid liver uptake. Under the conditions (a) that the tracer has been extracted totally by the liver and (b) that the liver perfusion does not change during the measurement, the uptake/time unit is only dependent on the colloid clearance rate (k-value):

Formula: $k\text{-value} = ln2/T_{1/2}(\text{min}^{-1})$

The clinical course was well documented especially considering the duration of initial hemorrhagic shock, transfusion volumes, fluid balance, and sepsis criteria (Table 2).

Statistics

For comparison of different time points within a group, a two-tailed t test for paired data was used. For comparison of different groups at the same point in time, a two-tailed Wilcoxon matched pair test was employed. In all instances, the null hypothesis was rejected at the $p < 0.05$ level. Data are reported as mean ± standard error of the mean unless otherwise specified.

Results

In a 2-year prospective study ten patients who suffered multiple trauma (five with additional liver trauma = +LT; five without liver trauma = −LT) were evaluated. The diagnoses of these patients are listed in Table 3. In spite of standardized resuscitation after trauma, two patients of the +LT group and one of the −LT group showed only delayed recovery from initial hemorrhagic shock, expressed as a high rectal/peripheral temperature difference, low urinary output, and decreased mean arterial pressure (<70 mmHg). In all cases a restitution was seen after 36–48 h. A significant increase in the overall fluid balance and transfusion volumes of these patients could not be seen.

Table 3. Diagnosis

1. Patients with blunt liver trauma	
T.A.	Liver rupture, multiple tears of the transverse colon, fractures to both legs below the knees
B.M.	Liver rupture, right-sided lung contusion with serial rib fractures, Malgaigne fracture
H.M.	Right-sided lung contusion, ruptures of liver and spleen, traumatic amputation of the right leg with severe décollement
W.I.	Lung contusion on both sides, ruptures of liver and spleen, Malgaigne fracture
B.J.	Left-sided lung contusion and serial rib fractures, ruptures of liver and spleen, fracture of the left acetabulum and sacrum
2. Patients without blunt liver trauma	
B.H.	Multiple fractures of the left humerus and radius and of the left femur. Open fractures of both tibiae
H.U.	Femoral fractures on both sides and fractures of the left humerus
D.J.	Right-sided tibial fracture, Malgaigne fracture, multiple tears of the descending colon, severe soft tissue decollement in the pelvic region
L.A.	Blunt abdominal trauma with rupture of the spleen, open tibial fractures on both sides
K.G.	Tibial fractures on both sides, left-sided femoral fracture and radius fracture

In the group with direct liver trauma (+LT) all intracellular hepatic enzymes were increased (Fig. 2) from the beginning. SGOT showed peak values after 24 h (153.6 ± 36.1). and SGPT and GLDH showed peak 3 days after trauma (158.1 ± 41.2; 168.3 ± 25.2). These parameters were normal or slightly increased in the −LT group during the entire time course.

The excretory function of the liver measured by γ-glutomyl transferase (γ-GT) and alkaline phosphatase (AP) was normal in both groups. The mean values are shown in Fig. 3. The increase in bilirubin was significantly ($p < 0.05$) different in the +LT/−LT groups; values being near controls in the −LT patients and showing a steady increase up to the 8th day in the group with direct liver trauma (+LT). This increase in total bilirubin levels in the +LT group (peak value at 55 ± 26.4 μmol/l) was mainly related to a direct, intrahepatic bilirubin load.

Liver synthesis was disturbed in all cases (Fig. 4). Cholinesterases (CHES) rapidly decreased in both groups during the 8-day period, first reaching control values at a mean of 11.3 days in the +LT group. Antithrombin synthesis was reduced in both groups, showing significantly lower values ($p < 0.05$) during the entire follow-up in the +LT group, with a minimum at the 5th day (66.7% ± 8.0%). Fibrinogen showed an initial minimum with a constant increase during the time course.

The results of liver scanning are shown in Fig. 5. Perfusion was significantly ($p < 0.01$) reduced in both groups, with an arterial portion in the −LT group of 50% ± 11.3% not reaching near-standard values before the

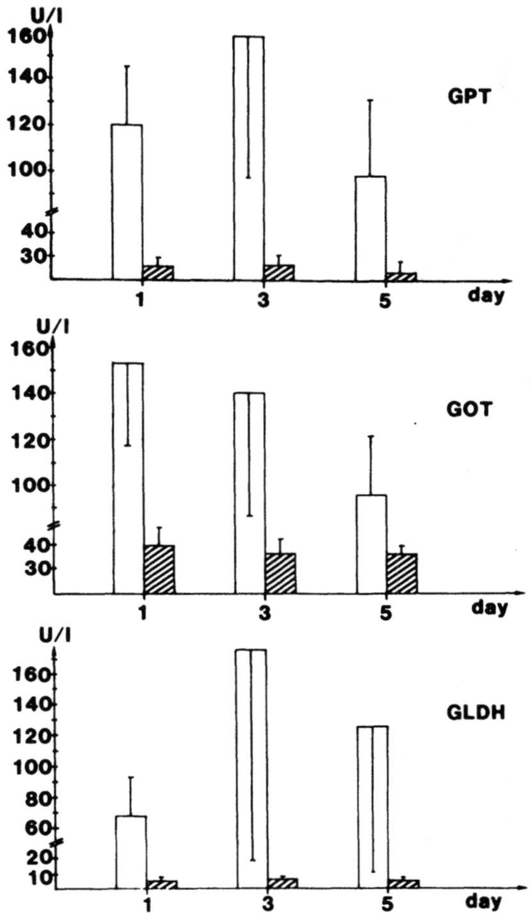

Fig. 2. Posttraumatic course of the intracellular hepatic enzymes (SGOT, SGPT, GLDH) in the groups with and without direct liver trauma

third measurement. In the group with blunt liver trauma (+LT) this disturbance was significantly higher, with an average arterial perfusion reaching 73.9% in the initial 24 h.

The disturbance of RES clearance was identical in both groups (Fig. 5) with highly pathologic values immediately posttrauma ($k = 0.45 \pm 0.12$ min in the +LT group and 0.47 ± 0.08 min in the −LT group). A restitution was seen in the −LT group on the 5th day, whereas in the +LT group RES function remained pathologic during the entire period of follow-up.

According to the defined criteria, a higher incidence of sepsis could be found in the patients with significantly disturbed RES clearance (*k*-value, $\leqslant 0.6$) (Table 4). A relationship to the degree of liver perfusion (arterial perfusion fraction) could not be proved. Sepsis was seen in both the −LT and +LT groups, developing in a later time period in the −LT group.

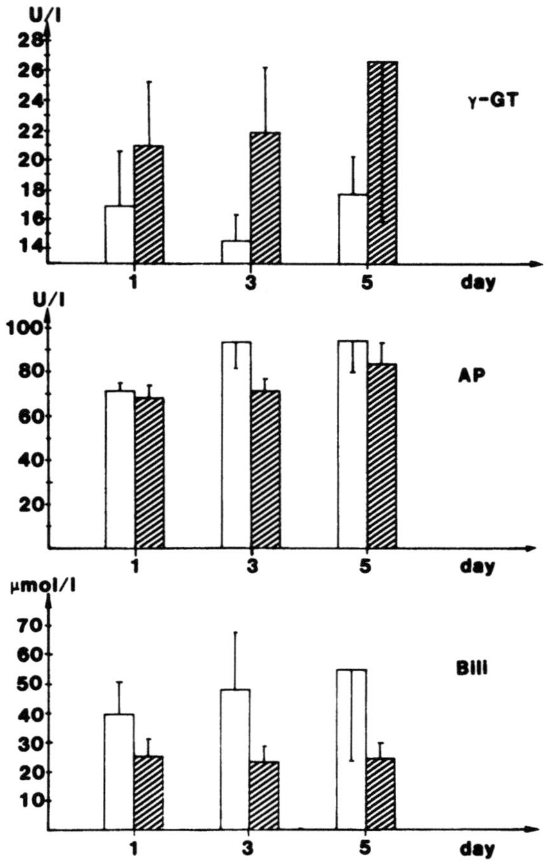

Fig. 3. Parameters measuring excretory function of the liver (γ-GT, AP, direct bilirubin) in the posttraumatic course

Table 4. Comparison of patients with and without sepsis

Patients		*k* values 1st	3rd	5th day	Arterial perfusion 1st	3rd	5th day	Liver trauma	Onset of sepsis (day)
With sepsis									
B.M.	*	0.48	0.53	0.75	76	85	40	+	6
H.M.	#	0.64	0.76	–	83	93	–	+	3
B.J.	*	0.36	0.59	–	86	85	–	+	5
H.K.	*	0.55	0.58	0.56	57	63	52	–	8
D.J.	*	0.80	0.54	0.45	40	53	42	–	8
Without sepsis									
T.A.	*	0.69	1.10	1.30	69	61	52	+	–
W.I.	#	0.63	1.00	1.15	69	65	60	+	–
B.H.	#	0.82	1.10	0.80	43	43	34	–	–
L.A.	*	0.60	0.88	0.50	95	93	86	–	–
K.G.	*	0.60	1.20	0.90	74	65	52	–	–

*, survivors; #, non-survivors

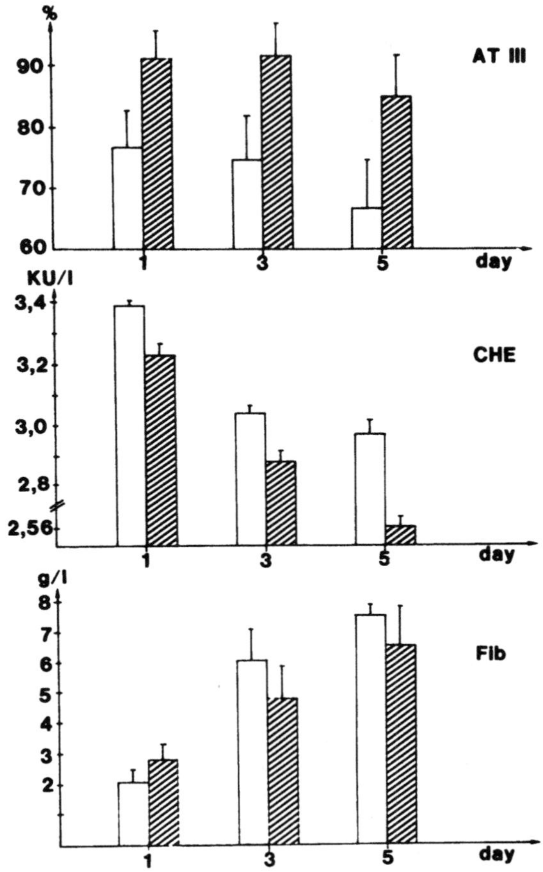

Fig. 4. Parameters representing the liver synthesis capacity in the posttraumatic course (CHE, AT III, fibrinogen)

Discussion

Our 2-year prospective study investigated ten patients to document the extent of liver dysfunction in multiple trauma victims. The influence of blunt liver trauma was included in the investigation. The intention was to clarify potential interactions between trauma, posttraumatic liver dysfunction, and onset of sepsis in the initial phase after trauma (1 week). The number of patients was limited since liver scan examination in mechanically ventilated intensive care unit patients is extremely difficult and costly.

The severity of injury was identical in these patients, differing only in the extent of blunt liver trauma. Although the initial treatment was standardized and the patients were all transferred primarily to our hospital, in three cases, delayed recovery from posttraumatic shock was seen. We explained this prolonged period of stabilization in two cases by the extreme decrease in body temperature before resuscitation, in one case by an 8-h rescue time (mining

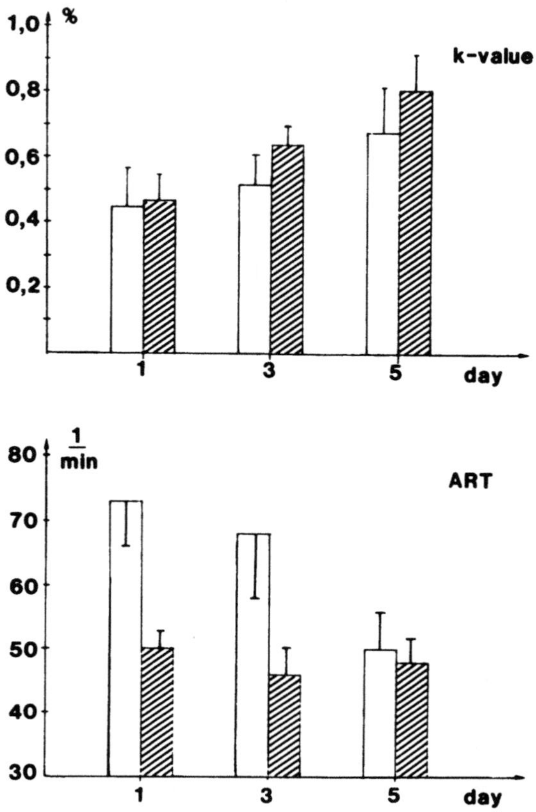

Fig. 5. Arterial liver perfusion and RES clearance measured at three time periods after trauma (1st, 3rd and 5th day) for the group with (+LT) and without (−LT) liver trauma

accident). A significant difference in liver perfusion in these patients compared with the others (without prolonged shock recovery) could not be found.

An increase in intracellular hepatic enzymes was seen exclusively in the +LT group in our study. An elevation of these enzymes in multiple trauma victims with blunt liver trauma has been described previously [1, 3, 6, 7]. Apparently initial perfusion changes lead to a temporary phase of liver ischemia (Fig. 5), which results in destruction of hepatocytes and liberation of intrahepatic enzymes [1, 5, 7]. In this regard especially SGOT seems to be a sensible parameter for assessment of initial anoxia. In our study SGOT shows a similar course to the deteriorated liver perfusion. SGPT and GLDH have delayed peak values (3rd day) with strong variances, depending on the degree of blund liver trauma.

The excretory function of the liver (γ-GT, AP) shows only discrete changes following multiple trauma. Increases in enzyme levels are said to be mostly moderate and irregular in appearance [1, 7]. The elevation of bilirubin seen in our study could not be correlated to a cholestatic component. Possibly it is the result of an increasing hepatic failure depending on the degree of the initial perfusion disturbances. The fraction of conjugated bilirubin was variable [1, 3]. Both higher levels of bilirubin and perfusion changes were seen in the +LT group in our study. Hepatic dysfunction and therefore bilirubinemia may be compounded by other insults, for instance, sepsis [1, 8, 10]. Bilirubin levels then rise as a reaction of both hemolysis and hepatocellular damage [1, 7].

Portal venous blood normally contributes 60%–80% of total hepatic blood flow and probably 70% of the liver oxygen requirements. In traumatic shock, portal venous flow falls to a greater extent than hepatic arterial flow and the liver relies more on the arterial supply for oxygen. This reduces the actual oxygen saturation of the liver and leads to necrosis of the centrilobular cells. Reduced venous flow in the liver (Fig. 5) (increased arterial fraction) could be shown especially in the +LT group in our study. Disturbances in perfusion lead to a higher rate of liver dysfunction in this group (Figs. 3, 4). A correlation, however, between the rate of sufficient liver perfusion and the degree of RES function, as has been postulated by other authors, could not be found in our study [1, 9]. Both the +LT and −LT group show the same pathologic RES clearance immediately after trauma, combined with a significantly different perfusion rate. This means that RES phagocytosis is apparently independent of changes of liver perfusion. Others relate the disturbances of RES function after trauma mainly to the loss of so-called opsonins [4, 8–10]. These are needed to discriminate foreign or destroyed particulate material, which is supposed to be phagocytized by the Kupffer cells of the liver RES. This loss of a sufficient opsonin concentration firstly results from a disturbed synthesis in the liver and secondly also from an increased consumption in the initial phase after trauma [4, 10].

A decrease in RES function which is seen in both groups in our study results in an insufficient clearance of particulate and bacterial matter. Especially endotoxin and other bacterial substances circulate longer in the blood circulation after RES blockade, as we know from experimental studies. This is supposed to lead to a higher susceptibility to sepsis [4, 9, 10], as we demonstrated in our study. A low k-value was combined in all cases with septic complications in the posttraumatic course. These results, however, do not allow conclusions to be drawn on the possible correlation between the development of a posttraumatic RES function and the onset of posttraumatic sepsis.

Conclusions

Liver function deteriorates immediately after multiple trauma. Perfusion is already initially disturbed after trauma and especially in the group with blunt liver injuries. This leads to a prolonged period of inefficient liver oxygen uptake, to necrosis of liver cells, and therefore to the liberation of intracellular hepatic enzymes. The temporary phase of liver ischemia is possibly associated with a higher rate of late liver dysfunction, which we saw especially in the increased bilirubin levels and disturbed synthesis of, for instance, antithrombin III and CHE. We were able to see an initial deterioration of RES clearance which was independent of the rate of perfusion, especially in the group without liver trauma. The disturbances of RES function were paralleled by the incidence of posttraumatic septic complications. These possibly develop in relation to the disturbed RES clearance of endotoxin and other bacterial substances.

Summary

Dysfunction syndromes of lung and kidney following multiple trauma are well known. The pathomechanisms relating disturbances of hepatic blood flow, liver cell integrity, and the function of the RES after trauma, however, have not yet been clarified. In our study liver function showed an immediate deterioration after multiple trauma. Perfusion was disturbed immediately after the insult and especially in the group with blunt liver injuries (+LT). This possibly leads to a prolonged period of inefficient liver oxygen uptake, necrosis of liver cells, and thereby to the liberation of intracellular enzymes, as shown in this study. In addition we were able to see an initial deterioration of the RES clearance, which was independent of the rate of perfusion, especially in the group without liver trauma (−LT). The disturbances of RES function were paralleled by the incidence of posttraumatic septic complications. These possibly develop in relation to the disturbed RES clearance of endotoxin and other bacterial substances.

References

1. Champion HR, Jones RT, Trump BF, et al. (1976) A clinicopathologic hepatic dysfunction following shock. Surg Gynecol Obstet 142:657–663
2. Gratz KF, Schober O, Schwarzrock R (1987) Nuklearmedizinische Untersuchungen in der Transplantatchirurgie. Nuklearmedizin 10:47–59
3. Kaku N (1987) Short-term and long-term changes in hepatic function in 60 patients with blunt liver injury. J Trauma 27:607–609
4. Kaplan JE, Saba TM (1976) Humoral deficiency and reticuloendothelial depression after traumatic shock. Am J Physiol 230:7–14
5. Mela L, Bacalzo LV, Miller LD (1971) Defective oxidative metabolism of rat liver mitochondria in hemorrhagic and endotoxin shock. Am J Physiol 220:571–577
6. Moyer E, Cerra F, Peters D, et al. (1981) Multiple systems organ failure. VI. Death predictors in the trauma-septic state – the most critical determinants. J Trauma 21:862–869
7. Norton L, Moore G, Eisenman R (1975) Liver failure in the postoperative patient: the role of sepsis and immunologic deficiency. Surgery, 78:6–13

8. Nunes G, Blaisdell FW, Margaretten W (1970) Mechanism of hepatic dysfunction following shock and trauma. Arch Surg 100:546–556
9. Rogers DE (1960) Host mechanisms which act to remove bacteria from the blood stream. Bacterial Rev 24:50–66
10. Scovill WA, Saba TM, Kaplan JE, et al. (1976) Deficits in reticuloendothelial humoral control mechanisms in patients after trauma. J Trauma 11:898–904

CD3$^+$, CD4$^+$, CD8$^+$ and B Lymphocyte Numbers in Blood and Bronchoalveolar Lavage Fluid from Trauma Patients with and without ARDS

E. Kreuzfelder[1], M. Maghsudi[2], R. Funk[1], and O. Thraenhart[1]

Introduction

It is generally recognized that trauma-associated changes in the immune response are highly complex and that, therefore, major problems such as the potential causes of injury-induced immune defects and the nature of these defects are unsolved [3]. This holds true especially concerning the description of the immunological situation of trauma patients with the adult respiratory distress syndrome (ARDS) since there is a lack of published results of numbers of T and B lymphocytes in ARDS. Therefore, we undertook a prospective study to evaluate the role of the immune system in the development of ARDS in trauma patients, measuring the numbers of CD3$^+$, CD4$^+$, CD8$^+$, and B lymphocytes in blood and bronchoalveolar lavage fluid (BALF).

Methods

Measurements were taken once a day up to 14 days after hospital admission.

Enumeration of Blood Cells

Blood mononuclear cells were isolated using Vetren blood samples (1 ml Vetren 200 + 19 ml blood) layered over Ficoll-Paque (Pharmacia) (Ficoll-separated cells). After washing, the number of Ficoll-separated cells was adjusted to 7.5×10^6 cells/ml. Of this cell suspension, 20 μl was then

[1] Institute for Medical Virology and Immunology, University Medical School, Hufelandstr. 55, W-4300 Essen 1, FRG
[2] Department of Trauma Surgery, Hannover Medical School, Konstanty-Gutschow-Str. 8, W-3000 Hannover 61, FRG

J.A. Sturm (Ed.)
Adult Respiratory Distress Syndrome

incubated for 60 min at 4°C together with 20 μl of each of the selected monoclonal antibodies. The following monoclonal antibodies were selected for evaluation: OKT3 (CD3, total T lymphocytes), OKT4 (CD4, helper T lymphocytes), and OKT8 (CD8, cytotoxic T lymphocytes). The OKT series of monoclonal antibodies are products of Ortho and were used in a 1:15 dilution. Following the initial incubation period with the primary antibody, the cells were washed and incubated for 60 min with a fluorescein isothiocyanate (FITC) conjugated goat anti-mouse immunoglobulin (Medac) secondary antibody. The labeled cells were analyzed on the Epics C flow cytometer (Coulter Electronics) as described previously [5].

To estimate the number of B lymphocytes, 0.2 ml Ficoll-separated cell suspension was incubated for a 60 min at 4°C together with 0.2 ml FITC-conjugated anti-human immunoglobulin (Behring). The labeled cells were examined using a Zeiss fluorescence microscope as described previously [5].

Enumeration of BALF Cells

Cells contained in about 7 ml BALF were collected by centrifugation and dispersed in 0.5 ml phosphate-buffered saline. A quantity of 0.2 ml suspension was used to determine the B lymphocyte number whereas the residual volume was divided into three aliquots with about 0.1 ml volume to estimate T lymphocyte numbers. B and T lymphocyte numbers were determined using the above-mentioned procedures and the microscopic technique. Since the number of lymphocytes was generally low, we did not estimate every lymphocyte type in every BALF sample.

Statistics

To ascertain differences between the ARDS and non-ARDS patient groups, Wilcoxon's two-sample tests were performed. If time intervals were analyzed, the median over time of each individual patient was calculated at first, and then distributions of medians in both groups were compared. Level of significance was set at alpha = 0.05 (two-tailed test).

Results

Relative numbers of peripheral blood CD4$^+$ cells were significantly increased in the ARDS patient group compared with the results of the other patients immediately after hospital admission and during the following 48 h (Table 1, Fig. 1). Whereas numbers of CD4$^+$ cells of the non-ARDs group were unchanged over time, numbers of these lymphocytes from the ARDS patient

Table 1. B and T lymphocytes (antigens: CD3, CD4, CD8) in peripheral blood and BALF of trauma patients with and without ARDS during a 14-day time course after hospital admission

Time after admission	Cell population	Blood					Bronchoalveolar lavage fluid				
		+ARDS		−ARDS		*p* value	+ARDS		−ARDS		*p* value
0 h	B (%)	8	(3)	8	(6)	NS	ND		ND		ND
	$CD3^+$ (%)	61	(3)	45	(6)	NS	ND		ND		ND
	$CD4^+$ (%)	38	(4)	30	(6)	0.0243	ND		ND		ND
	$CD8^+$ (%)	26	(4)	11	(6)	0.0528	ND		ND		ND
	$CD4^+/CD8^+$	1.6	(4)	1.6	(6)	NS	ND		ND		ND
0–48 h	B (%)	10	(8)	12	(12)	NS	11	(4)	0	(6)	NS
	(cells/μl)	91	(3)	139	(5)	NS	ND		ND		ND
	$CD3^+$ (%)	53	(8)	38	(12)	0.0759	16	(4)	18	(7)	NS
	(cells/μl)	566	(3)	381	(5)	NS	ND		ND		ND
	$CD4^+$ (%)	39	(8)	31	(12)	0.0278	18	(4)	13	(6)	NS
	(cells/μl)	418	(3)	276	(5)	NS	ND		ND		ND
	$CD8^+$ (%)	15	(8)	11	(12)	NS	6	(4)	3	(6)	NS
	(cells/μl)	167	(3)	138	(5)	NS	ND		ND		ND
	$CD4^+/CD8^+$	2.6	(8)	2.4	(12)	NS	1.7	(3)	3.8	(3)	NS
4–14 days	B (%)	9	(10)	13	(13)	0.0349	3	(7)	3	(6)	NS
	(cells/μl)	77	(5)	239	(6)	0.0547	ND		ND		ND
	$CD3^+$ (%)	42	(10)	39	(13)	NS	14	(7)	3	(6)	NS
	(cells/μl)	445	(5)	726	(6)	NS	ND		ND		ND
	$CD4^+$ (%)	30	(10)	30	(13)	NS	7	(7)	3	(6)	NS
	(cells/μl)	354	(5)	513	(6)	NS	ND		ND		ND
	$CD8^+$ (%)	7	(10)	10	(13)	NS	2	(6)	0	(6)	NS
	(cells/μl)	111	(5)	172	(6)	NS	ND		ND		ND
	$CD4^+/CD8^+$	4.1	(10)	3.6	(13)	NS	3.0	(3)	1.4	(2)	ND

Figures in the table are medians and numbers of patients (in parenthesis). +ARDS, trauma patients with ARDS; −ARDS, trauma patients without ARDS; ND, not done; NS, not significant ($p > 0.05$); %, percentage of lymphocytes

group declined after the first 2 days and reached the values of the non-ARDS patient group at the end of the study period.

A trend toward increased values in the ARDS patients in comparison to the non-ARDS patient group was also seen in the case of $CD8^+$ lymphocytes immediately after admission and in the case of $CD3^+$ cells up to 48 h after admission (Table 1). In contrast, B lymphocyte numbers were lower in the ARDS patient group compared with the non-ARDS group during the time interval between 4 and 14 days after admission (Table 1). Bronchoalveolar lavage fluid cell numbers in the two groups were not different over the entire period (Table 1).

In comparison to median numbers of T lymphocytes from healthy individuals, all measured values of both patients groups were lower after the 14-days time course. Whereas numbers of $CD3^+$, $CD4^+$, and $CD8^+$ lymphocytes of the ARDS patients decline over time, numbers of these cells from non-ARDS patients were more stable over the entire period (Table 1).

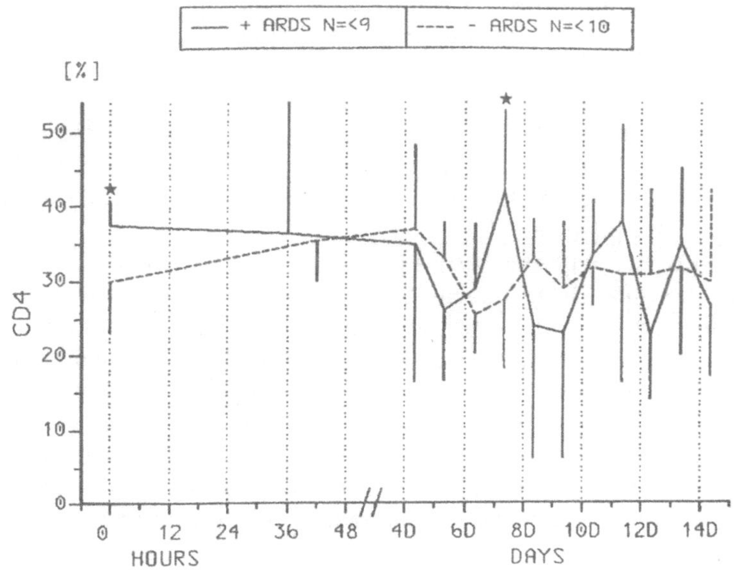

Fig. 1. Blood T lymphocyte (antigen, CD4) numbers in trauma patients with and without ARDS during a 14-day time course after hospital admission. Median values and pseudo standard deviations are shown. +ARDS, trauma patients with ARDS; −ARDS, trauma patients without ARDS; *N*, number of patients; *, significant ($p < 0.05$); %, percentage of lymphocytes

Initial values of $CD3^+$ and $CD4^+$ lymphocytes from the ARDS patients were normal in comparison to healthy individuals and $CD8^+$ cell numbers were even higher. In contrast to T lymphocytes, B lymphocyte numbers of the non-ARDS group increased up to 14 days after admission, whereas ARDS patient group values were unchanged (Table 1) but lower than normal values.

Discussion

In principle our results are in agreement with the published findings concerning the numbers of peripheral blood T lymphocytes following trauma: numbers of circulating $CD3^+$ and $CD4^+$ lymphocytes decline [4]. Astonishingly, median values of these T lymphocytes of the non-ARDS patients were low immediately after hospital admission and remain low in contrary to ARDS group medians, which were initially comparable to normal values [5] and declined over time. Furthermore, numbers of $CD8^+$ cells from the ARDS patients were higher than normal values immediately after admission and declined afterwards.

Although the functional significance of the relative normal immunological situation of the ARDS patients with regard to T lymphocyte numbers up to 2 days after hospital admission is unclear, we may speculate that this is related to the increased activation of other immunological systems, for instance, neutrophils and complement cascade from the ARDS patients. Since numbers of $CD4^+$ lymphocytes were increased immediately after hospital admission in blood of ARDS patients, measurement of these cells may provide a "... biochemical marker in either the blood or urine, which can herald the onset of ARDS with a reasonable degree of specificity and sensitivity" as Petty [6] wrote.

In contrast to the published results [4], B lymphocyte numbers increased over time in the non-ARDS patient group, whereas ARDS patient group values were unchanged over time. The decreased number of B lymphocytes from ARDS patients seems to have no serious functional consequences since serum immunoglobulin levels were not different between both patient groups over the entire period (see Maghsudi et al. this volume).

Since at the end of the entire period all measured cell numbers (with the exception of B lymphocyte numbers of non-ARDS patients) were low in comparison to healthy individuals, immunodeficiency seems to be the consequence of injury.

The only conclusion we may draw from the values of lymphocyte numbers estimated in BALF is that B and T lymphocyte numbers were low in both patient groups in comparison to normal values [1, 2].

Conclusion

Peripheral blood lymphocytes show an increase in $CD4^+$ cells up to 48 h after admission of trauma patients with ARDS in comparison to those trauma patients without ARDS. Since other immunological systems show signs of activation during the same period, we may speculate that this increased $CD4^+$ cell number also reflects activation and may be used as an early indicator for the development of ARDS. During the period between 4 and 14 days after hospital admission, all measured lymphocyte numbers (with the exception of B lymphocyte numbers of the non-ARDS patients) were low in comparison to healthy individuals, indicating a general state of immunodeficiency following trauma.

References

1. Crystal RG, Gadek JE, Ferrans VJ, Fulmer JD, Line BR, Hunninghake GW (1981) Interstitial lung disease: current concepts of pathogenesis, staging and therapy. Am J Med 70:542
2. Ginns LC, Goldenheim PD, Burton RC, Colvin RB, Miller LG, Goldstein G, Hurwitz C, Kazemi H (1982) T-lymphocyte subsets in peripheral blood and lung lavage in

idiopathic pulmonary fibrosis and sarcoidosis analysis by monoclonal antibodies and flow cytometry. Clin Immunol Immunopathol 25:11
3. Green DR, Faist E (1988) Trauma and the immune response. Immunol Today 9:253
4. Grob PJ, Holch M, Brunner W (1987) Posttraumatisches/postoperatives Immundefekt-syndrome, Schweiz Med Wochenschr 117:471
5. Kreuzfelder E, Shen G, Rodeck U, König E, Luboldt W, Keinecke HO, Brockmeyer N, Scheiermann N (1987) Relative and absolute numbers of human lymphocyte subpopulations. J Immunol Methods 97:251
6. Petty TL (1988) ARDS: refinement of concept and redefinition. Am Rev Respir Dis 138:724

IV Activation of Inflammatory Cells

Role of Leukotrienes in the Pathophysiology of ARDS After Polytrauma*

J. Knöller, W. Schönfeld, and W. König

Introduction

Adult respiratory distress syndrome is a severe complication with a high rate of mortality frequently observed in polytraumatized patients after bypass surgery, aspiration, and septicemia [4–6, 18, 19, 21]. Edema formation in the lung interstitium, destruction of the physiological endothelial and epithelial barrier, and inflammatory processes result in an impairment of the lung function. Different alterations in the humoral and cellular immunological systems are described; the complement cascade is activated, and the regular functions of the endothelial cells in the lung are disturbed. Several studies indicate a crucial role of granulocytes in the pathogenesis of lung destruction: The generation of O_2^- radicals and the release of proteases such as elastase could provoke damage of the endothelial layer. The majority of studies performed in humans deal with the clinically evident ARDS; therefore, data about the pathophysiologically relevant period before the onset of the disease process are still lacking. A further still unresolved problem is the relationship of ARDS and septicemia. Although there are often no bacteria detected in blood cultures, clinical signs of sepsis or endotoxinemia are frequently observed in patients with ARDS. Moreover, in the rat model the intravenous injection of endotoxins results in an irreversible lung injury in contrast to infusion with zymosan [17]. The latter activation provokes similar but reversible alterations [16].

The relationship between sepsis and lung complications especially after polytrauma suggests the involvement of inflammatory mediators. In this regard lipoxygenase products of the arachidonic acid cascade apparently are of major importance for the pathophysiology of ARDS [20, 23]. Arachidonic

* This work was supported by the Deutsche Forschungsgemeinschaft – "Grundmechanismen des posttraumatischen progressiven Lungenversagens" (Kö 427/8-3)

Department for Medical Microbiology und Immunology, Working Group for Defense Mechanisms against Infection, Ruhr University Bochum, Universitätsstr. 150, W-4630 Bochum, FRG

J.A. Sturm (Ed.)
Adult Respiratory Distress Syndrome

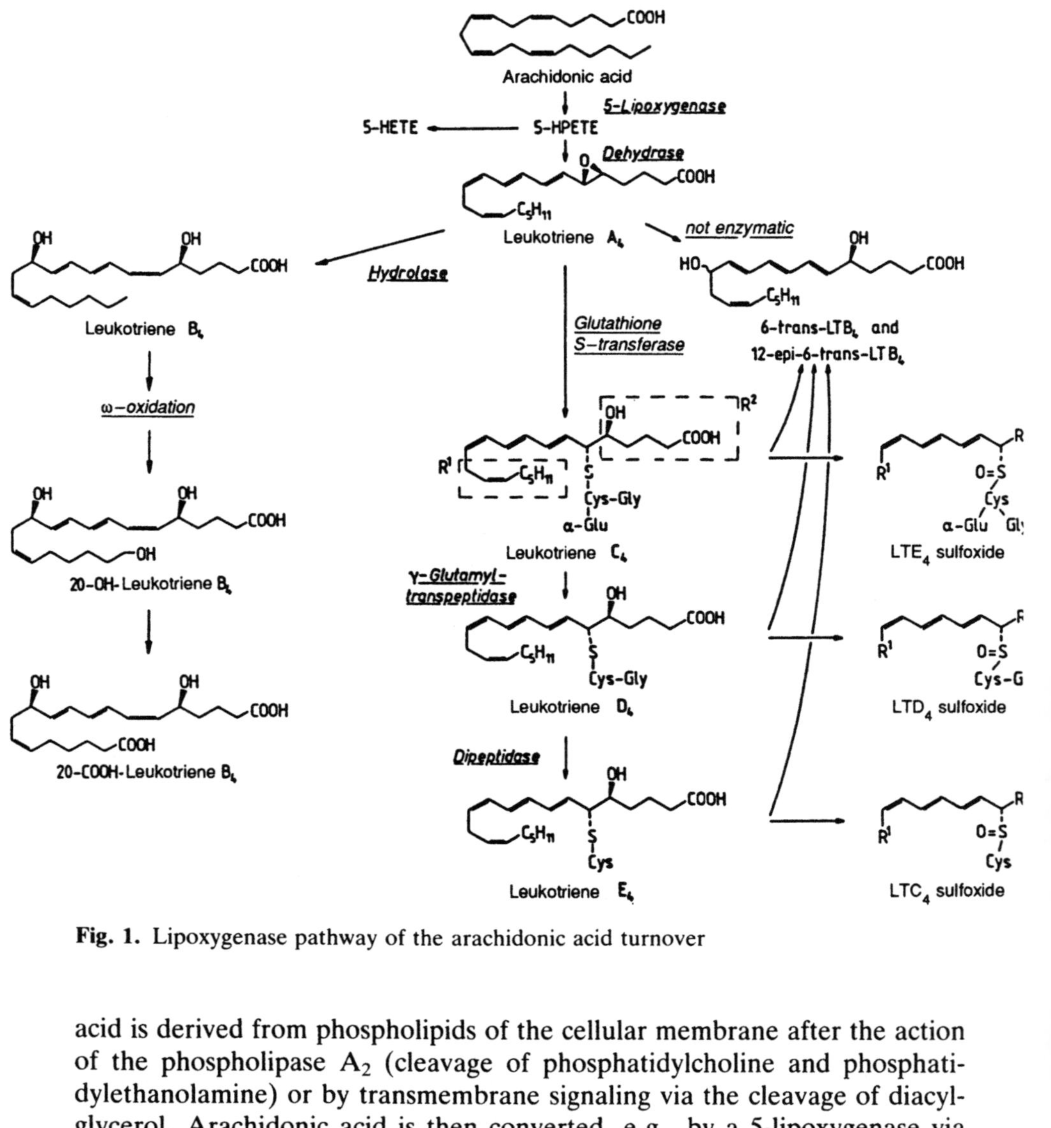

Fig. 1. Lipoxygenase pathway of the arachidonic acid turnover

acid is derived from phospholipids of the cellular membrane after the action of the phospholipase A_2 (cleavage of phosphatidylcholine and phosphatidylethanolamine) or by transmembrane signaling via the cleavage of diacylglycerol. Arachidonic acid is then converted, e.g., by a 5-lipoxygenase via 5-hydroperoxyeicosatetraenoic acid (5-HPETE) into leukotrienes (Fig. 1) or by the complex action of the cyclooxygenase into prostaglandins, thromboxanes, and prostacyclin. Lipoxygenase products – predominantly leukotrienes (LTs) – may contribute to different aspects of the disease process:

1. Leukotriene B_4 (LTB_4) is one of the most potent chemoattractants for granulocytes which acts via specific ligand-receptor activation. The resident lung macrophages have a high capability to generate LTB_4 [12, 13, 25] and may initiate chemotaxis.

2. Leukotriene B_4 is a potent stimulus which may lead to granulocyte sticking and aggregation within the lung capillary as well as to activation and degranulation.
3. Recently, the action of LTB_4 as a mediator involved in the intercellular signalling between lymphocytes and monocytes was thoroughly studied. Farrar and Humes [3] described that the release and action of interleukins-1 and -2 are mimicked by LTB_4. Furthermore, the proliferation of suppressor T cells by LTB_4 may also influence the outcome of inflammatory processes.
4. The vasoconstriction and contraction of endothelial cells caused by cysteinyl leukotrienes may result in the leakage of the arterial wall with edema formation.

Leukotrienes are produced predominantly by granulocytes, macrophages, and mast cells. LTB_4 is metabolized via ω-oxidation into 20-OH-LTB_4 [5(*S*), 12(*R*), 20-hydroxy-6, 14-*cis*-8, 10-*trans*-eicosatetraenoic acid] and 20-COOH-LTB_4 [5(*S*), 12(*R*)-dihydroxy-20-carboxy-6, 14-*cis*-8, 10-*trans*-eicosatetraenoic acid] by granulocytes and into the dihydro-LTB_4 by lung macrophages. Leukotriene C_4 (LTC_4) is converted into leukotriene D_4 (LTE_4) by the enzymatic action of γ-glutamyltranspeptidase and dipeptidases. Generation of leukotrienes is observed in vitro after stimulation with bacterial endo- and exotoxins, bacterial adhesins, and bacteria themselves, by immunological (e.g., anti-IgE, C5a, platelet aggregation factor (PAF)] and nonimmunological stimuli, e.g., the calcium ionophore [1, 10]. It was the purpose of this study to evaluate the role of lipoxygenase products for the pathophysiology of the ARDS. LTC_4 levels were determined in plasma as well as in BALs and the generation of leukotrienes from peripheral granulocytes was monitored.

Materials and Methods

Sample Preparation for Radioimmunoassay

The samples (1 ml plasma or 4 ml BAL) were deproteinized with acetonitrile/methanol (50/50 v/v, 8 ml) and the supernatant lyophylized. The evaporate was suspended in Tris buffer (600 μl, pH 7.0, 0.1% gelatine). The recovery of cysteinyl leukotrienes and LTB_4 by this method was higher than 80%–90% as determined with radioactive-spiked samples. A polyclonal rabbit antiserum specific for LTC_4 was used for the detection of immunoreactive LTC_4 as previously described [22]. The LTC_4 antiserum was used at a dilution of 1:5000, and cross-reactivity against LTD_4, LTE_4, and LTB_4 was less than 10%, 4%, and 1%, respectively. No cross-reaction was obtained with arachidonic acid, prostaglandins, and glutathione. Analysis was performed of 200 μl of the samples in duplicate, and the concentration of LTC_4 was determined by external standardization with synthetic leukotrienes (a generous gift from Dr. Rokach, Merck, Frosst, Canada).

Stimulation of Granulocytes

Peripheral granulocytes were isolated according to the method of Boyum as described previously [22]. In brief, heparinized blood (20 ml) was separated by Ficoll-metrizoate gradient centrifugation followed by dextran sedimentation to eliminate erythrocytes. The granulocyte-containing fraction was washed twice with phosphate-buffered saline (PBS) buffer. The granulocytes (1×10^7) were incubated with the calcium ionophore A23187 (Sigma, Munich, FRG) at a concentration of 7.3 μM for 5 min and 20 min at 37°C. In addition, experiments were carried out using arachidonic acid and opsonized zymosan as stimuli. After incubation the cells were immediately spun down (10000 *g*, 1 min) and the supernatant deproteinized in 2 ml acetonitrile/methanol (50/50 v/v). The samples were stored at −70°C for 24 h and centrifuged (1200 *g*, 10 min, 4°C). The supernatant was evaporated to dryness and resolved in 600 µl methanol/water (30/70, v/v).

High-Performance Liquid Chromatography Analysis

Leukotriene analysis in the cell supernatants was performed by high-performance liquid chromatography (HPLC) as described elsewhere [7]. The technical equipment was purchased from Milton Roy (Constametric III, LCD Milton Roy, Hasselroth, FRG). HPLC processing, peak area integration, and determination of retention time were performed with the Nelson Analytical Chromatography System 2600 (Nelson Analytical, Mannheim, FRG). A two-step gradient system was used at 40°C; a mixture of acetonitrile/methanol-/water (30/20/50 v/v) served as solvent A to which 2.5 g KH_2PO_4 and 0.4 g ethylenediaminetetracetic acid (EDTA)/l water was added. The pH was adjusted to 5.0 with H_3PO_4. Solvent A separated the following lipoxygenase products within 35 min with an α-factor of >1.1:20-COOH-LTB_4, 20-OH-LTB_4, LTC_4, LTD_4, LTE_4, 6-*trans*-LTB_4 [5(*S*), 12(*R*)-dihydroxy-6,8,10(all *trans*)-14-*cis*-eicosatetraenoic acid], 12-epi-6-*trans*LTB_4 [5(*S*),12(*S*)-dihydroxy-6,8,10(all *trans*)-14-*cis*-eicosatetraenoic acid], LTB_4, 5*S*-12*S*-di-HETE [5(*S*),12(*S*)-dihydroxy-6-*cis*-8-*trans*-10-*trans*-14-*cis*-eicosatetraenoic acid]. After 35 min a solvent switch was performed to solvent B (acetonitrile/methanol/water 50/30/20 v/v, pH 5.0, 0.2 g EDTA and 1 g KH_2PO_4/l water) to elute the 5-HETE, 12-HETE, and 15-HETE from the column. The wavelength was set at 280 nm (leukotrienes) and 235 nm (HETEs). The detection limit ranged from 0.2 to 0.5 ng. The substances were identified by external standardization of synthetic substances (generous gift from Dr. Rokach, Merck Frosst, Canada).

Statistics

Statistical significance was determined by Student's *t* text for independent means.

Results

Plasma Levels

Figure 2 shows the median values for LTC_4 levels measured in plasma of both patient groups, which were evaluated together (Fig. 2) and separately for the Hannover (Fig. 3, upper panel) and Essen (Fig. 3, lower panel) centers. A comparison of the patients from Essen with or without respiratory failure yielded no difference between the two patient groups. Within the group 1 of patients from Hannover (patients without respiratory failure) LTC_4 levels were about 2 ng/ml plasma. In contrast high levels of extravascular lung water correlated with a significant increase in LTC_4 up to 5 ng/ml in group 2. The clinical symptoms within this group became evident on days 3–4 after trauma.

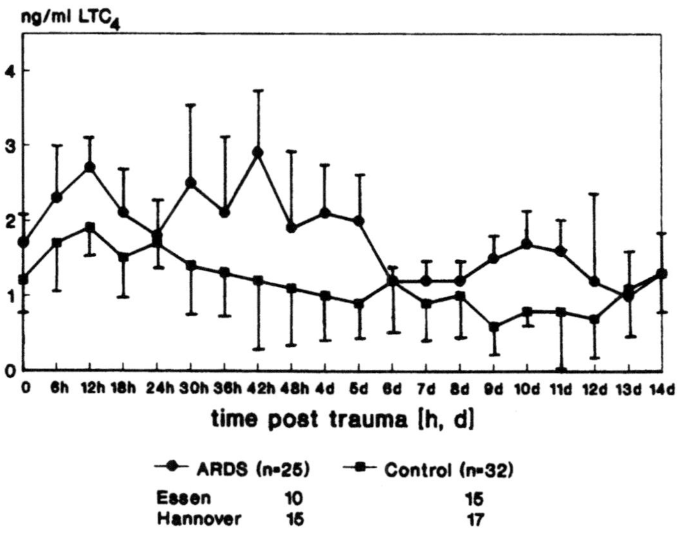

Fig. 2. Leukotriene C_4 levels (median values ± SEM) in plasma as determined by radioimmunoassay (RIA)

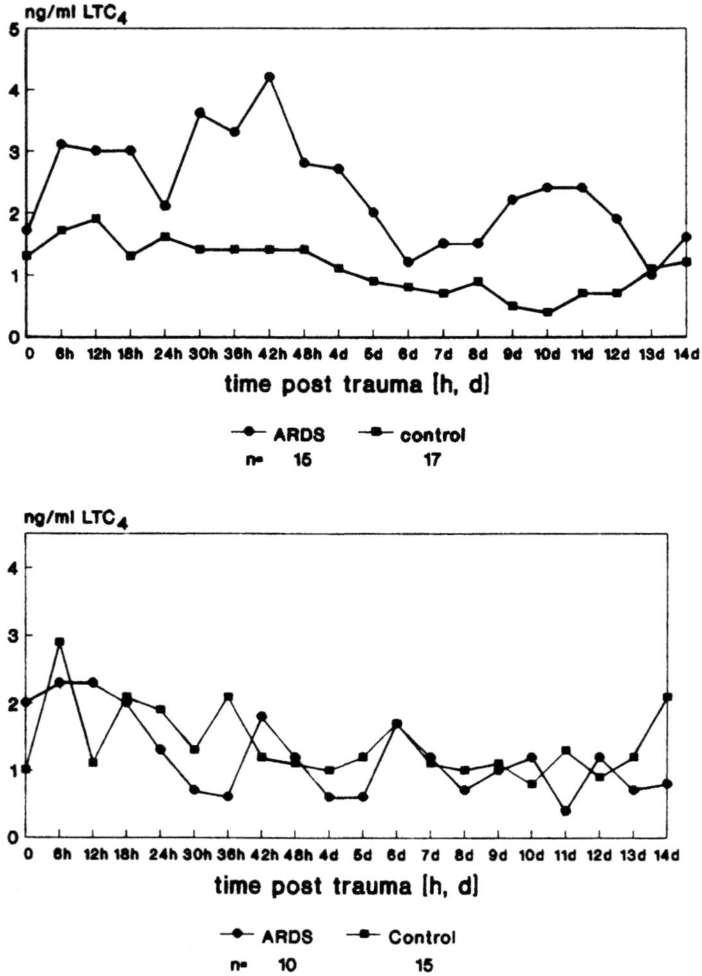

Fig. 3. Leukotriene C_4 levels (median values) in plasma of the patients from Hannover (*upper panel*) and Essen (*lower panel*)

Bronchoalveolar Lavages

The involvement of cysteinyl leukotrienes in the pathophysiology of ARDS in clearly suggested by the BAL data. The lavages were performed on subjects in four different groups: (1) 10 healthy volunteers with no history of allergic diseases or lung dysfunction, (2) polytraumatized patients ($n = 15$) with no lung complication who did not enter the study because they did not meet the criteria, (3) polytraumatized patients of the study without ARDS (control group), and (4) polytraumatized patients with ARDS ($n = 11$). Repeated lavage of the bronchoalveolar space did not lead to an impairment of lung

Table 1. Detection of cysteinyl leukotrienes in the BAL fluid (Essen)

Patient	Eosinophils	ARDS *N*	Positive	Patient	Eosinophils	Control *N*	Positive
401	ND	3	3	402	ND	1	–
404	ND	3	3	403	ND	5	–
406	ND	3	–	405	ND	–	–
410	ND	4	4	407	ND	–	–
414	++	17	3	408	ND	3	–
418	++	23	9	409	ND	3	–
422	+++	21	4	412	ND	6	–
425	+	25	6	416	+	10	6
428	+	17	5	419	–	12	–
431	+	15	9	420	++	12	–
432	+++	13	7	423	–	20	–
				424	–	10	–
				427	+	21	–
				429	–	15	5
				430	–	–	–

			Total		
ARDS	144	58	Control	126	11
positive	40%			9%	

N, number of lavages; *Positive*, number of lavages in which LTC_4 levels rose above the detection limit of the radioimmunoassay; *ND*, not determined

function as determined by continuous control of the pO_2 and pCO_2 either in the ARDS group or in the control group. Neither in polytraumatized patients without ARDS nor in the BAL of healthy volunteers were LTC_4, and LTE_4 detected by radioimmunoassay as well as HPLC analysis.

In the ARDS group, however, 41% of all lavages (58 out of 144, $n = 11$) showed formation of the cysteinyl leukotrienes (Table 1). The levels of LTC_4 ranged from 0.2 to 6 ng/ml. The data were combined and divided into four periods (Fig. 4), which cover the initial posttraumatic phase without symptoms of ARDS, the onset of clinical signs of ARDS which lasts from 48 h posttrauma up to day 4, and the period after the 4th day. LTC_4 was detected even within the first 48 h posttrauma.

Generation and Metabolism of Leukotrienes by Granulocytes

The elevated levels of cysteinyl leukotrienes in plasma and BAL fluid during ARDS raises the question of the origin of leukotrienes. We therefore analyzed the capacity of the peripheral granulocytes to synthesize cysteinyl leukotrienes as well as LTB_4. In nine patients these cells were isolated repeatedly after trauma and the generation of lipoxygenase products was analyzed by HPLC. These data were compared with the generation and metabolism of lipoxygenase products from peripheral cells of healthy

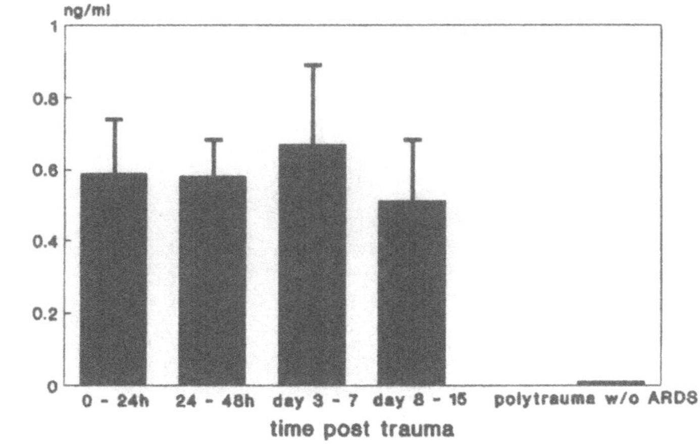

Fig. 4. Levels of cysteinyl leukotrienes in the BAL. Columns represent mean values ± SD (ng/ml lavage fluid) of the lavages in which the amount of LTC_4 rose above the detection limit of the RIA (50 pg LTC_4)

volunteers ($n = 8$). As is seen from Fig. 5, the predominant production of LTB_4 is observed after calcium ionophore stimulation. Substantial amounts of the nonenzymatic products of the LTA_4-6-*trans* isomers, i.e., 6-*trans* and 12-epi-6-*trans* isomers, and a further lipoxygenase product, the 5*S*-12-*S*-di-HETE are additionally generated. The 5- and 12-HETE are detected in

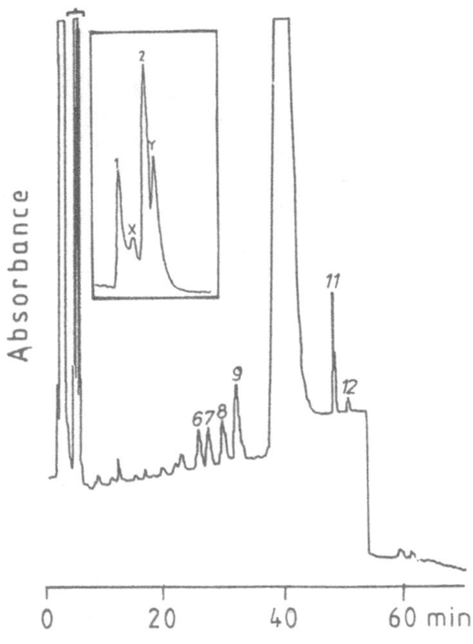

Fig. 5. High-performance liquid chromatography analysis of a cell supernatant (PMNs, 1×10^7) from a polytraumatized patient stimulated with the calcium ionophore for 20 min: 6-*trans*-LTB_4 (*6*), 12-epi-6-*trans*-LTB_4 (*7*), LTB_4 (*8*), 5*S*, 12*S*-di-HETE (*9*), 12-HETE (*11*), 5-HETE (*12*). Attenuation settings of the UV photometers were 0.005 absorbance units full scale at 280 and 235 nm. *Insert*, extended ω-oxidation region of Fig. 5 (*marked by brace*): 20-COOH-LTB_4 (*1*), 20-OH-LTB_4 (*2*)

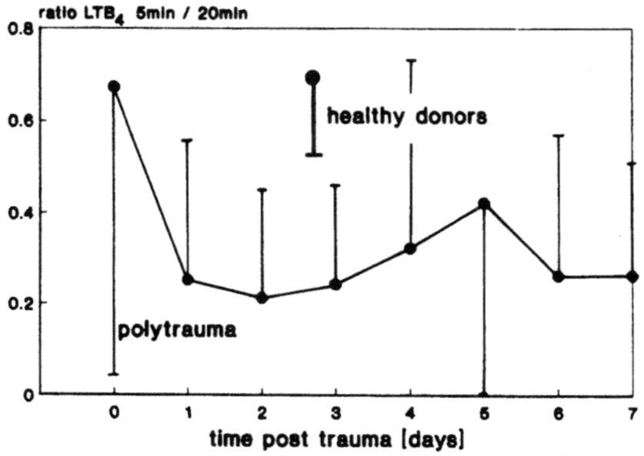

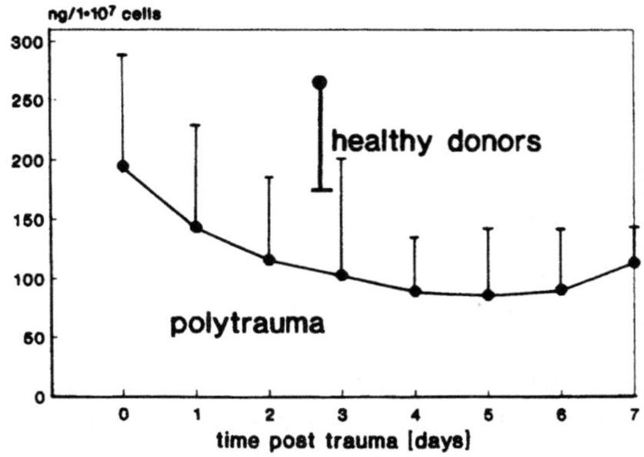

Fig. 6. *Upper*, ratio of LTB_4 levels in the supernatants of stimulated granulocytes (1×10^7) after 5 min versus 20 min of stimulation with the calcium ionophore (healthy donors $n = 8$, polytraumatized patients $n = 8$; mean ± SD). *Lower*, combined amounts of LTB_4 and its ω-oxidized metabolities after stimulation with the calcium ionophore (5 min, 37°C); mean ± SD of nine polytraumatized patients and of eight healthy donors

quantities of about 100 ng/1 × 10^7 cells. Parallel to the synthesis of LTB_4, inactivation into 20-OH- and 20-COOH-LTB_4 is observed. The cell subset of the granulocyte fraction in the healthy volunteers consists of more than 99% pure granulocytes, the amount of eosinophils ranging between 0% and 3%.

In contrast to these data an altered generation and metabolization profile of lipoxygenase products is found in polytraumatized patients. Figure 6 shows the combined amounts of LTB_4, 20-OH-, and 20-COOH-LTB_4 in the stimulated cell supernatants of all polytraumatized patients, as well as the ratio of LTB4 after stimulation with the calcium ionophore for 5 and 20 min, respectively. All patients survived the trauma. A rapid decrease in the formation of LTB_4 and its metabolites after stimulation can be observed within 24 h after trauma, which slowly turns to normal levels during the subsequent days. Parallel to the decrease of the enzymatically synthesized

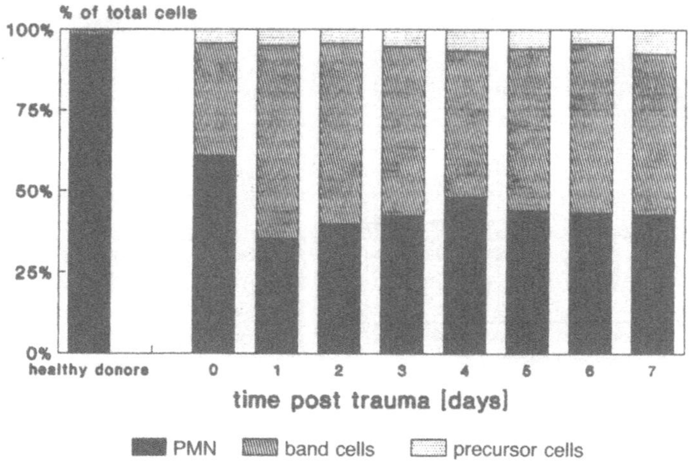

Fig. 7. Distribution of polymorphonuclear granulocytes, band cells, and precursors in the peripheral granulocytes fraction (mean of $n = 8$ healthy donors and $n = 8$ polytraumatized patients)

lipoxygenase products, reduced concentrations of the nonenzymatic isomers 6-*trans* and 12-epi-6-*trans*-LTB_4 are observed. These data indicate a reduced capacity of the granulocyte fraction to synthesize lipoxygenase products and suggest an inhibition beyond the level of the LTA_4, which is the precursor of the leukotrienes. Stimulation experiments in three patients indicated that the availability of free arachidonic acid is decreased. Exogenously added arachidonic acid led to increased production of leukotrienes after stimulation even during the period of poor responsiveness are compared with the levels after stimulation with the calcium ionophore in the absence of exogenous arachidonic acid.

To investigate the relationship between these alterations and differences in the cellular distribution of the granulocyte fraction, we compared the differential blood cell count with leukotriene synthesis and metabolism (Fig. 7). Band cells and myelocytes were predominantly observed in the post-traumatic period. However, there is no correlation between the amount of band cells in the peripheral blood and the differences in the metabolism of arachidonic acid. In addition, the neutropenia and neutrophilia do not correlate with the changes in the lipoxygenase pathway.

In two patients with clinical symptoms of ARDs, the typical atlerations of the LTB_4, generation and metabolism as obtained for the other polytraumatized patients could be observed. In addition, the stimulation of peripheral granulocytes leads to an elevated production of cysteinyl leukotrienes. Figure 8 shows the individual data of two patients. During the clinical symptoms of ARDS an increase in LTC_4 production was obtained. The LTC_4 levels ranged between 30 and 80 ng/1 $\times$ 10^7 cells after 5 min of stimulation. LTC_4 levels up

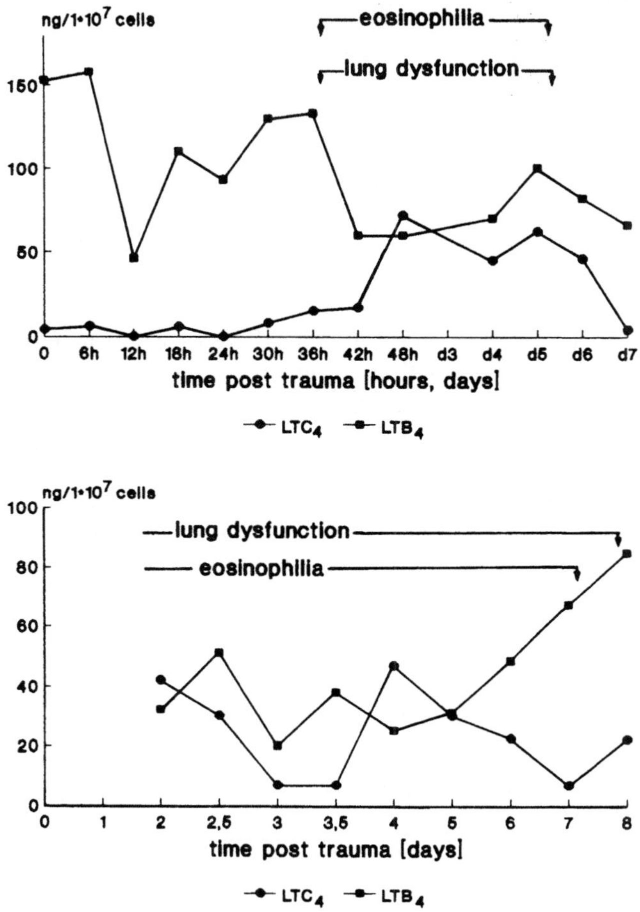

Fig. 8. Leukotriene C_4 and LTB_4 levels in the stimulated cell supernatants (calcium ionophore, 5 min, 37°C) of two polytraumatized patients with ARDS; *eosinophilia*, more than 5% eosinophils in the granulocyte fraction; *lung dysfunction*, period of respiratory distress

to 325 ng/1 × 10^7 granulocytes were detected after a stimulation period of 20 min (data not shown). A comparable profile for LTC_4 production was obtained in a severely burned patient suffering from ARDS (LTC_4 levels up to 180 ng/1 × 10^7 granulocytes, data not shown). These amounts are significantly elevated compared with polytraumatized patients without ARDS (levels between 5 and 10 ng/1 × 10^7 cells). In parallel, LTC_4 levels in the ARDS patients decreased with the improvements in clinical signs. When the cellular distribution of the peripheral granulocyte fraction was analyzed in the three patients, evidence was provided for an involvement of eosinophils in ARDS. All three patients showed eosinophilia (up to 18%) during the period of elevated production of LTC_4.

Discussion

In recent years the involvement of low molecular weight mediators such as leukotrienes in the process of different inflammatory processes has been established. Especially the pathophysiology of different lung disorders is obviously influenced or even provoked by these mediators. Our data clearly suggest an involvement of lipoxygenase products in the pathophysiology of ARDS. In this study, ARDS is defined predominantly as an elevation of the extravascular lung fluid. This elevation is caused by a general disturbance of the permeability in the endothelial barrier of the lung. This mechanism allows the extravasation of protein-rich lung fluid which is commonly supposed to cause the impaired ventilation and gas exchange between the alveolus and the capillary system of the lung. Parallel studies by Kreuzfelder et al. [11] performed on the same patients showed that the mechanisms of edema formation are not only localized in the lung but also in the kidney. These data argue for a combined effect of different mediators and cells on the endothelial wall of the blood vessels. The question arises whether edema formation can be related to production of biologically active substances. in this regard cysteinyl leukoctrienes are involved in edema formation as shown in the in vitro experiments.

Two aspects of the involvement of leukotrienes with regard to the pathophysiology of ARDS have been studied: concentrations of LTC_4 within plasma and BAL were determined by a specific radioimmunoassay; furthermore, stimulation experiments were carried out to elucidate the origin of the leukotrienes produced.

Elevated concentrations of LTC_4 were detected in the with plasma of ARDS patients of only one center (Hannover), whereas the ARDS patients of the second center (Essen) showed no differences compared with the control group.

In the BAL significant differences between both patients groups (ARDS versus control) were established. Recently, Stephenson et al. [26] confirmed these results; they reported elevated levels of LTC_4 in the BAL of ARDS patients as first reported by Matthay et al. [15]. No leukotrienes were detected in healthy volunteers as well as in the lavages of polytraumatized patients without ARDS.

The rapid elevation of LTC_4, levels in our study above the detection limit within hours posttrauma suggests that cysteinyl leukotrienes are involved in the early events of endothelial leakage. However, elevated levels of cysteinyl leukotrienes in the BAL are not specific for ARDS; these mediators were also detected in asthma and cystic fibrosis with no signs of damage of the capillary/endothelial barrier. Our stimulation experiments indicated that the alterations of the lipoxygenase pathway in peripheral granulocytes explain the different effects of elevated LTC_4 levels in ARDS compared with allergic disorders.

Several cascades of the humoral and cellular immune system are activated by polytrauma such as the complement system, blood-clotting system, and fibrinolytic processes; furthermore thrombopenia, neutrophilia, and neutropenia are observed. Our studies indicate that neutrophil granulocytes are altered as to their capacity to generate a chemotactic potential: the synthesis of LTB_4 is decreased and the inactivation process (ω-oxidation) of LTB_4 is increased. These phenomena are comparable to the findings in severely burned patients suffering from post burn wound sepsis [2, 8, 9]. In polytraumatized patients the alterations are observed within the first 48 h posttrauma in contrast to burned patients, in whom sepsis was commonly evident during the 2nd week post-burn [9]. These data provide evidence for a common mechanism of neutrophil dysfunction in polytrauma and post burn sepsis. It is known that sepsis or septic conditions are associated with polytrauma, e.g., blunt trauma may reduce the normal blood supply of the gut. This leads to an impaired intestinal function; bacteria and bacterial toxins may cross the natural barrier and enter the systemic blood system. Bacteria, endo-, and exotoxins are able to induce leukotriene synthesis from granulocytes; furthermore, preincubation of cells from healthy donors with these stimuli leads to an impaired generation of LTB_4 and an increased ω-oxidation in vitro when the cells were subsequently challenged with the calcium ionophore [1]. These in vitro studies correlate with the in vivo findings of severly burned and polytraumatized patients.

Despite the evidence of the influence of sepsis and septic conditions on the function of neutrophils, their involvement in the pathophysiology of ARDS has to be questioned: A correlation between granulocyte dysfunction and their appearance in the BAL is described in ARDS. In addition several animal models of acute lung injury indicate the crucial role of neutrophil granulocytes in this disease. However, animal models differ from the (human) ARDS disease process with regard to the period and underlying mechanisms of the acute lung injury. In addition, our own data obviously support the hypothesis that neutrophil granulocytes are only unspecifically altered and involved in the disease process: In the BAL of polytraumatized patients without ARDS, granulocytes are also present in the ARDS group. Moreover, the alterations of the lipoxygenase pathway in neutrophil granulocytes are comparable in the polytraumatized patients with and without ARDs. Finally, the elevated levels of LTC_4 in the BAL and its increased production from the peripheral cells of the ARDS patients cannot be explained solely by the influx of neutrophil granulocytes. The produce predominantly LTB_4 rather than LTC_4.

Different cell sources may contribute to the formation of LTC_4. Mast cells of the lung as well as macrophages are able to synthesize LTC_4. However, our own data indicate that only minute amounts of LTC_4 are generated by lung macrophages which preferentially produce LTB_4 [25]. The interaction between granulocytes which release LTA_4 and platelets which are able to convert the granulocyte-derived LTA_4 into LTC_4 may occur [14]. The appearance of platelets in the bronchoalveolar space, however, is only possible in profound leakages of the endothelial/epithelial barrier. An interaction of endothelial cells and granulocytes must also be considered which by the same mechanisms may contribute to the generation of LTC_4.

The patients of the ARDS group had significantly elevated levels of eosinophils in the BAL fluid and peripheral blood. These cells produce LTC_4 after stimulation with the calcium ionosphore, zymosan, and complement. The cellular experiments on three patients with ARDS further strengthen the hypothesis that eosinophils are involved in LTC_4 production and in the pathophysiology of the ARDS. Similar findings were also described by Venge et al. [27]. The occurrence of eosinophils is therefore suggestive of a more specific phenomenon in ARDS than the involvement of neutrophil granulocytes. Moreover, these findings associated with ARDS can be clearly distinguished from the results associated with sepsis, in which eosinophilia and LTC_4 production are absent.

Further studies are required to elucidate the interaction of eosinophils, macrophages, and granulocytes in the peripheral blood and in the bronchoalveolar space. In addition, the consequences and causes of the eosinophilia in comparison to other lung disorders such as asthma require investigation.

Summary

In this prospective study we investigated the role of leukotrienes in the pathophysiology of adult respiratory distress syndrome (ARDS) of polytraumatized patients. In patients with (n = 10 out of 11) and without (n = 2 out of 16) ARDS, LTC_4 levels in the bronchoalveolar lavage (BAL) were determined by a specific radioimmunoassay. The clinical symptoms of ARDS correlate with a peripheral and bronchoalveolar eosinophilia. Cysteinyl leukotrienes were detected in 58 out of 144 lavages. The levels ranged between 0.6 and 6 ng/ml. In healthy volunteers (n = 10) and polytraumatized patients (n = 35) leukotriene amounts were below the detection limits. Stimulation of peripheral granulocytes with the calcium ionophore A23187 from polytraumatized patients (n = 9) indicated a reduced capacity to generate a chemotactic potential: The synthesis of LTB_4 was reduced and the ω-oxidation into 20-OH- and 20-COOH-LTB_4 increased within hours after trauma lasting for the whole period of 7 days monitored. These findings are comparable to alterations previously described in severely burned patients with post burn wound sepsis. A similar profile was obtained in four patients with ARDS; in addition, concomitant to the symptoms of ARDS in these patients a significantly elevated production of LTC_4 was observed from peripheral granulocytes.

Our data clearly suggest an involvement of lipoxygenase products in the pathophysiology of ARDS. In the BAL significant differences between both patient groups (ARDS versus control) could be established. No leukotrienes were detected in healthy volunteers. The occurrence of eosinophils of concomitant with a release of LTC_4 is suggestive of a more specific phenomenon in ARDS than the involvement of neutrophil granulocytes.

Our data provide evidence that cysteinyl leukotrienes derived predominantly from eosinophils are involved in the pathophysiology of ARDS, whereas the alterations of the lipoxygenase pathway in neutrophil granulocytes are more specific for the underlying septic conditions in polytraumatized patients.

References

1. Bremm KD, König W, Thelestam M, Alouf JE (1987) Modulation of granulocyte functions by bacterial exo- and endotoxins. Immunology 62:363
2. Brom J, Köller M, Schönfeld W, Knöller J, Erbs G, Miller FE, König W (1988) Decreased expression of leukotriene B_4 receptor sites on polymorphonuclear granulocytes of severely burned patients. Prostaglandins Leukotrienes Essential Fatty Acids 34:153
3. Farrar WL, Humes JL (1985) The role of arachidonic acid metabolism in the activities of interleukin 1 and 2. J Immunol 135:1153
4. Fowler AA, Hamman RF, Zerbe GO, Benson KN, Hyers TM (1985) Adult respiratory distress syndrome – prognosis after onset. Am Rev Respir Dis 132:472
5. Hyers TM, Fowler AA (1986) Adult respiratory distress syndrome: causes morbidity and mortality. Fed Proc 45:22
6. Kaplan RL, Sahn SA, Petty TL (1979) Incidence and outcome of the respiratory distress syndrome in gram-negative sepsis. Arch Intern Med 139:867
7. Knöller J, Schönfeld W, Köller M, Henseler T, König W (1988) Arachidonic acid metabolites from polymorphonuclear leukocytes of healthy donors, severely burned patients and cystic fibrosis. J Chromatogr 427:199
8. Köller M, Schönfeld W, Knöller J, Bremm KD, König W, Spur B, Crea A, Peters W (1985) The metabolism of leukotrienes in blood plasma studied by high performance liquid chromatography. Biochim Biophys Acta 833:128
9. Köller M, König W, Brom J, Raulf M, Groß-Weege W, Erbs G, Müller F (1988) Generation of leukotrienes from polymorphonuclear granulocytes of severely burned patients. J Trauma 28:733
10. König W, Bremm KD, Scheffer J, Kritschker B, Schönfeld W, Theobald K (1986) Generation of mediators of inflammation (histamine, leukotrienes) from various cells by bacterial products. In: Falmagne P, Alouf JE, Fehrenbach FJ, Jeljaszewicz J, Thelestam M (eds) Bacterial protein toxins. Fischer, Stuttgart, p. 131
11. Kreuzfelder E, Joka T, Keinike H-O, Obertacke U, Schmit-Neuerburg K-P, Nakosteen JA, Scheiermann N (1987) Adult respiratory distress syndrome as a specific manifestation of a general permeability defect in trauma patients. Am Rev Respir Dis 136:288
12. Laviolette M, Coulombe R, Picard S, Braquet P, Borgeat P (1986) Decreased leukotriene B_4 synthesis in smokers' alveolar macrophages in vitro. J Clin Invest. 77:54
13. Martin TR, Altman LC, Albert RK, Henderson WR (1984) Leukotriene B_4 production by human alveolar macrophage: a potential mechanism for amplifying inflammation in the lung. Am Rev Respir Dis 129:106
14. Maclouf JA, Murphy RC (1988) Transcellular metabolism of neutrophil-derived leukotriene A_4 by human platelets. A potential source of leukotriene C_4. J Biol Chem 263:174

15. Matthay MA, Eschenbacher WL, Goetzl EJ (1984) Elevated concentrations of leukotriene D_4 in pulmonary edema fluid of patients with the adult respiratory distress syndrome. J Clin Immunol 16:479
16. Meyrick BO (1986) Endotoxin-mediated pulmonary endothelial cell injury. Fed Proc 45:19
17. Meyrick BO, Brigham KL (1984) The effect of a single infusion of zymosan-activated plasma on the pulmonary microcirculation of sheep. Am J Pathol 114:32
18. Montgomery AB, Stager MA, Carrico CJ, Hudson LD (1985) Causes of mortality in patients with the adult respiratory distress syndrome. Am Rev Respir Dis 132:485
19. Murray JF (1977) Mechanisms of acute respiratory failure. Am Rev Respir Dis 115:1071
20. Parker CW (1987) Lipid mediators produced through the lipoxygenase pathway. Annu Rev Immunol 5:63
21. Pepe PE, Potkin RT, Holtman Reus D, Hudson LD, Carrico CJ (1982) Clinical predictors of the adult respiratory distress syndrome. Am J Surg 144:124
22. Raulf M, Stüning M, König W (1986) Metabolism of leukotrienes by L-γ-glutamyltranspeptidase and dipeptidase from human polymorphonuclear granulocytes. Immunology 55:135
23. Salmon JA, Higgs GA (1987) Prostaglandins and leukotrienes as inflammatory mediators. Brit Med Bull 43(2):285
24. Schönfeld W, Knöller J, Brom J, Raulf M, Köller M, Joka T, König W (1987) Altered arachidonic acid metabolism in granulocytes of polytraumatized patients. Prostaglandins Leukotrienes Med 27:227
25. Schönfeld W, Schlüter B, König W (1988) Leukotriene generation and metabolism in isolated human lung macrophages. Immunology 65:529
26. Stephenson AH, Lonigro AJ, Hyers TM, Webster RO, Fowler AA (1988) Am Rev Respir Dis 138:714
27. Venge P, Dahl R, Fredens K, Peterson CGB (1988) Epithelial injury by human eosinophils. Am Rev Respir Dis 138:S54

Specific Proteins of Inflammatory Cells and α_1-Proteinase Inhibitor in Alveolar Epithelial Lining Fluid of Polytraumatized Patients: Do They Indicate Posttraumatic Lung Failure?

M. Jochum[1]
With experimental data from A. Dwenger[2] and W. Machleidt[3]

Introduction

Despite numerous hints that activated inflammatory cells may trigger lung injury, the causative role especially of the polymorphonuclear (PMN) granulocytes (neutrophils) to promote enhanced microvascular permeability in acute respiratory distress syndrome (ARDS) is still a matter of debate [22, 25, 27, 28, 31]. In the early 1980s, Hammerschmidt et al. [11] demonstrated that complement-mediated neutrophil sequestration in pulmonary capillaries leading to lung vascular endothelial injury was a common feature of patients suffering from acute respiratory distress syndrome (ARDS). Meanwhile, however, a wealth of basic information exists indicating that neutrophil activation occurs to a similar extent in high-risk patients who do not, however, eventually develop ARDS [21]. Moreover, signs of ARDS have been described in neutropenic patients, thus calling into question whether neutrophils are required in the generation of ARDS [19]. Yet, the latter observations may be taken as an indirect evidence for the importance of other inflammatory cells, e.g., activated alveolar macrophages [7], in disturbing the alveolar barrier from the epithelial side of the alveoli, at least in neutropenic patients.

Although the primary role of both types of phagocytes (invading neutrophils, sessile lung macrophages) in the development of ARDS still deserves further clarification, the potentially harmful armament of these cells released during cell activation in response to an inflammatory event (e.g., multiple trauma) is beyond doubt. This potent cellular equipment for causing tissue injury in the microenvironment of the phagocytes include elastolytic proteinases (e.g., neutrophil elastase, macrophage-derived cathepsin B) and

[1] Department of Clinical Chemistry and Clinical Biochemistry, Surgical Clinic, City, University of Munich, Nußbaumstr. 20, W-8000 Munich 2, FRG
[2] Department of Clinical Biochemistry, Hannover Medical School, Konstanty-Gutschow-Str. 8, W-3000 Hannover 61, FRG
[3] Institute of Physiological Chemistry, Physical Biochemistry and Cell Biology, University of Munich, Goethestr. 33, W-8000 Munich 2, FRG

J.A. Sturm (Ed.)
Adult Respiratory Distress Syndrome

highly destructive oxygen species [7, 18]. The production of the most effective molecules of the latter – hypochlorous acid, chloramines and hydroxyl radicals – is greatly enhanced during phagocytosis by the catalytic action of the neutrophil lysosomal proteins, myeloperoxidase [18] and lactoferrin [17]. Moreover, extracellularly released lactoferrin is known to increase the adhesiveness of neutrophils to pulmonary endothelial cells, thereby prolonging the destructive action of the phagocytes on the vascular permeability barrier [30].

The harmful efficacy of proteolytic and oxidative substances discharged to the extracellular milieu is normally restricted to and abolished in the close vicinity of phagocytizing cells by numerous proteinase inhibitors [29] and antioxidants [20]. During an overshooting activation process, e.g., caused by a serious trauma event, the local anti-oxidative capacity seems to be overcome, especially in the lung, thereby enabling also the oxidative inactivation of proteinase inhibitors [29]. In this respect α_1-proteinase inhibitor (α_1PI), by far the most effective inhibitor of the neutrophil serine proteinase elastase, is highly sensitive to oxidative destruction [29, 18]. In addition, this inhibitor molecule can easily be degraded by cysteine proteinases (cathepsin B, L) and a metalloproteinase released from activated alveolar macrophages [29]. Just recently, the proteolytic inactivation of α_1PI by a neutrophil metalloproteinase has been also demonstrated [8]. Interestingly, the α_1PI, which is probably degraded proteolytically in the epithelial lining fluid (ELF) of the lung, is inactive against elastase [26, 32], but has proved to be a potent neutrophil chemoattractant [4] and may thus augment the elastase burden of the lung during an inflammatory process.

The increase of the lung's permeability due to the proteolytic/oxidative destruction of the endothelial–epithelial barrier in the early phase of ARDS is characterized by the influx of plasma proteins into the ELF [12]. Whereas this stage of the disease may be reversible, the later fibrotic phase [3] is often associated with a lethal outcome due to an irreversible gas exchange disturbance. As shown recently, activated lung macrophages seem to play an essential role in stimulating fibroblasts to enhanced collagen synthesis via the production of a platelet-derived growth factor-like substance [5]. In addition, the diminished regulatory function of destroyed alveolar epithelial cells also promotes fibroblast activity and, thus, fibrosis [1]. The extracellular occurrence of the procollagen-III-peptide (P-III-P) in the ELF can be taken as a clear indication of such an intensified fibrotic process [6].

Up to now, the evaluation of biochemical changes in the ELF drawn by the broncho-alveolar lavage (BAL) technique [24] has been widely applied to gain more insight into the pathomechanisms taking place during lower respiratory tract inflammation [10, 13, 25, 26, 31, 32]. However, convincing clarification of the significance of the different biochemical factors under discussion as inflammatory mediators has been hampered by the lack of close-meshed follow-up determinations after an event (multiple injuries, septicemia, etc.) which suddenly renders a person a high-risk ARDS patient. Therefore, the aims of our present study were as follows:

- Firstly, to find out whether daily determinations of specific proteins released from inflammatory cells into the ELF of severely injured patients can contribute to elucidate the importance of these cellular products for the development of posttraumatic ARDS.
- Secondly, to examine whether one or more of these biochemical inflammation markers can predict the onset as well as the severity of a posttraumatic ARDS course.

To achieve these aims, three neutrophil lysosomal proteins — elastase, myeloperoxidase, and lactoferrin — as well as the macrophage-derived proteinase cathepsin B, the fibroblast product P-III-P, and the proteinase inhibitor α_1PI were determined in BAL fluid samples drawn daily from multiply injured patients over a generally 14 days posttraumatic observation period.

Methods

Study Population

Multiply injured patients ($n = 27$; Injury Severity Score >40 points) from two surgical centers (17 subjects from Essen, 10 from Hannover) were included in this study with a prospectively fixed observation period of 14 days. The persistent rise of extravascular lung water (EVLW) to above 10 ml/kg body weight about 3–4 days after admission was taken as a reliable sign of an increase in pulmonary microvascular permeability. According to this feature, 12 patients had to be classified as "ARDS" subjects, the other 15 as a "non-ARDS" group [16]. Two of the ARDS patients died within 8 days, and three individuals 12 days post trauma, whereas the three nonsurviving patients in the non-ARDS collective died on the 9th and 12th and after the 14th posttraumatic day, respectively.

In addition, ten healthy subjects served as controls for comparative measurements of the test parameters.

Sampling Procedure

Bronchoalveolar Lavage Fluid (BALF). To obtain ELF from the alveoli, BAL was performed by instilling 100 ml 0.9% saline in 20-ml aliquots via a fiberoptic bronchoscope as described previously [15, 16]. In about half of the traumatized patients, this procedure was carried out daily, whereas due to logistic conditions in the other injured patients, performance of BAL was feasible only every 2nd day up to the patient's death or the end of the 14-day observation period. The healthy individuals were subjected to one BAL each on three successive days [15].

After withdrawal (recovery of more than 60% of the instilled saline), cellular components and fluid phase of the combined lavage suspensions were immediately separated by centrifugation [15, 16]. The unconcentrated BALF (on average containing more than 60-fold diluted ELF) was then kept frozen at −70°C until determination of specific proteins and urea.

Citrated Plasma. At each performance of BAL, venous blood was drawn simultaneously from a central line, processed to citrated plasma and deep-frozen at −70°C until selected plasma components had been assayed.

Protein Determinations

The neutrophil lysosomal proteins elastase (complexed with α_1PI), myeloperoxidase, and lactoferrin in BALF and plasma samples were determined by specific enzyme-linked immunoassays (established in the Biochemical Department of E. Merck, Darmstadt, FRG) as indicated elsewhere [14].

To quantify proteolytically active neutrophil elastase in BALF, one part of each BALF sample was incubated with normal plasma containing enough α_1PI for total elastase inhibition and then reassayed for an increase in the elastase–α_1PI complex. After subtracting the amount of the complex added with the normal plasma and correcting for the dilution effect, a rise of more than 10% in elastase–α_1PI complex over the complex concentration already present in the untreated portion of the same BALF sample was taken as reliable proof for the occurrence of proteolytically active elastase in the alveolar epithelial environment.

The macrophage-derived lysosomal cysteine proteinase cathepsin B was quantified only in pilot measurements as described by Assfalg-Machleidt et al. [2] by estimating the enzyme-catalyzed cleavage of a convenient fluorogenic substrate.

Determination of the fibroblast product P-III-P was carried out with a commercially available radioimmunoassay (RIA-gnost Prokollagen-III-Peptid, Behringwerke, Marburg, FRG).

The immunologically detectable amount of α_1PI was measured using a nephelometric method as described by Dwenger et al. [9].

Urea Measurement and Correction of the Dilution Effect in BALF

Urea concentrations in corresponding BALF and plasma samples were enzymatically determined as described elsewhere [9]. These measurements were performed to correct the concentrations of the protein components quantified in BALF samples to their original amount in the ELF. Since it is suspected that urea diffuses without restriction between the blood/air compartments of the lung, the ratio of the urea concentration between blood and BALF is supposed to indicate the dilution of ELF by saline. According to

Rennard et al. [23] the following calculation was applied to evaluate concentrations (C) of various proteins in ELF:

$$c_{\text{protein in ELF}} = \frac{c_{\text{protein in BALF}} \times c_{\text{urea in plasma}}}{c_{\text{urea in BALF}}}$$

Diagrams

Data are presented as follow-up curves, either for an individual subject or as mean ± SEM for the two study groups (ARDS; non-ARDS) if not otherwise stated.

Statistical analysis was performed using the Mann-Whitney U-test.

Results

BALF Data of Healthy Subjects

BAL repeated daily in healthy subjects triggered a distinct influx of PMN granulocytes (mean number of cells/ml BALF was 5700 in the first lavage and 27600 in the third lavage) to the alveolar space and a significant release of lysosomal proteins, which indicated local neutrophil activation. This was confirmed not only by the increase in extracellular complexed elastase from an average concentration of 0.77 µg/ml ELF (first BAL) (range: 0.37–1.0) up to 4.2 µg/ml ELF (third BAL) (range: 2.2–6.9), but also by the rise in the specific amount of the elastase complex from 4.8 ng up to 10.4 ng/1000 PMN cells. Yet, no proteolytically active elastase could be demonstrated in any of these BALF samples. Remarkably, the concentration of complexed elastase in the ELF of healthy subjects was approximately tenfold that of normal plasma levels (80 ng/ml)

The lysosomal neutrophil proteins, myeloperoxidase and lactoferrin, were discharged in a similar manner, although in a somewhat lower amount in the case of myeloperoxidase (up to 4.2 µg/ml ELF in the third BAL) and a clearly higher amount in the case of lactoferrin (up to 17.2 µg/ml ELF in the third BAL) than elastase. Since the release of such quantities of neutrophil proteins did not entail any pathological pulmonary disturbances (e.g., influx of blood proteins) in the volunteers, an extracellular concentration of 7 µg complexed elastase or myeloperoxidase as well as 20 µg lactoferrin/ml ELF might be suggested as the upper physiologically tolerable limit.

The average immunologically determined concentration of 200 µg/ml ELF of the main elastase inhibitor, α_1PI, corresponds to about 10% of the plasma level. This level did not change during repeated BAL procedures, thus indicating the absence of an increase in pulmonary permeability. Interestingly, this inhibitor amount equals maximally to only about a 140-fold molar excess over the extracellular concentration of the elastase measurable in the ELF under physiological conditions, whereas in the plasma of healthy subjects, it is more than 10000-fold.

With the assay system applied (lower detection limit: 1 ng/ml) no P-III-P could be demonstrated in the BALF samples of the healthy volunteers.

Due to logistic conditions, BALF samples had not been available for the evaluation of normal values of the macrophage proteinase cathepsin B in the ELF.

BALF Data of Traumatized Patients

As shown in Fig. 1, a repeated release of elastase (measured as the total amount of complexed elastase after the addition of inhibitorily active α_1PI) up to more than 60-fold normal values could be seen in all patients during the whole observation period, with a tendency to larger amounts on days 4–6 post trauma. This period was generally associated with the manifestation of the increase in the amount of EVLW in the ARDS group. Surprisingly, however, the neutrophil proteinase was discharged to an even higher, though not statistically different, degree in the non-ARDS patients. The same held

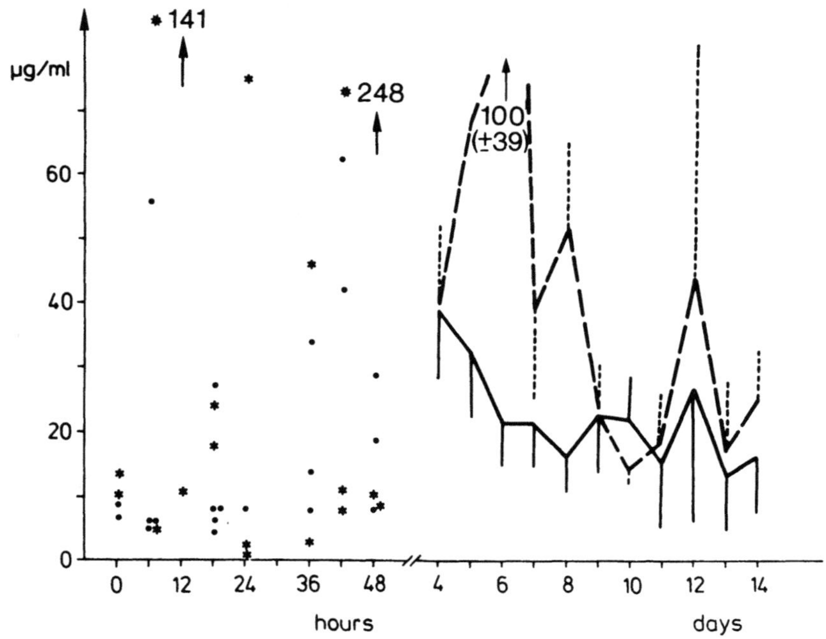

Fig. 1. Posttraumatic course of the overall released neutrophil elastase (E), measured as E–α_1PI complex after the addition of inhibitorily active α_1-proteinase inhibitor (α_1PI) to the alveolar epithelial lining fluids (ELF) of ARDS (*solid line*; *asterisk*; $n \leq 12$) and non-ARDS (*broken line*; *circle*; $n \leq 15$) patients. Data are given as individual measurements in the early, and as mean ± SEM in the later posttraumatic phase

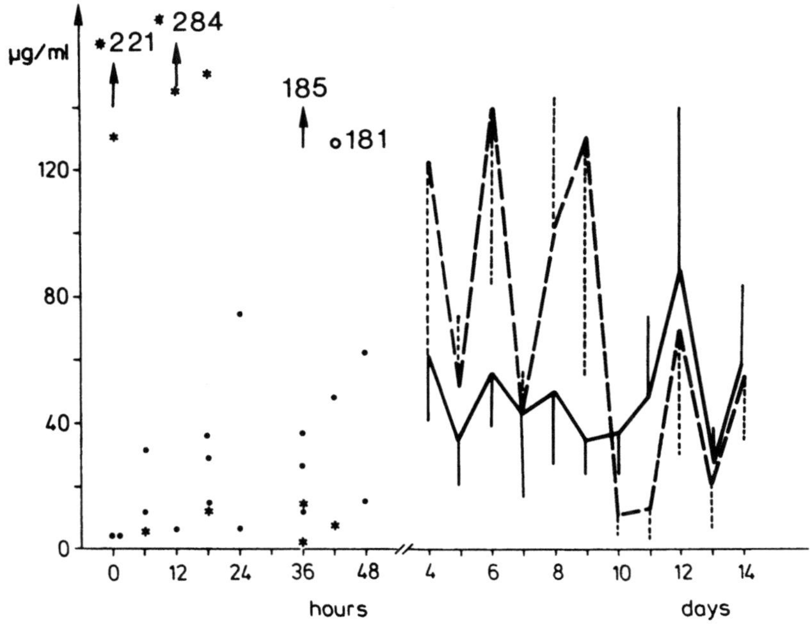

Fig. 2. Posttraumatic course of neutrophil lactoferrin in the alveolar epithelial lining fluids (ELF) of ARDS (*solid line*; *asterisk*; $n \leqslant 7$) and non-ARDS (*broken line*; *circle*; $n \leqslant 10$) patients. Data are given as individual measurements in the early, and as mean ± SEM in the later posttraumatic phase

true for myeloperoxidase (not depicted here) and lactoferrin (Fig. 2). The simultaneous release of all three lysosomal proteins, especially during the manifest elevation of EVLW, is exemplarily shown in Fig. 3. The data are from a patient who finally overcame the ARDS phase.

Sequential mean α_1PI concentrations were distinctly more elevated above normal in the ELF of the ARDS collective (on an average between 600 and 1200 µg/ml) than in the non-ARDS group who generally showed a 1.5- to 3-fold (300–600 µg/ml) increase (Fig. 4). Despite scarce data available for the first 48 h post trauma, α_1PI concentrations well above 300 µg/ml ELF in 6 of 12 ARDS patients and 2 of 15 non-ARDS patients indicate a very early trauma-induced pulmonary capillary permeability leakage which was clearly more pronounced in the ARDS group. This is confirmed by the observation that during the early posttraumatic phase, α_1PI in the ELF of ARDS patients reached concentrations which were already as high as in the later course of the disease. In contrast, the plasma levels of α_1PI were clearly lower at the beginning of the observation period (below 2000 µg/ml) and increased up to fivefold (to approximately 6000 µg/ml) within 6 days after the traumatic event (Fig. 5; in the graphs, the plasma α_1PI levels of traumatized patients not subjected to BAL for clinical reasons are also included). Assuming that with an intact blood/air barrier the influx of α_1PI to the

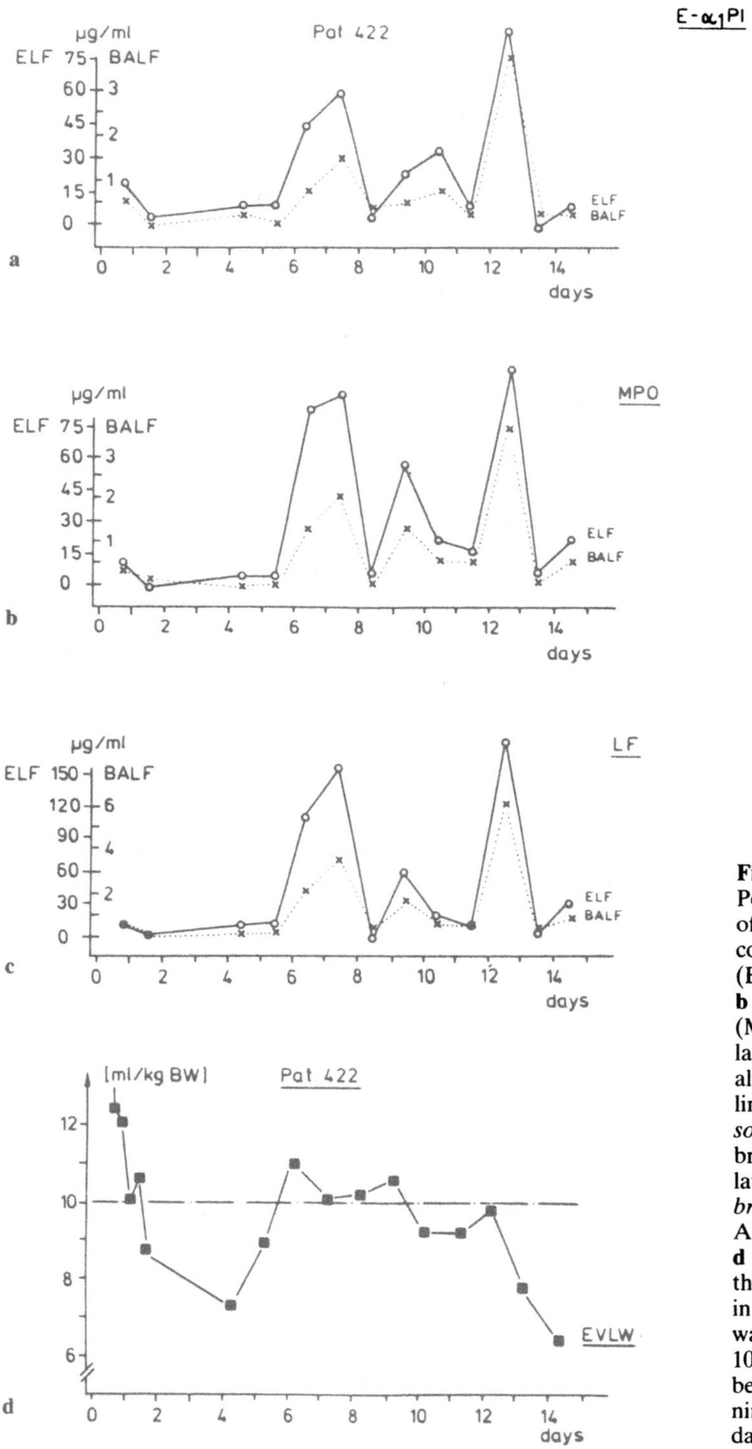

Fig. 3a–d. Posttraumatic courses of neutrophil **a** complexed elastase (E-α_1PI), **b** myeloperoxidase (MPO), and **c** lactoferrin (LF) in the alveolar epithelial lining fluids (ELF; *solid line*) and the bronchoalveolar lavage fluids (BALF; *broken line*) of an ARDS patient. **d** ARDS is indicated by the manifest elevation in extravascular lung water (EVLW) above 10 ml/kg body weight between the fifth and ninth posttraumatic day

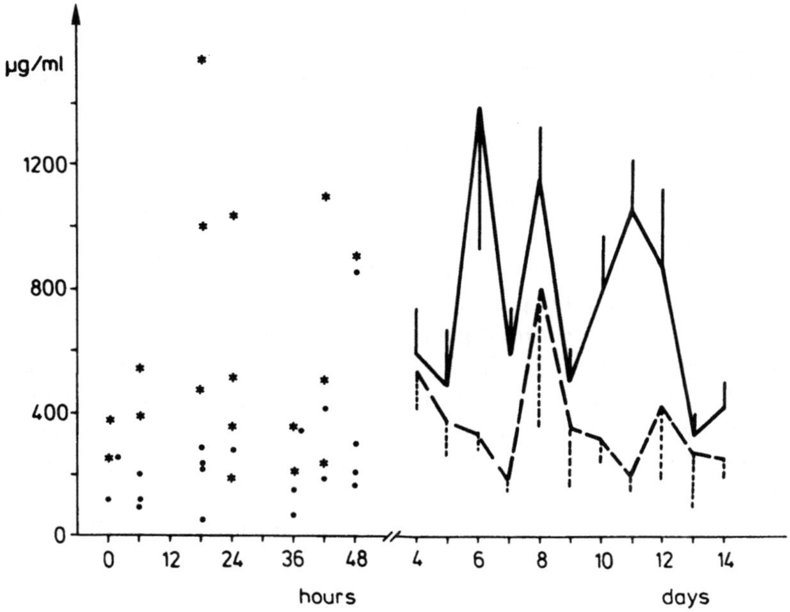

Fig. 4. Posttraumatic course of α_1-proteinase inhibitor (α_1PI) in the alveolar epithelial lining fluids (ELF) of ARDS (*solid line*; *asterisk*; $n \leqslant 12$) and non-ARDS (*broken line*; *circle*; $n \leqslant 15$) patients. Data are given as individual measurements in the early, and as mean ± SEM in the later posttraumatic phase.

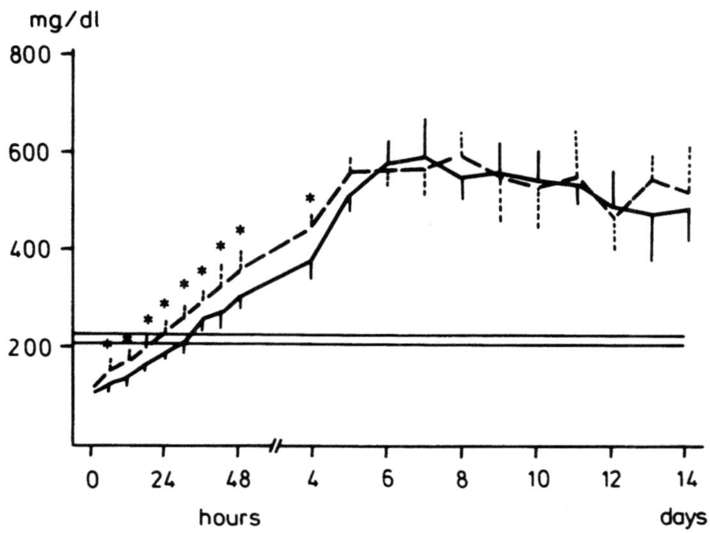

Fig. 5. Posttraumatic course of α_1-proteinase inhibitor (α_1PI) in plasma samples of ARDS (*solid line*; $n \leqslant 26$) and non-ARDS (*broken line*; $n \leqslant 31$) patients. Data (including those of patients not subjected to bronchoalveolar lavage for clinical reasons) are given as mean ± pseudostandard error (PSE). *Asterisks* mark significant differences between the two patient groups ($p < 0.05$)

alveolar epithelial compartment approaches at most 10% of the blood level, an early and/or late pulmonary permeability increase could be seen in 11 of the 12 ARDS patients, whereas such a disturbance could be verified only in 3 of the 15 non-ARDS subjects.

Taking 300 μg α_1PI/ml ELF – if reached within 48 h post trauma – as a threshold level for the prognosis of later ARDS, the following predictive parameters were calculated: 63% for sensivity, 71% for specificity, 80% for the positive predictive value, and 58% for the negative predictive value.

Although the immunologically measurable α_1PI concentration was highly elevated in the ELF of ARDS patients, the molar excess of α_1PI over the total amount of released elastase varied generally in the later posttraumatic phase only between 8.6- to 39.6-fold (Fig. 6) compared with about 140-fold under normal conditions. This reduced ratio does not seem to be enough to inactivate the whole amount of elastase discharged from the stimulated invading neutrophils. As shown in Fig. 7a, up to 30% of the released elastase could be detected as an active enzyme in the ARDS group. Moreover, due to the lower amount of α_1PI in the ELF of non-ARDS subjects and the clearly

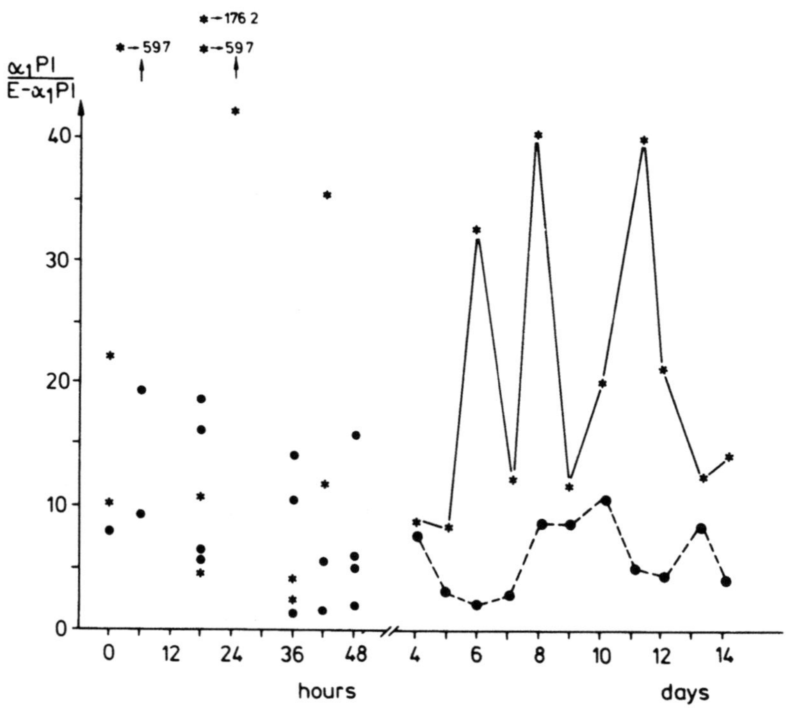

Fig. 6. Posttraumatic course of the calculated molar ratio of α_1-proteinase inhibitor to the overall released neutrophil elastase (see Fig. 1) in alveolar epithelial lining fluids (ELF) of 12 ARDS (*solid line*; *asterisk*) and 15 non-ARDS (*broken line*; *circle*) patients. In the ELF of healthy subjects this ratio is approximately 140-fold. Data are given as individual ratios in the early, and as ratio of mean values in the later posttraumatic phase

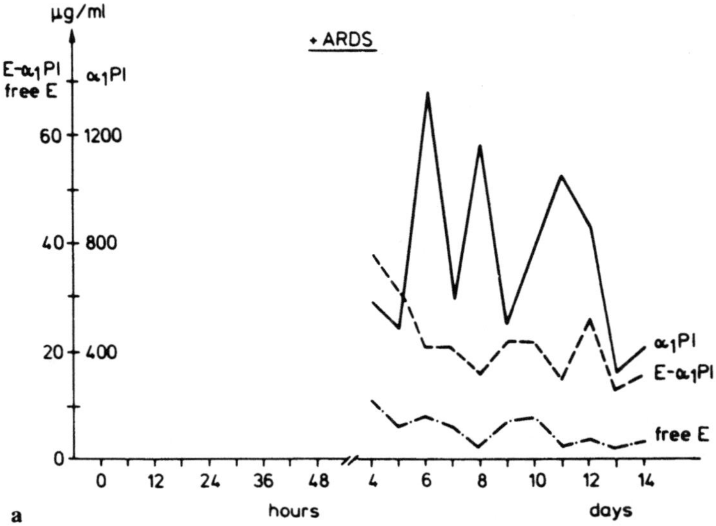

a

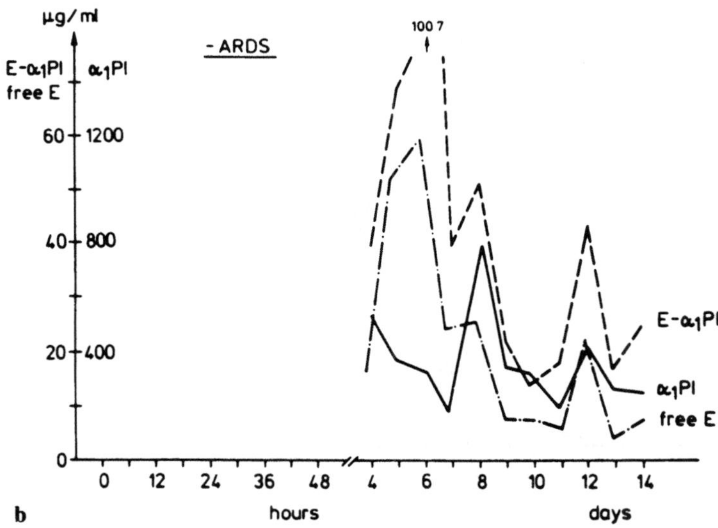

b

Fig. 7a,b. Posttraumatic courses of overall released neutrophil elastase (E-α_1PI; see Fig. 1.), proteolytically active elastase (*free E*) and α_1-proteinase inhibitor (α_1PI) in the alveolar epithelial lining fluids (ELF). Data are given as means for **a** 12 ARDS patients and **b** 15 non-ARDS patients in the later posttraumatic phase

higher release rate of elastase especially in the later posttraumatic phase, the molar surplus of α_1PI in these subjects was only 1.9- to 12.8-fold (Fig. 6). This might be responsible for the observation that, on average, more than 50% of the extracellular neutrophil proteinases were not inhibited by the locally available epithelial α_1PI (Fig. 7b) in the non-ARDS collective.

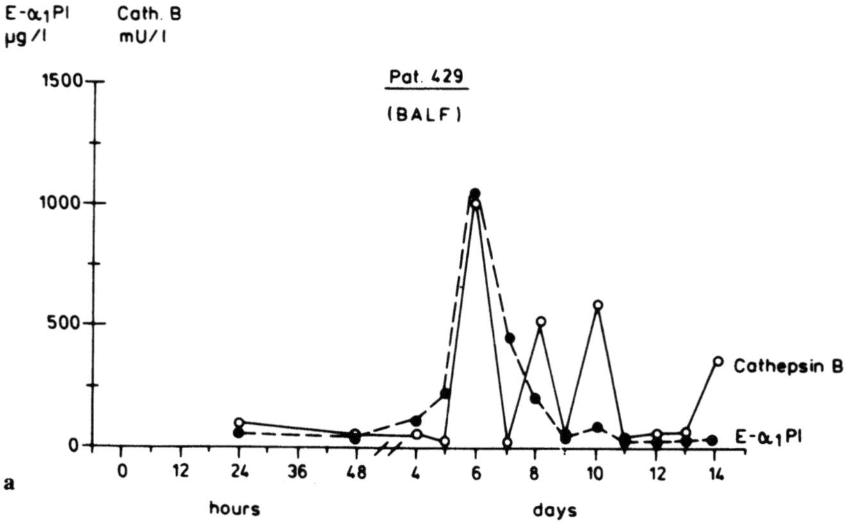

a

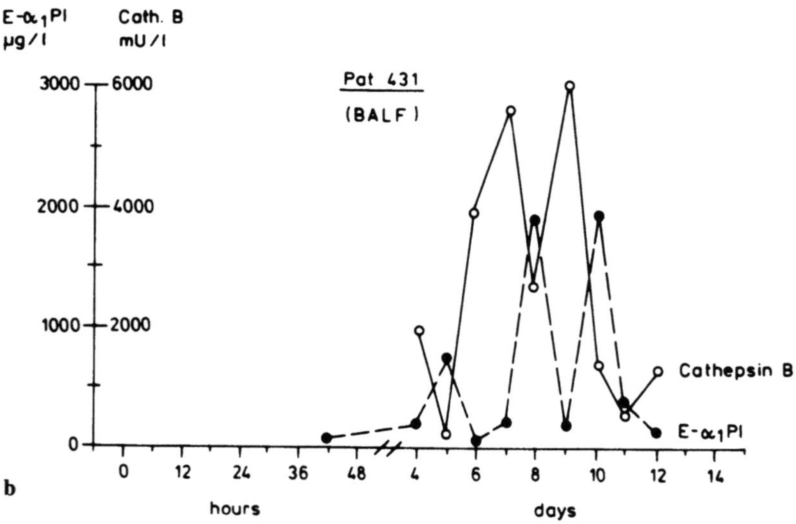

b

Fig. 8a,b. Individual posttraumatic courses of overall released neutrophil elastase measured as E-α_1PI complex and macrophage-derived cathepsin B in the bronchoalveolar lavage fluids (BALF) of individual patients. **a** Pat. 429 without ARDS, and **b** Pat. 431 with ARDS

Due to logistic conditions, the release of the alveolar macrophage-derived cysteine proteinase cathepsin B could be determined only in pilot measurements. Fig. 8 depicts the discharge pattern of cathepsin B compared with that of neutrophil elastase in the BALF of a non-ARDS (Pat. 429) and an ARDS subject (Pat. 431), respectively. Both proteinases showed a re-

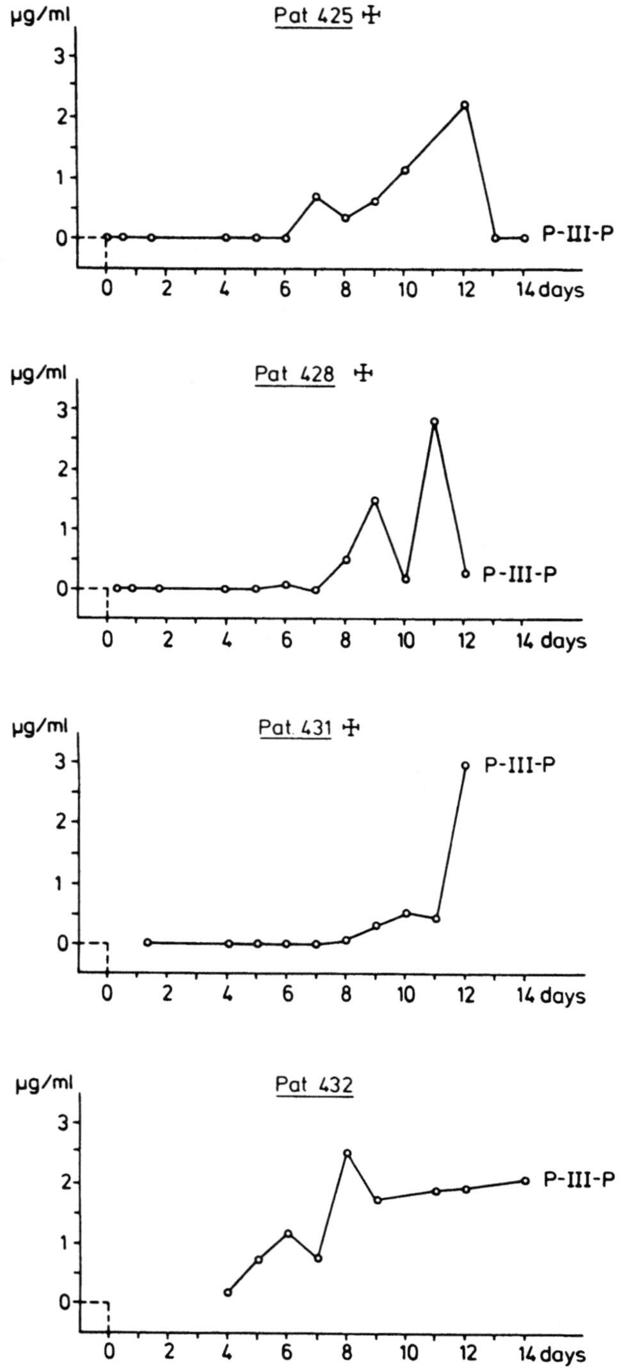

Fig 9. Individual posttraumatic courses of the procollagen-III-peptide (P-III-P) in the alveolar epithelial lining fluids (ELF) of four ARDS patients. Three patients (+) did not survive the organ failure

peated, though not congruent, release which indicates more or less permanent posttraumatic activation of the phagocytic cells. In contrast to the above-given elastase data (combined in mean values for each study group), the diagrams of the individual patient's data point to a distinctly lower stimulation of both types of phagocytes in the non-ARDS subject.

For measuring the fibrosis marker P-III-P, sequential BALF samples had been available only from a subgroup of the study population (6 ARDS and 7 non-ARDS subjects from Essen). Up to the 4th posttraumatic day, P-III-P was not elevated above the lower detection limit (1 ng/ml) of the applied assay in any of the BALF specimens. Between the 4th and 9th posttraumatic days, P-III-P started to increase in all ARDS patients reaching maximum values of 2.2–4.9 μg/ml ELF. Because of the small number of and great individual variation in the data, it is not feasible to present these as mean values. Therefore, four separate diagrams are depicted in Fig. 9. In contrast to the high and longer lasting (more than 5 days) elevation of P-III-P in all ARDS subjects, in 4 of the 7 non-ARDS patients, no P-III-P could be detected in any of the BALF samples drawn daily during the whole observation period. The other three subjects exhibited only a short-term (2–3 days) slight P-III-P increase (maximum values: 0.2–0.6 μg/ml ELF) in the late posttraumatic phase. Although P-III-P levels above 1 μg/mg ELF were always associated with ARDS, they did not predict the outcome of the disease.

Discussion

In the present study, we intended to contribute to the understanding of the ambiguous role of PMN granulocytes in the pathogenesis of ARDS by measuring extracellularly released neutrophil proteins in BALF samples drawn daily from polytraumatized high-risk patients. The conversion of the protein concentrations quantified in BALF to the actual amounts present in alveolar ELF by using the plasma/BALF concentration ratio of urea [23] was expected to allow a sufficiently exact follow-up observation of the locally discharged neutrophil products.

Applying this method, in healthy volunteers the amount of neutrophil lysosomal constituents, elastase, myeloperoxidase, and lactoferrin, which could be determined in ELF, was five- to tenfold the amount found in plasma levels measured simultaneously. This may be taken as a clear hint of considerable, intensive, local activation of PMN granulocytes, which occurs even under physiological conditions. Although repeated BAL was associated with an increased alveolar influx and stimulation of neutrophils, the quantity of proteolytically and oxidatively active cell products released thereby did not apparently disturb the blood/air barrier. Likewise, the amount of α_1PI, though only available in a 140-fold molar surplus over elastase as compared to a more than 10000-fold excess in plasma, seemed to be enough to achieve complete inactivation of its discharged target enzyme. From the given results we may conclude that concentrations up to 7 μg complexed elastase/ml ELF are without pathophysiological relevance.

Moreover, taking the rise in EVLW as an unequivocal sign of ARDS [16], it became obvious in our study that even neutrophil movement into the airspaces of patients at high risk did not necessarily cause an increase in alveolar capillary membrane permeability. Although these results are in agreement with those reported by others [21], some paradoxical phenomenons shown here deserve further explanation.

As outlined, the amounts of neutrophil lysosomal proteins repeatedly discharged into the ELF of non-ARDS patients were distinctly higher than those in ARDS subjects, whereas in the latter cases the local plasma-derived α_1PI was clearly elevated, especially in the early posttraumatic phase. Considering the recent findings of Dwenger et al. and Zilow et al. (see this volume), this discrepancy may be explained as follows. The severe traumatic event triggered the influx of neutrophils to the alveolar environment of all patients at risk to develop ARDS. During adhesion to the endothelial layer and the subsequent passage through the alveolar capillary barrier, the cells of patients who eventually developed ARDS could have been considerably more activated, probably by the neutrophil-stimulating complement components, C3a and C5a, which were present in clearly augmented amounts in the circulation of such patients.

Thereby, the aggressive neutrophil substances, which were also released in higher quantities into the circulation, may have contributed to the more or less simultaneous destruction of the pulmonary endothelial and epithelial cell layer, giving rise to increased permeability not necessarily associated with an elevation in EVLW. This early disturbance of the blood/air barrier is, however, reflected by the significantly higher ELF concentrations of plasma-derived α_1PI found in ARDS patients than those found in non-ARDS patients and healthy volunteers.

Since preactivated neutrophils, which had invaded the epithelial compartment, had evidently exhausted their lysosomal protein equipment, they may have responded to supplementary local stimuli (bacteria, cell debris, complement split products, etc.) only with a diminished release of cellular constituents. In addition, in the later posttraumatic course a growing portion of immature granulocytes with a distinctly lower content of lysosomal proteins appeared in the circulation of ARDS patients and was stimulated to pass the alveolar capillary barrier. This altogether may have been responsible for the generally lower amount of neutrophil proteins present in ELF of ARDS than in that of non-ARDS subjects.

In the later course of ARDS (from the 4th posttraumatic day onwards) the epithelial wall seemed to be sealed again by fibrotic processes, as is partly demonstrated by the appearance of the fibroblast product P-III-P in ELF specimens, whereas the endothelial layer continued to be progessively destroyed. This pathological situation was now associated with a manifest increase in EVLW in the ARDS patients. Despite reparative processes on the epithelial side of the alveoli, the repeated influx of plasma-derived α_1PI well above the regular 10% ELF/plasma ratio of this protein can be taken as a further indication that the blood/air barrier was still disturbed.

In contrast, in non-ARDS subjects a similar permanent pulmonary impairment could not be verified, neither by a persistent influx of α_1PI nor by the rise in EVLW. Here, an early transitory inflow of α_1PI into the alveolar space distinctly exceeding the physiological 10% ELF/plasma ratio was followed later by a two- to threefold elevation in ELF-α_1PI, which can be explained by the simultaneously rising plasma concentration of the inhibitor as an acute phase protein.

Although the α_1PI concentration was far above the normal value in all ELF specimens of the traumatized patients, this was apparently not sufficient to inhibit all neutrophil elastase released in the local epithelial milieu of the alveoli. Therefore, the obviously deficient inhibitory capacity of α_1PI may have been caused by two synergic effects. On the one hand, despite the increase of α_1PI in ELF, the inhibitor amount equalled only a considerably lower molar surplus (in general two- to 40-fold) over its released target enzyme compared to the 140-fold excess found under physiological conditions. This by itself might give rise to a locally incomplete proteinase inhibition. On the other hand, the simultaneously discharged neutrophil lysosomal proteins myeloperoxidase and lactoferrin – both of which are known to be involved in oxidatively destructive processes [18, 17] – as well as the macrophage-derived cathepsin B, presumably together with the even more potent α_1PI-degrading cathepsin L and metalloproteinases (for references see [8]), may have contributed to an additional decrease in the elastase inhibitory capacity, which was not previously sufficient. Applying special assay systems, both oxidatively and proteolytically inactivated α_1PI could be demonstrated by Schraufstatter et al. [26] in some individual BALF samples drawn only once during manifest ARDS courses. Moreover, these authors also detected active elastase despite the presence of a surplus of immunologically quantified α_1PI in those BALF specimens. As shown recently, proteolytically degraded α_1PI is a potent neutrophil chemoattractant [4] and may thus augment neutrophil influx to the alveolar spaces, resulting there in an increased elastase burden during a pathophysiological situation. However, other authors have not been able to demonstrate elastase activity against high molecular weight protein substrates in BALF samples of ARDS patients [13, 32]. This might be for two reasons: first an insufficiently sensitive assay system, which probably did not allow detection of small amounts of free elastase in the highly diluted BALF samples, and second, the lack of enough sequentially drawn BALF specimens during the development and manifestation of ARDS. As pointed out here, the repeated release of phagocyte constituents in to the alveolar space requires a close-meshed sampling procedure to enable sufficient insight into the local inflammatory cell-induced pathomechanisms.

Although the distinctly higher amount of free elastase in the BALF specimens of non-ARDS patients could be due to an augmented local elastase/α_1PI imbalance, these observations seem to contradict the importance which is generally assumed for this neutrophil enzyme in the development of ARDS. In this respect, our findings support data published by other authors (for review of literature see [21]) indicating an equivalent or even higher influx and activation of neutrophils in high-risk patients not generating ARDS. Yet, it should be kept in mind that both the ARDS and non-ARDS patients required artificial ventilation throughout the observation period. This indicates persistent lung failure in all severely traumatized subjects. Therefore, the considerably higher amounts of neutrophil products released to the alveolar compartments of both patient groups may indeed have contributed to lung dysfunction in comparison with the situation evaluated in healthy volunteers. Moreover, as it can be deduced from the high standard deviations of mean, the presentation of data combined in mean values for each group may have concealed somehow the individual situation. This is exemplarily depicted in Figs. 3 and 8. The diagrams demonstrate the existence of a clear correlation between the augmented release of phagocyte constituents and elevated EVLW. However, the definition of ARDS as an increase of EVLW above 10 ml/kg body weight [16] might not be reliable enough to classify exactly the degree of severity of lung function disturbances, because those subjects are excluded whose inflammatory cell-induced pulmonary dysfunction is already indicated by a smaller elevation in EVLW. Therefore, final proof of presumed pathomechanisms awaits further follow-up studies with higher numbers of a homogeneous (e.g., only traumatized) high-risk patients collective, which may allow an exact classification of lung dysfunctions according to various clinical and biochemical parameters.

Regarding the second aim of our study, of the inflammation markers measured so far, only α_1PI in amounts above 300 µg/ml ELF in the early posttraumatic phase heralded the later onset of ARDS with a clinically acceptable degree of sensitivity and specificity. These findings are in agreement with results published by Fowler et al. [10] who could also show permeability changes in patients at high risk for ARDS prior to development of the syndrome. Moreover, manifestation of ARDS was clearly confirmed in our study by ELF concentrations of the fibrosis parameter P-III-P exceeding 1 µg/ml. Yet, neither this nor the other inflammation markers determined here were able to indicate the outcome of the disease.

Conclusion

Daily drawn BALF samples of multiply injured patients and healthy volunteers allowed us to confirm a significantly higher influx of neutrophils into the alveolar space as well as an increased local discharge of phagocyte (neutrophil; macrophage) constituents (elastase, myeloperoxidase, lactoferrin; cathepsin B) in subjects at high risk to develop ARDS. Hence, these aggressive components of inflammatory cells may indeed contribute to the occurrence of lung dysfunctions in all severely traumatized patients.

Taking EVLW elevation above 10 ml/kg body weight as an unambiguous sign of ARDS manifestation, in patients showing this sign 3–4 days post trauma, the permeability increase of the blood/air barrier was heralded much earlier (within 48 h after the traumatic event) by the enhanced inflow of plasma-derived α_1PI to the alveolar epithelial environment. ELF concentrations of α_1PI above 300 µg/ml in this initial posttraumatic phase predicted the later occurrence of ARDS with a clinically acceptable degree of sensitivity (63%) and specificity (71%). Moreover, concentrations of the fibrosis marker, P-III-P, exceeding 1 µg/ml ELF confirmed ARDS manifestation. However, none of the inflammation markers studied indicated the outcome of posttraumatic lung dysfunctions.

Acknowledgement. We are very grateful to Prof. Dr. H. Fritz for helpful discussions. P-III-P test kits were kindly supplied by the Radiochemical Department of Behringwerke AG.

References

1. Adamson IY, Young L, Bowden D (1988) Relationship of alveolar epithelial injury and repair to the production of pulmonary fibrosis. Am J Pathol 130:377
2. Assfalg-Machleidt I, Jochum M, Klaubert W, Inthorn D, Machleidt W (1988) Enzymatically active cathepsin B dissociating from its inhibitor complexes is elevated in blood plasma of patients with septic shock and some malignant tumors. Biol Chem Hoppe Seyler 369 [Suppl]: 263
3. Auler JO, Cahlheiros DF, Brentani MM, Santello JL, Lemos PC, Saldiva PH (1986) Adult respiratory distress syndrome: evidence of early fibrogenesis and absence of glucocorticoid receptors. Eur J Respir Dis 69:261
4. Bander MJ, Rice AG, Griffin GL, Senior RM (1988) α_1-Proteinase inhibitor is a neutrophil chemoattractant after proteolytic inactivation by macrophage elastase. J Biol Chem 263:4481
5. Brody AR, Bittermann PB (1988) The lung matrix and inflammation: Part II. Biochemical and molecular mechanisms of fibrogenesis: Implications of environmental lung disease. Am Rev Respir Dis 138:1056
6. Cantin AM, Boileau R, Begin R (1988) Increased procollagen III aminoterminal peptide – related antigens and fibroblast growth signals in the lungs of patients with idiopathic pulmonary fibrosis. Am Rev Respir Dis 137:572
7. Chapman HA Jr, Stone OL (1984) Comparison of live human neutrophil and alveolar macrophage elastolytic activity in vitro. J Clin Invest 74:1693
8. Desrochers PE, Weiss SJ (1988) Proteolytic inactivation of alpha-1-proteinase inhibitor by a neutrophil metalloproteinase. J Clin Invest 81:1646
9. Dwenger A, Schweitzer G, Regel G (1986) Bronchoalveolar lavage fluid and plasma proteins, chemiluminescence response and protein contents of polymorphonuclear leukocytes from blood and lavage fluid in traumatized patients. J Clin Chem Clin Biochem 24:73

10. Fowler AA, Hyers TM, Fisher BJ, Bechard DE, Centor RM, Webster RO (1987) The adult respiratory distress syndrome. Cell populations and soluble mediators in the air spaces of patients at high risk. Am Rev Respir Dis 136:1225
11. Hammerschmidt DW, Weaver LJ, Hudson LD, Craddock PR, Jacobs HS (1980) Association of complement activation and elevated plasma-C5a with adult respiratory distress syndrome: pathophysiologic relevance and possible prognostic value. Lancet 1:947
12. Holter JF, Weiland JE, Pacht ER, Gadek JE, Davis WB (1986) Protein permeability in adult respiratory distress syndrome. J Clin Invest 78:1513
13. Idell S, Kucich U, Fein A, Kueppers F, James HL, Walsh PN, Weinbaum G, Colman RW, Cohen AB (1985) Neutrophil elastase-releasing factors in bronchoalveolar lavage from patients with adult respiratory distress syndrome. Am Rev Respir Dis 132:1098
14. Jochum M, Fritz H (1989) Pathobiochemical mechanisms in inflammation. In Faist E, Ninnemann JL, Green DR (eds) Immune consequences of trauma, shock and sepsis. Springer, Berlin Heidelberg New York Tokyo, p 165
15. Joka Th, Nakhosteen JA, Obertacke U, Herrmann J, Coenen Th, Brand M, Jochum M, Zilow G, Dwenger A, Kreuzfelder E (1988) Beeinflußt die bronchoalveoläre Lavage das Milieu in der Alveole? Prax Klin Pneumol 42:705
16. Kreuzfelder E, Joka Th, Keinecke H-O, Obertacke U, Schmit-Neuerburg K-P, Nakhosteen JA, Paar D, Scheiermann N (1988) Adult respiratory distress syndrome as a specific manifestation of a general permeability defect in trauma patients. Am Rev Respir Dis 137:95
17. Nemet K, Simonovitis I (1985) The biological role of lactoferrin. Haematologia 18:3
18. Nowak D (1988) The comparative study of reactive oxygen species generated by polymorphonuclear leukocytes as α_1-proteinase inhibitor inactivators. Possible application for antioxidant prevention of emphysema. Arch Immunol Ther Exp 36:723
19. Ognibene FP, Martin SE, Parker MM (1986) Adult respiratory distress syndrome in patients with severe neutropenia. N Engl J Med 315:547
20. Pacht ER, Davis WB (1988) Role of transferrin and ceruloplasmin in antioxidant activity of lung epithelial lining fluid. J Appl Physiol 64:2092
21. Parsons PE, Worthen GS, Moore EE, Tate RM, Henson PM (1989) The association of circulating endotoxin with the development of the adult respiratory distress syndrome. Am Rev Respir Dis 140:294
22. Regel G, Dwenger A, Seidel J, Nerlich ML, Sturm JA, Tscherne H (1987) Die Bedeutung der neutrophilen Granulozyten bei der Entstehung des posttraumatischen Lungenversagens. Unfallchirurg 90:99
23. Rennard SJ, Basset G, Lecossier D, O'Donnell KM, Pinkston P, Martin PG, Crystal RG (1986) Estimation of volume of epithelial lining fluid recovered by lavage using urea as a marker of dilution. J Appl Physiol 60:532
24. Reynolds HY (1987) State of the art: bronchoalveolar lavage. Am Rev Respir Dis 135:250
25. Rinaldo JE (1986) Mediation of ARDS by leukocytes. Chest 89:590
26. Schraufstatter I, Revak SD, Cochrane CG (1984) Biochemical factors in pulmonary inflammatory disease. Federation Proc 43:2807
27. Shale DJ (1987) The adult respiratory distress syndrome – 20 years on. Thorax 42:641
28. Thommasen HV (1985) The role of the polymorphonuclear leukocyte in the pathogenesis of the adult respiratory distress syndrome. Clin Invest Med 8:185
29. Travis J, Salvesen GS (1983) Human plasma proteinase inhibitors. Am Rev Biochem 52:655
30. Varani J, Fligiel SEG, Till GO (1985) Pulmonary endothelial cell killing by human neutrophils. Possible involvement of hydroxyl radical. Lab Invest 53:565
31. Weiland JE, Davis WD, Holter JF, Mohammed JR, Dorinsky PM, Gadek JE (1986) Lung neutrophils in the adult respiratory distress syndrome. Clinical and pathophysiologic significance. Am Rev Respir Dis 133:218
32. Wewers MD, Herzyk DJ, Gadek JE (1988) Alveolar fluid neutrophil elastase activity in the adult respiratory distress syndrome is complexed to alpha-2-macroglobulin. J Clin Invest 82:1260

V Endothelial and Epithelial Mechanisms of Injury

Plasma and Bronchoalveolar Lavage Fluid Proteins as Markers of Increased Lung Permeability in ARDS as a Result of Multiple Trauma

A. Dwenger, G. Schweitzer, and M. Funck

Introduction

Bronchoalveolar lavage (BAL) can be used as a means for investigating the inflammatory and immue processes of the human lung. BAL fluids were obtained from ARDS patients in order to study the pathomechanisms of this syndrome [5–8]. Accuracy and reproducibility of the BAL technique and protein measurements seemed to depend on the choice of a suitable reference substance. Urea is now considered to be the accepted reference [11, 12]. Although increased protein permeability of the lung is well documented in ARDS, little information is available as to the actual distribution of plasma proteins in various sizes between blood and epithelial lining fluid (ELF) in this disorder [4] and no information is available on the time course of this distribution. In addition, patients at risk who do not subsequently develop ARDS have not been studied. Therefore, the aim of the present study was to evaluate the extent and time course of lung permeability alterations in multiply traumatized patients with ARDS predisposition in comparison with normals by means of protein and urea measurements in plasma and BAL fluid. Another goal was to determine a predictor system for ARDS.

Methods

Study Population

Citrated venous blood and bronchoalveolar lavage fluid (BALF) of 27 multiply traumatized patients (Injury Severity Score >30 points; 12 ARDS and 15 non-ARDS patients) were obtained daily or every 2nd day for up to 8 days after trauma and processed as previously described [2].

Department of Clinical Biochemistry, Hannover Medical School, Konstanty-Gutschow-Str. 8, W-3000 Hannover 61, FRG

J.A. Sturm (Ed.)
Adult Respiratory Distress Syndrome

Extravascular Lung Water Measurement

The extravascular lung water (EVLW) was determined according to previous descriptions [9].

Urea Measurement

In plasma and BALF, urea concentrations were determined enzymatically as described previously [2].

Protein Measurements

In plasma and BALF, lactate dehydrogenase (LDH) was determined with the test combination "LDH opt. UV-test" (Boehringer, Mannheim, FRG), total protein (TP) with the biuret method, albumin (ALB) with bromocresol green, elastase (ELA)-α_1-proteinase inhibitor (PI) by enzyme immunoassay with the test combination "PMN elastase" (Merck, Darmstadt, FRG), cholinesterase (CHE) with a test combination (substrate: butyrylthiocholine, Boehringer, Mannheim, FRG), β-*N*-acetylglucosaminidase (β-NAG) spectrofluorometrically with a fluorogenic substrate according to Yatziv et al. [14], α_1-proteinase inhibitor (α_1-PI), transferrin (TRF), ceruloplasmin (CER), and α_2-macroglobulin (α_2-M) immunological-nephelometrically using reagent sets, protocols, and instrumentation of Immuno Diagnostika GmbH, FRG.

Calculations

The protein concentrations/activities of the ELF were calculated by:

$$C_{ELF} = C_{BALF} \cdot C_{plasma\text{-}urea}/C_{BALF\text{-}urea},$$

the ELF/plasma ratios by

$$R = C_{ELF}/C_{plasma}$$

and the distribution coefficients (DCs) according to

$$DC = C_{plasma}/C_{plasma\text{-}urea}/C_{BALF}/C_{BALF\text{-}urea},$$

and according to Bell et al. [1] and Holter et al. [4]:

$$DC = C_{plasma}/C_{plasma\text{-}TP}/C_{BALF}/C_{BALF\text{-}TP}$$

Statistical analysis was performed by the Mann-Whitney *U* test.

To demonstrate time dependency of the parameters measured the data obtained every 2 days were combined for calculation due to the small number of cases. For calculation of ARDS prognosis from initial ELF/plasma ratios,

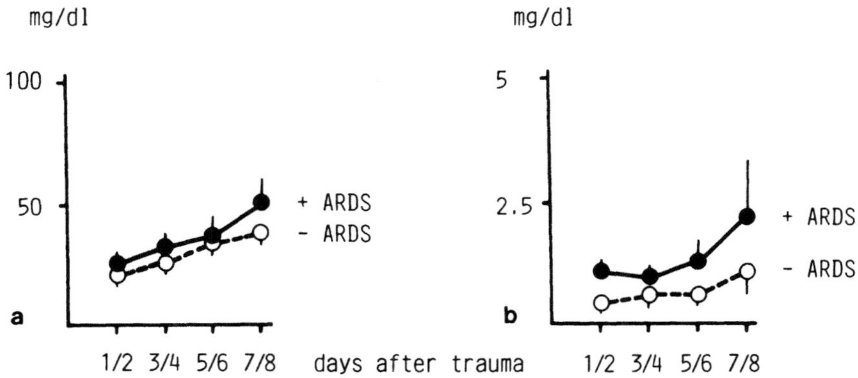

Fig. 1a,b. Posttraumatic courses of urea concentrations in plasma (**a**) and BALF (**b**) of 12 ARDS and 15 non-ARDS patients. $\bar{x} \pm$ SEM

sensitivity and specificity were demonstrated by the cumulative frequency distribution function.

Results

In Fig. 1, the posttraumatic courses of the urea concentrations in plasma (Fig. 1a) and BALF (Fig. 1b) are depicted for ARDS and non-ARDS patients, showing a time-dependent twofold increase in the plasma of ARDS patients which is paralleled by a twofold increase in BALF. To demonstrate the necessity of correcting BALF protein concentrations for acute-phase effects, the posttraumatic courses of the BALF concentration (a), the ELF concentration (b), and the ELF/plasma ratio of α_1-PI for ARDS and non-ARDS patients are shown in Fig. 2. Figure 3 indicates the posttraumatic courses of ELF/plasma ratios of α_1-PI (a), albumin (b), transferrin (c), and ceruloplasmin (d), whereas Fig. 4 shows such ratios for cholinesterase (a), α_2-macroglobulin (b), and total protein (c). In Fig. 5, the posttraumatic courses of the LDH activity (a) in the ELF are shown as well as the ELA-α_1-PI complex concentration (b) and the β-*N*-acetylglucosaminidase activity (c). Figure 6 demonstrates that there was no correlation between the ELF albumin concentrations and the corresponding EVLW values. Figure 7 is a diagrammatic representation of the endothelial-epithelial border showing the alterations in albumin concentrations in plasma, interstitium, and ELF for (a) intact endothelium and epithelium, (b) damaged endothelium and intact epithelium, and (c) intact endothelium and damaged epithelium, which were then compared with the albumin concentrations actually measured in ARDS patients, non-ARDS patients, and normals. According to Bell et al. [1], Holter et al. [4], Marcy et al. [11], and Rennard et al. [12], the interrelation-

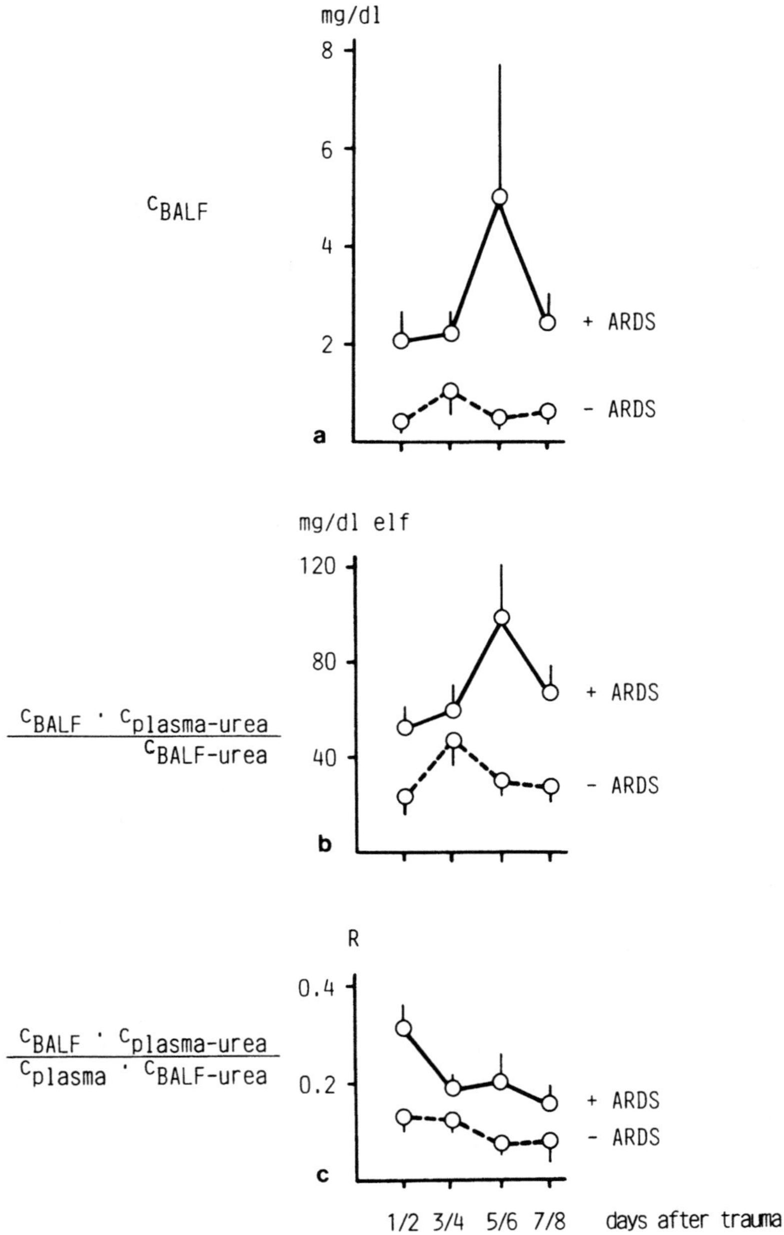

Fig. 2a–c. Posttraumatic courses of BALF concentration (**a**), ELF concentration (**b**), and ELF/plasma ratio (**c**) of α_1-PI in 12 ARDS and 15 non-ARDS patients. $\bar{x} \pm$ SEM

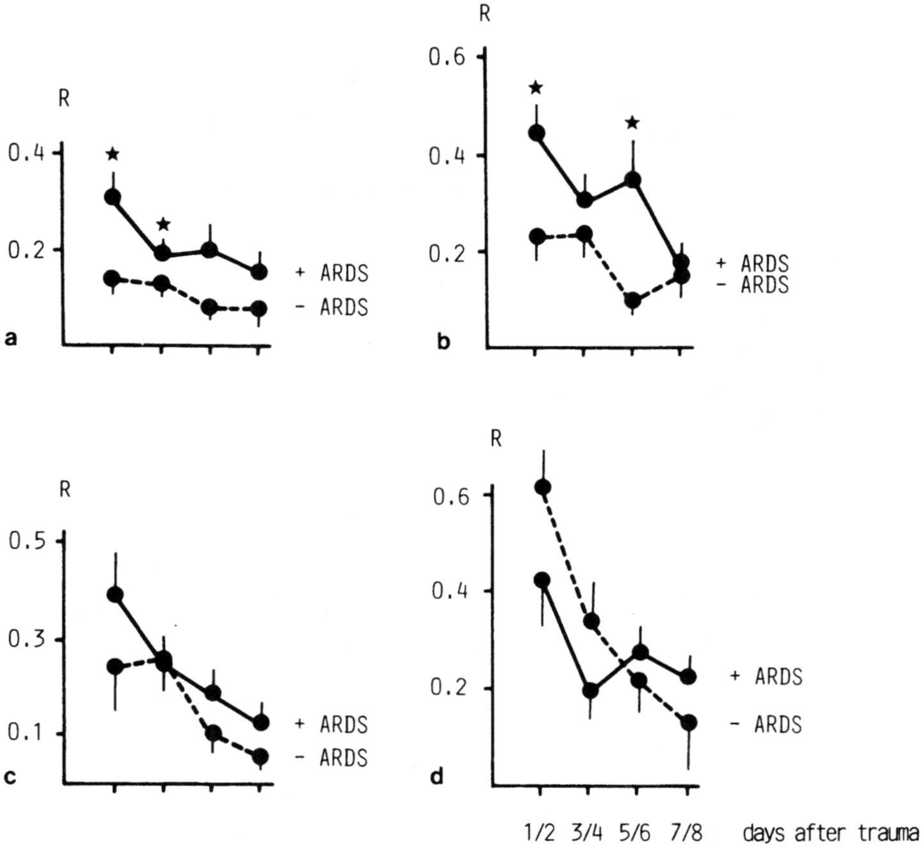

Fig. 3a–d. Posttraumatic courses of ELF/plasma ratios R of α_1-PI (**a**), albumin (**b**), transferrin (**c**), and ceruloplamin (**d**) of 12 ARDS and 15 non-ARDS patients. $\bar{x} \pm$ SEM. $^*p < 0.05$

ship between the distribution coefficient, DC, and the ELF/plasma ratio, R, using urea as an internal reference substance is demonstrated in Fig. 8, as well as the dependence of R and DC on the molecular weights of proteins. A comparison between urea and total protein as an internal reference for the calculation of ELF protein concentrations is given in Fig. 9. Figure 10 depicts R and DC of ARDS patients, non-ARDS patients, and normals for three different-sized proteins, transferrin (90 000 Da), cholinesterase (348 000 Da), and α_2-macroglobulin (820 000 Da), summarizing all the data obtained through the 8th day after trauma. By subdividing these data in Fig. 10 into four groups from days 1 and 2 up to days 7 and 8, the initial loss of the protein size selectivity of the blood/air barrier could be seen for ARDS and non-ARDS patients in comparison with normals (Fig. 11). In Fig. 12, the posttraumatic development of the EVLW is shown. As possible indicator of ARDS development the measurement of initial α_1-PI concentrations in ELF and

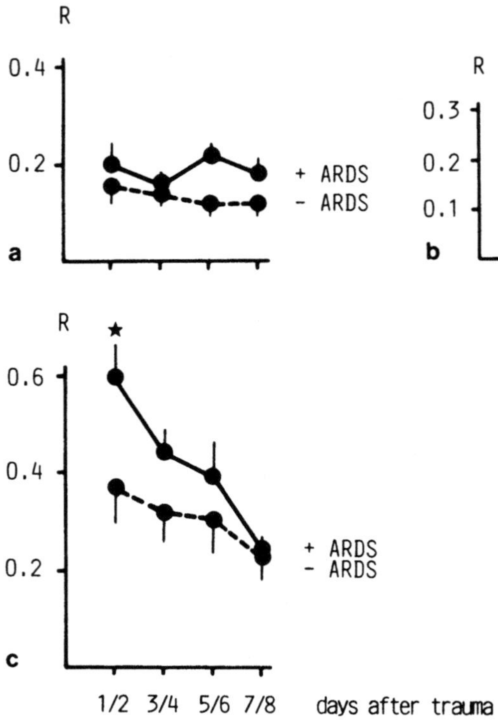

Fig. 4a–c. Posttraumatic courses of ELF/plasma ratios R of cholinesterase (**a**), α_2-macroglobulin (**b**), and total protein (**c**) of 12 ARDS and 15 non-ARDS patients. $\bar{x} \pm$ SEM. $^{*}p < 0.05$

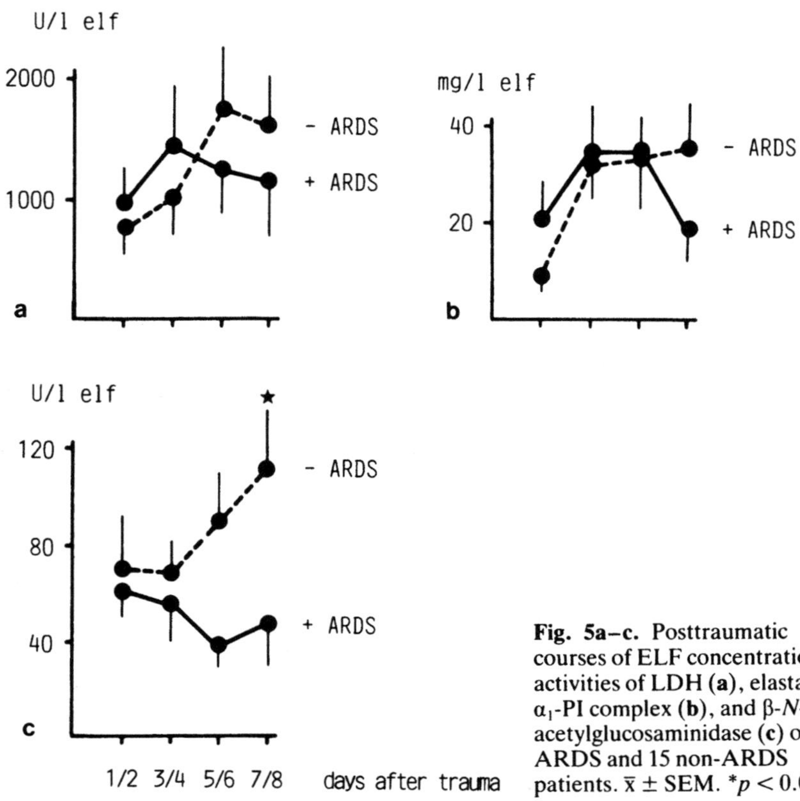

Fig. 5a–c. Posttraumatic courses of ELF concentrations/activities of LDH (**a**), elastase-α_1-PI complex (**b**), and β-*N*-acetylglucosaminidase (**c**) of 12 ARDS and 15 non-ARDS patients. $\bar{x} \pm$ SEM. $^{*}p < 0.05$

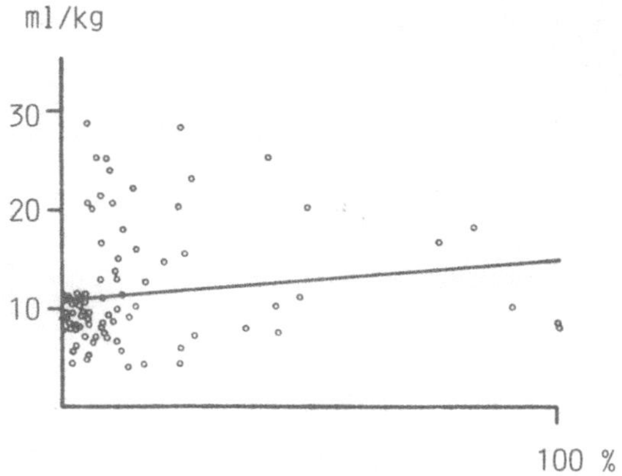

Fig. 6. Regression plot of ELF albumin concentrations (highest value = 100%) and corresponding EVLW values (ml/kg) of 12 multiply traumatized patients. $y = Ax + B$; $r = 0.1164$; $B = 11.2493$; $A = 0.0316$

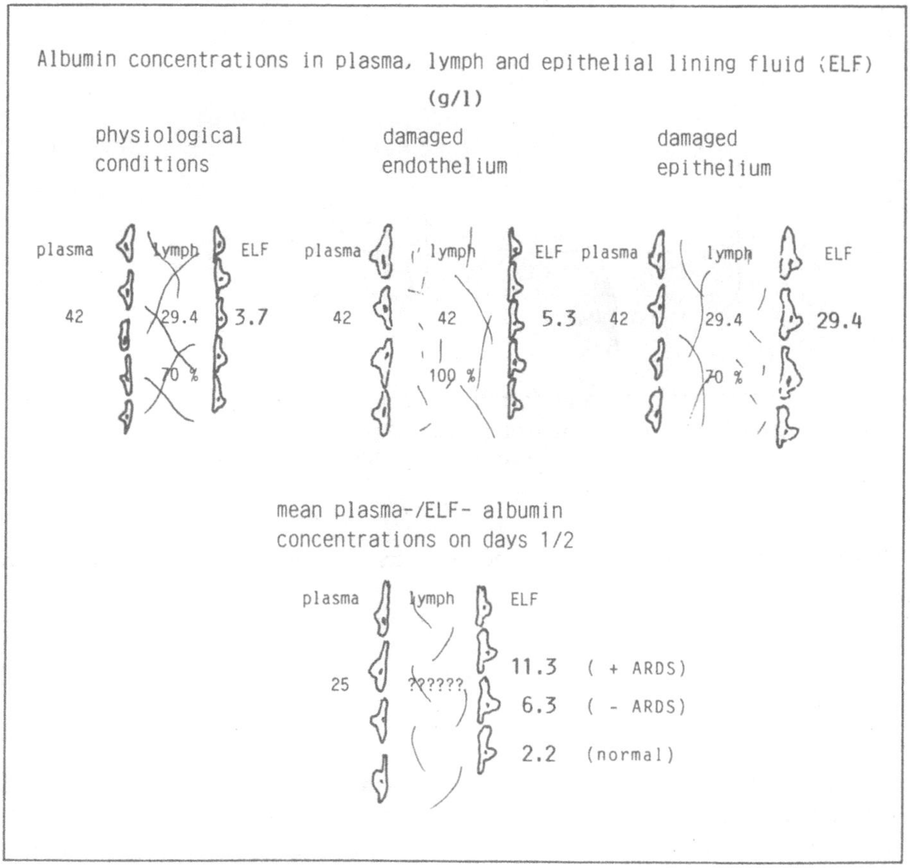

Fig. 7. Endothelial-interstitial-epithelial wall

c = concentration of a protein component in plasma and BALF

$$\text{distribution coefficient} \quad DC = \frac{c_{plasma} / c_{plasma\text{-}TP}}{c_{BALF} / c_{BALF\text{-}TP}} \qquad (1, 4)$$

$DC_{high} \;\hat{=}\;$ increasing restriction from ELF

$DC_{low} \;\hat{=}\;$ increasing accumulation in ELF

$$DC = \frac{c_{plasma} / c_{plasma\text{-}urea}}{c_{BALF} / c_{BALF\text{-}urea}} \qquad R = \frac{c_{ELF}}{c_{plasma}}$$

$$c_{ELF} = \frac{c_{BALF} \cdot c_{plasma\text{-}urea}}{c_{BALF\text{-}urea}} \qquad (11, 12)$$

$$R = \frac{c_{BALF} \cdot c_{plasma\text{-}urea}}{c_{plasma} \cdot c_{BALF\text{-}urea}} = \frac{c_{BALF} / c_{BALF\text{-}urea}}{c_{plasma} / c_{plasma\text{-}urea}} = \frac{1}{DC}$$

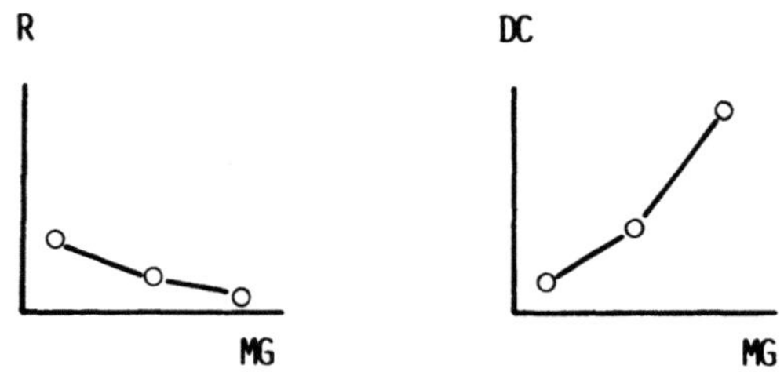

Fig. 8. Relationship between the ELF/plasma ratio, R, and the distribution coefficient, DC, as well as their plots versus molecular weight MG

plasma enabled the sensitivity and specificity of prognosis to be calculated (Fig. 13).

Discussion

Current results confirmed the validity of using urea as an internal reference substance since it can freely diffuse across biological membranes [12]. During the posttraumatic course, the plasma urea concentrations of the ARDS group increased twofold up until the 8th day following trauma, and this increase was reflected in the BAL fluid of this patient group. Therefore, the BALF protein concentrations were corrected for the inevitable alterations

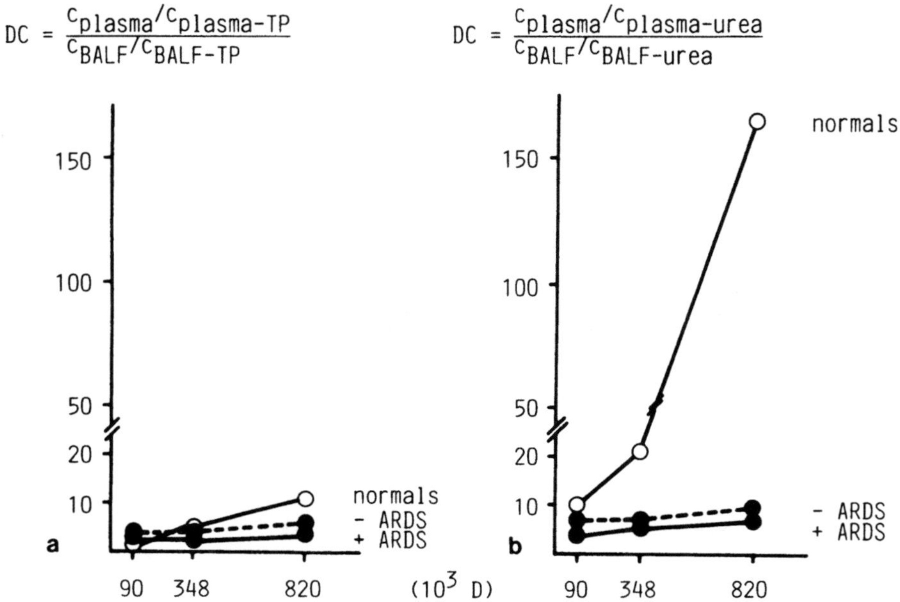

Fig. 9a,b. Mean distribution coefficients. DC, calculated with respect to TP (**a**) and to urea (**b**) of 12 normals, 12 ARDS, and 15 non-ARDS patients for transferrin (90 000 Da), cholinesterase (348 000 Da), and α_2-macroglobulin (820 000 Da)

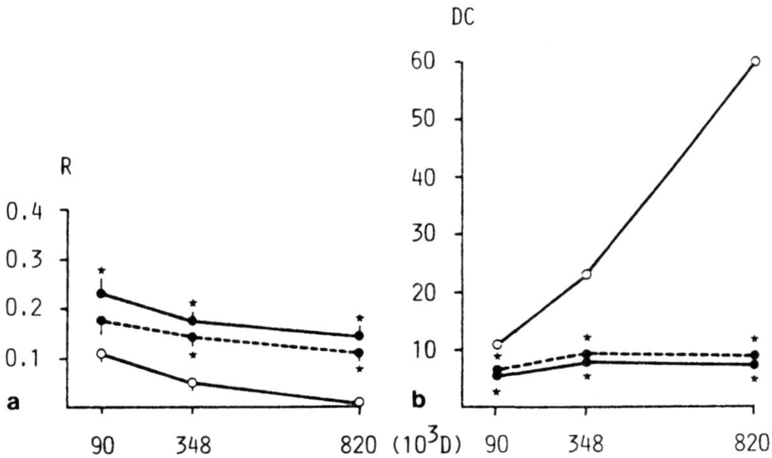

Fig. 10a,b. Mean ELF/plasma ratios R (**a**) and mean distribution coefficients DC (**b**) using urea as an internal reference substance of 12 normals (○——○), 12 ARDS (●——●), and 15 non-ARDS (●------●) patients for transferrin, cholinesterase, and α_2-macroglobulin; data were collected and analyzed through the 8th day after trauma. $^*p < 0.05$ for +ARDS or −ARDS versus normals

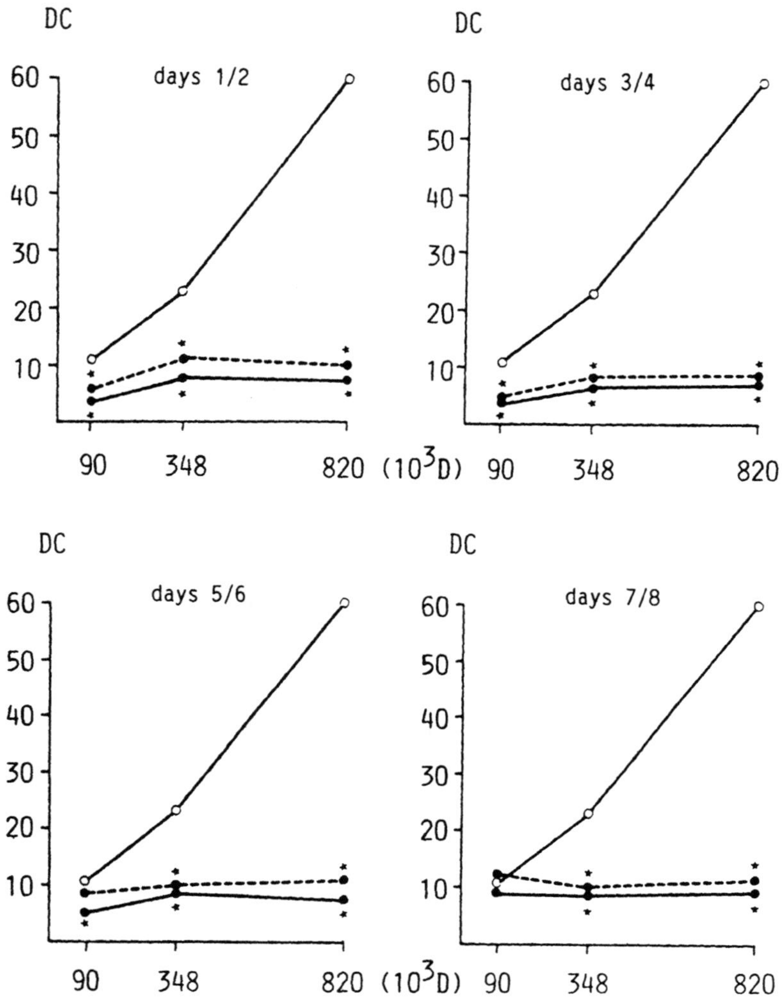

Fig. 11. Mean distribution coefficients from Fig. 10 after subdivision into four equa periods. $^{*}p < 0.05$ for +ARDS or −ARDS versus normals

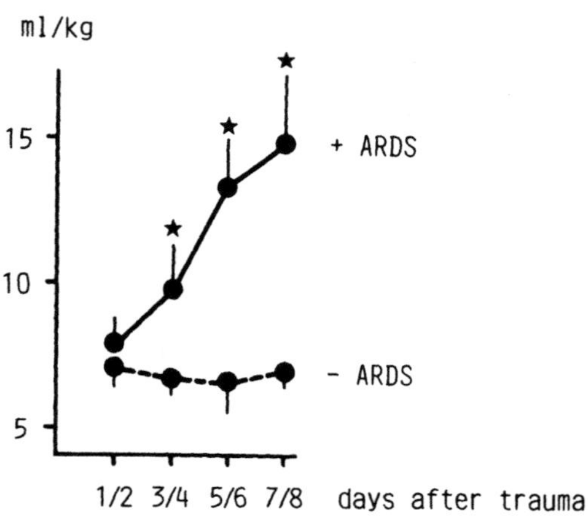

Fig. 12. Posttraumatic courses of EVLW values of six ARDS and six non-ARDS patients

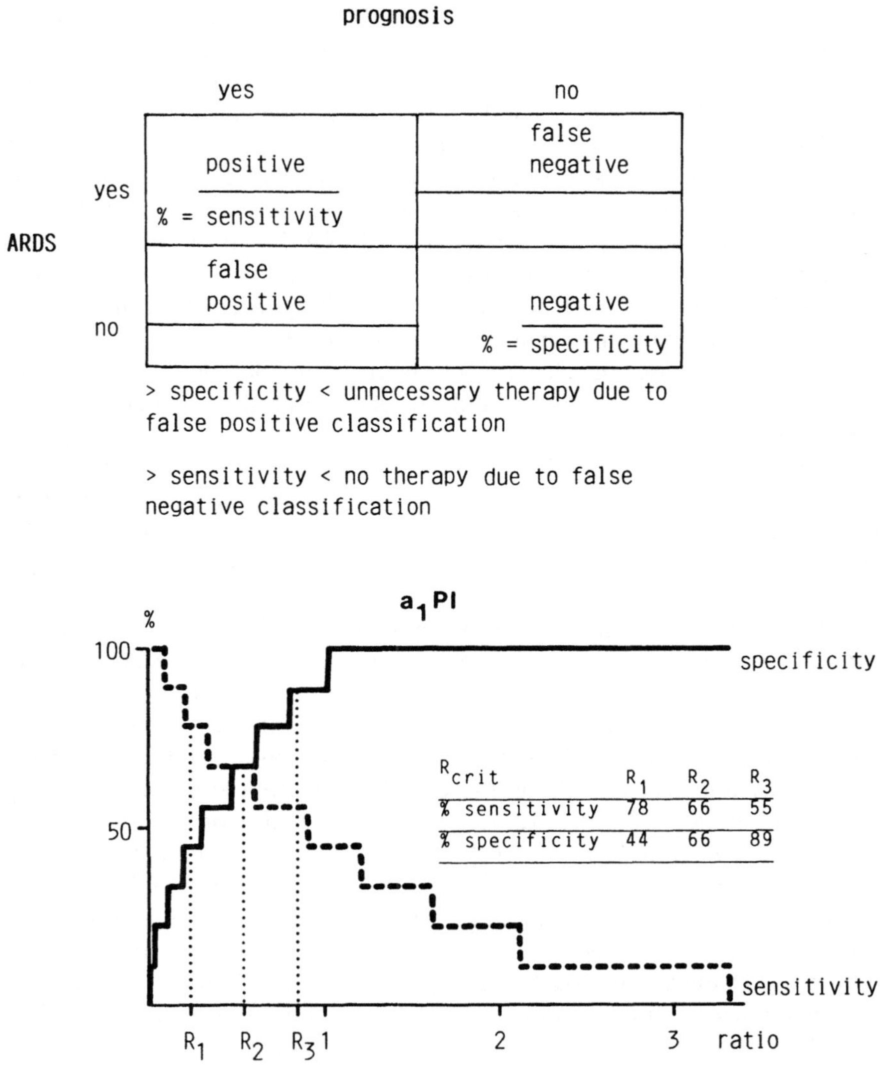

Fig. 13. A prognostic system for ARDS by ELF/plasma ratios of α_1-PI

of the BAL procedure by the use of plasma and BALF urea concentrations for the calculation of the ELF protein concentrations. These were then divided by the corresponding plasma protein concentrations to obatin the ELF/plasma ratios. By this method, misinterpretations were avoided which could be caused by increased BALF protein concentrations as a result of an increased plasma protein concentration (e.g., by acute-phase effects) rather than by a pathological permeability increase.

In BALF, two types of proteins were found: (a) type I proteins, which were synthesized intravascularly and reached the alveoli by diffusion across the endothelial and epithelial wall, and (b) type II proteins which were predominantly released from mobile cells present in or having invaded the alveoli, e.g., elastase from neutrophils, β-*N*-acetylglucosaminidase from neutrophils and macrophages and LDH from all alveolar cell types.

The posttraumatic course of the LDH activity in ELF indicated that the extent of alveolar cell damage was similar in ARDS and non-ARDS patients but there was a slight tendency toward increasing activity in the non-ARDS groups. This tendency was elucidated in the β-NAG courses, which increased for non-ARDS patients in comparison with the nearly constant time course for ARDS patients. This behavior indicated the participation of lysosome-containing cells other than neutrophils, presumably macrophages, since the extracellular release of elastase by neutrophils demonstrated a nearly identical degree of phagocytosis and cell damage of alveolar neutrophils for ARDS and non-ARDS patients.

Concerning type I proteins, the posttraumatic courses of the ELF/plasma ratios showed a generalized behavior, the ratios of ARDS patients being (occasionally significantly) higher in comparison with the ratios of non-ARDS patients, and the ratios of both patients groups indicating a time-dependent decrease.

Accordingly, the question arose as to how a decrease of the alveolar protein concentration with the observed concomitant EVLW increase, especially in ARDS patients, could be explained.To answer this question, we have to consider some different states of the blood/air barrier, concerning the albumin concentration of three different compartments as indicated in Fig. 7. Under physiological conditions there is 42 g/l plasma albumin and 29.4 g/l lymph albumin. Of this, 12.6% is in the ELF, or 8.8% of 42 g/l, corresponding to 3.7 g/l [10, 12]. Now, we can consider two extreme situations: (a) in the case of total structural damage of the endothelial wall there is also 42 g/l lymph protein present and 12.6% of this is in the ELF, namely 5.3 g/l, (b) in the case of total epithelial damage, lymph and ELF albumin concentrations would become equal to be 29.4 g/l. In the actual albumin concentrations determined in ELF, we found 11.3 g/l in ARDS and 6.3 g/l in non-ARDS patients in comparison with 2.2 g/l in normals with respect to the lower plasma albumin concentrations of the patients in the initial posttraumatic phase of 48 h, indicating that there must be simulataneous damage to endothelial *and* epithelial structures in the initial posttraumatic course. In the following time course, the epithelial wall seemed to be tightened by fibrotic and reparative processes (time-dependent decrease of alveolar protein concentrations) in ARDS and non-ARDS patients, whereas the endothelial wall seemed to be repaired (non-ARDS patients) or progressively destroyed (ARDS patients) as seen by the EVLW courses. Nearly identical results were obtained from albumin extravasation scintigraphy [13], indicating an early increase in pulmonary capillary permeability after severe multiple trauma on the second posttraumatic day followed by an EVLW increase on day 6 after trauma. This also agreed with our findings of a lack of correlation between the ELF concentrations of a permeability marker such as albumin and the corresponding EVLW values. In summary, the ARDS development could not be seen from the alveolar protein concentration courses.

To obtain insight into the loss of the sieve function and its time dependency, the ELF/plasma ratios, Rs, and, especially the distribution coefficients, DCs, were calculated and plotted versus the molecular weights of different proteins. In this context, urea was more suitable and reliable as an internal reference substance in comparison with total protein values as used by other authors [1, 4], as was seen in Fig. 9. Total protein concentrations as an internal reference did not fulfill the basic requirements of identical behavior in physiological and pathological situations, since the total protein diffusion is dependent on the integrity of the barrier. This does not hold true for urea.

By summarizing all the data obtained through the eighth posttraumatic day, there was a directly proportional relationship between the DCs and the molecular weights for normals from 90000 Da up to 820000 Da, which was lost in the ARDS and non-ARDS patients [3, 4]. Apparently, the discriminatory ability of the sieve did not exist for proteins with molecular weights lower than about 100000 Da, since there was no dependence on the DCs for α_1-PI and albumin. But, in the high molecular range the DCs for ARDS and non-ARDS patients decreased to low values as they were observed for the low molecular range, indicating the loss of the sieve function, especially for high molecular weight proteins. After subdivision of the data into four equal time periods of 2 days duration from days 1 and 2 up to days 7 and 8, the initial permeability increase was observed with no essential alterations for up to day 8 after trauma for ARDS and non-ARDS patients. From these results, some doubts arose as to the value of long-term BALF protein measurements because of the reparative tightening of the epithelial wall. However, in the initial posttraumatic phase, namely on day 1 or days 1 and 2, (occasionally significant) differences between the ELF/plasma ratios of low molecular weight proteins for ARDS and non-ARDS patients were observed. Therefore, the ELF/plasma ratios of α_1-PI from days 1 and 2 were used to try to establish a prognosticative system. It was determined that the critical α_1-PI-ELF/plasma ratio should not exceed 0.24, giving a sensitivity of 78% and, therefore, preventing false-negative classifications of ARDS patients who therefore would not receive necessary therapy. On the other hand, 44% of non-ARDS patients would be classified as false positive and receive unnecessary therapy that might cause deleterious side effects.

Conclusion

In conclusion, the current results were considered in the context of the pathogenesis, diagnosis, and prognosis of adult respiratory distress syndrome.

After multiple trauma, patients at risk for ARDS showed a permeability increase for low and high molecular sized proteins of the endothelial-interstitial-epithelial wall early after the traumatic event (within 48 h), which was higher for patients who developed ARDS in comparison to patients who did not. This development could be predicted by the measurement of the initial ELF/plasma ratios for low molecular size proteins, e.g., for α_1PI with 78% sensitivity and 44% specificity.

Due to the posttraumatic "sealing" of the alveolar epithelium, BALF protein concentrations decreased in spite of the progressive increase in interstitial/alveolar edema. Therefore, BALF protein measurements were of no diagnostic or prognostic importance, except during the initial posttraumatic phase.

References

1. Bell DY, Haseman JA, Spock A, McLennan G, Hook GGR (1981) Plasma proteins of the bronchoalveolar surface of the lungs of smokers and nonsmokers. Am Rev Respir Dis 124:72
2. Dwenger A, Schweitzer G, Regel G (1986) Bronchoalveolar lavage fluid and plasma proteins, chemiluminescence response and protein contents of polymorphonuclear leukocytes from blood and lavage fluid in traumatized patients. J Clin Chem Clin Biochem 24:73
3. Dwenger A, Regel G, Joka T, Sturm JA, Tscherne H, Schmit-Neuerburg KP (1988) Loss of protein size selectivity of the alveolar epithelium after polytrauma. J Clin Chem Clin Biochem 26:739
4. Holter JF, Weiland JE, Pacht ER, Gadek JE, Davis WB (1986) Protein permeability in the adult respiratory distress syndrome. Loss of size selectivity of the alveolar epithelium. J Clin Invest 78:1513
5. Hunninghake GW, Gadek JE, Kawanami O, Ferrans VJ, Crystal RG (1979) Inflammatory and immune processes in the human lung in health and disease: evaluation by bronchoalveolar lavage. Am J Pathol 97:149
6. Idell S, Cohen AB (1985) Bronchoalveolar lavage in patients with the adult respiratory distress syndrome. Clin Chest Med 6:459
7. Joka T, Nakhosteen JA, Obertacke U, Herrmann J, Coenen T, Brand M, Jochum M, Zilow G, Dwenger A, Kreuzfelder E (1988) Beeinflußt die bronchoalveoläre Lavage das Milieu in der Alveole? Prax Klin Pneumol 42:705
8. Lee CT, Fein AM, Lippman M, Holtzmann H, Kimbel P, Weinbaum G (1981) Elastolytic activity in pulmonary lavage fluid from patients with adult respiratory distress syndrome. N Engl J Med 304:192
9. Lewis FR, Elings VB (1982) The measurement of extravascular lung water by thermalgreen dye indicator dilution. Ann NY Acad Sci 384:394
10. Lindena J, Trautschold I (1983) Enzymes in lymph: a review. J Clin Chem Clin Biochem 21:327
11. Marcy TW, Merrill WW, Rankin JA, Reynolds HY (1987) Limitations of using urea to quantify epithelial lining fluid recovered by bronchoalveolar lavage. Am Rev Respir Dis 135:1276
12. Rennard SI, Basset G, Lecossier D, O'Donnell KM, Pinkston P, Martin PG, Crystal RG (1986) Estimation of volume of epithelial lining fluid recovered by lavage using urea as marker of dilution. J Appl Physiol 60:532

13. Sturm JA, Wisner DH, Oestern H-J, Kant CJ, Tscherne H, Creutzig H (1986) Increased lung capillary permeability after trauma: a prospective clinical study. J Trauma 26:409
14. Yatziv S, Kahane I, Abeliuk P, Cividalli G, Rachmilewitz EA (1979) "Lysosomal" enzyme activities in red blood cells of normal individuals and patients with homozygous β-thalassaemia. Clin Chim Acta 96:67

Lung Capillary Leak After Severe Trauma: A Prospective Clinical Study

J.A. Sturm[1], D.H. Wisner[2], H.-J. Oestern[1], C.-J. Kant[1], H. Tscherne[1], H.-C. Pape[1], U. Lehmann[1], and H. Creutzig[3]

Introduction

According to our current understanding, the development of interstitial edema is the most important feature of the adult respiratory distress syndrome (ARDS). It is not known whether such increased permeability occurs immediately after trauma or is instead largely associated with the later development of a sepsis-like syndrome. However, knowing when it occurs is of critical importance if suspected biochemical and cellular factors are to be correlated with lung damage. Trying to determine whether trauma leads to a lung capillary permeability increase via the activation of neutrophils, for example, requires an understanding of when this permeability increase first occurs and how it subsequently develops.

Currently there is no good parameter for quantifying lung capillary permeability. In general, the clinical parameters of lung function used are the oxygenation quotient (OQ; Horovitz 1974) compliance, shunt fraction (Q_S/Q_T), and the alveolar-arterial difference in the partial pressure of oxygen (A-aDO_2). It is not known whether there is a delay between increases in capillary permeability and the subsequent reflection in gross measures of pulmonary function. The parameters mentioned above are sometimes heavily influenced by other variables (i.e., the influence of positive end expiratory pressure (PEEP) on compliance).

Extravascular lung water (EVLW) measurement has been suggested as a useful reflection of pulmonary vascular permeability, but opinion is divided on the correlation of increased permeability and increased EVLW. It is also not known whether compensatory mechanisms in the lung may mask increases in pulmonary permeability. So far, no prospective studies of EVLW have been performed in a large group of severely injured patients.

[1] Department of Trauma Surgery, Hannover Medical School, Konstanty-Gutschow-Str. 8, W-3000 Hannover 61, FRG
[2] Department of Surgery, University of Davis, Sacramento
[3] Department of Nuclear Medicine, Hannover Medical School, Konstanty-Gutschow-Str. 8, W-3000 Hannover 61, FRG

J.A. Sturm (Ed.)
Adult Respiratory Distress Syndrome

Sugerman et al. (1980) described a method for directly determining the degree of pulmonary capillary permeability with scintigraphic measurements of the extravasation of radiolabeled albumin. To date, however, studies have only been performed in a limited number of patients with pulmonary dysfunction; prospective investigations have not been undertaken, nor have patients been selected on the criterion of major trauma.

In this study, it was our purpose to answer the following questions:

1. When does the permeability damage occur?
2. Which relationship exists between permeability changes and the development of interstitial edema?

Materials and Methods

The inclusion criterion for the study was severe injury, i.e., more than 30 points on the polytrauma score (PTS). Patients with severe head injury (less than 8 points on the Glasgow coma scale on admission) were excluded, as were those with late hospital transfer (>120 min after trauma) (Tables 1

Table 1. Polytrauma score

Site of injury	Score	Site of injury	Score
Head		Pelvis	
1° Head injury	4	Simple pelvic fracture	3
2° Head injury	8	Multiple pelvic fracture	9
3° Head injury	12	Pelvic urogenital injury	12
Simple facial fracture	2	Spinal fracture	3
Severe facial fracture	4	Spinal cord injury	3
		Crushed pelvis	15
Abdomen		Extremities	
Ruptured spleen	9		
Ruptured liver/spleen	13–18	Central hip fracture/dislocation	12
Extensive liver injury	13–18	Simple femur fracture	8
Bowel, mesentery, kidney, or pancreas injury	9	Comminuted femur fracture	12
		Tibia/fibula fracture	4
		Knee, patella, ankle, radius, ulna fracture	2
Thorax			
Sternal, 1–3 rib fracture	2	Scapula, humerus fracture	4
>3 rib fractures (unilateral)	5	Vascular injury associated with elbow/knee injury	4
>3 rib fractures (bilateral)	10		
Hemo-, pneumo-thorax		Above-elbow/above-knee amputation	8
Lung contusion (unilateral)	7		
Lung contusion (bilateral)	9	Below-elbow/below-knee amputation	8
Unstable chest wall	3		
Aortic rupture	7	Each open 2°/3° fracture	4
		Large soft tissue injury	2

Table 2. Study admission criteria

1. polytrauma score greater than 50
2. Glasgow coma scale greater than 8 on admission
3. Age 14–65 years
4. Time between accident and primary care less than 60 min
5. Time between accident and arrival at hospital less than 120 min
6. No albumin, dextrans, or other colloids received
7. No steroids, barbiturates, or proteinase inhibitors received
8. No patients operated upon for head injury
9. No patients in whom extracorporeal circulation was used
10. No patients transferred from other facilities

and 2). Patients initially treated at other institutions and subsequently transferred to us were also excluded. All of our patients were blunt trauma victims. During initial resuscitation and operative intervention, extensive blood samples and hemodynamic measurements were taken. These were continued on a regular basis for the duration of the 14-day study period. The investigations and measurements made and their frequency are shown in Table 3.

Within 6 h of injury, both a pulmonary artery catheter and an EVLW catheter (Edwards Model 96B-020-5F, Am. Edwards Labs, Irvine, CA, USA) were placed. Pulmonary artery catheters were placed via either an internal jugular or a subclavian approach, and EVLW catheters via the femoral artery. All patients required mechanical ventilation on admission. Levels of inspired oxygen concentration (FiO_2), PEEP, and inspiratory to expiratory ratio (I:E) were adjusted to ensure an arterial oxygen concentration (PaO_2) of at least 80 mmHg when possible. Tidal volume and ventilatory rates were

Table 3. Blood study protocol

Study performed	Frequency
Electrolytes, blood urea nitrogen	Every 6 h for 48 h, then every
Prothrombin time/partial thromboplastin time, platelet count	12 h, for 14 days
Specialized clotting studies (e.g., antithrombin III)	Twice daily for 14 days
Blood gases (arterial and venous)	Daily for 14 days
Creatinin clearance	
Endotoxin	Every other day for 14 days
	Admission, days 2, 4, 8, and 12
Differential white blood cell count	Admission, days 4, 8, and 12
Cytotoxicity	
Lysosomal enzymes	
Proteinase inhibitors, fibronectin	
Glucose, pyruvate, lactate	
Prostaglandin, thromboxane	
Monocyte, granulocyte function tests	
Lymphocyte function tests	

generally set to yield arterial CO_2 values no greater than 35–40 mm Hg. Volume ventilators were used in all cases, but high-frequency ventilation was not employed in any patient.

Both arterial and mixed venous blood samples were drawn for blood gas determinations at 6-h intervals for the first 48 h and subsequently at 12-h intervals for a total of 14 days. Arterial pressure, pulmonary artery pressure, central venous pressure, pulmonary artery wedge pressure, and cardiac output (CO) were determined according to the same time schedule as used for blood gas determinations. Peak inspiratory and plateau pressures, FIO_2, and PEEP levels at the time of measurement were also recorded. Chest X-rays were also taken every 6 h for the first 48 h and subsequently at 12-h intervals for a total of 14 days. CO was measured in threefold at each measurement time by injecting 10 ml iced saline at 0°C via the central venous port of the pulmonary artery catheter. A commercially available bedside CO computer (HMV 7905, Hoyer GmbH., Bremen, FRG) connected to the thermistor of the pulmonary artery catheter was used to calculate CO by thermodilution. The cardiac index was subsequently calculated from the averaged value of CO with standard nomograms for body surface area in adults, using admission values for height and body weight.

Table 4 lists the various parameters measured as possible indicators of lung permeability as well as the frequency with which they were studied. The OQ is a derived value determined by dividing the PaO_2 by the FIO_2. Dynamic compliance (DC) was determined with the aid of a VRP respiratory monitor (Research Development Corporation, San Francisco, CA, USA). The A-aDO_2 and the Q_S/Q_T percentage were calculated using formulas for patients receiving less than 100% oxygen.

EVLW was determined by the double indicator thermodilution technique as refined for bedside use by Lewis and Sturm (Lewis and Sturm 1979; Sturm et al. 1979). Indocyanine green (Cardio-Green, 10 ml of a 2.5% solution; Hynson, Westcott, and Dunning, Baltimore, MD, USA) and iced saline were the indicators for intravascular and total lung water, respectively. A lung water computer (Edwards Model 9310, Edwards Laboratories, Santa Ana, USA) was used for bedside determinations and calculations. EVLW was determined in triplicate and averaged. These averaged values were then

Table 4. Measures of pulmonary capillary permeability

Measure	Frequency
Oxygenation quotient (OQ)	Every 6 h for 48 h then every 12 h for 14 days
Dynamic compliance (DC)	
Alveolar-arterial difference in the partial pressure of oxygen (A-aDO_2)	Within 24 h of admission, then daily when possible
Shunt fraction percentage ($Q_S/Q_T \times 100$)	
Extravascular lung water (EVLW)	
Albumin extravasation scintigraphy (SI)	

normalized by dividing by the admission body weight, and EVLW values are thus reported as milliliter per kilogram body weight.

The extravasation of labeled albumin was determined scintigraphically using a modified version of the method developed by Sugerman et al.(1980). It was done whenever possible within the first 24 h after trauma and then subsequently on a daily basis. The study required transport of patients to the nuclear medicine department, therefore not all patients were studied within the first 24 h or on a daily basis. The imaging technique used was always the same. Patients were placed under a gamma camera (ZLC 370, Siemens Gamma Sonics, FRG) and care was taken not to alter either the patient's position or any of the ventilatory parameters during the course of the extravasation study. After positioning, 0.1 mg of human albumin (CIS, St. Quentin, France) labeled with 5–7 mCi of technetium-99m was injected through the central venous port of the pulmonary artery catheter. The initial 300 s after injection were used to designate *regions of interest* in the heart and both lungs. Pulmonary regions of interest were 30 cm^2 in size and taken from the lateral part of the lung. Scanning was then done at 10-s intervals for

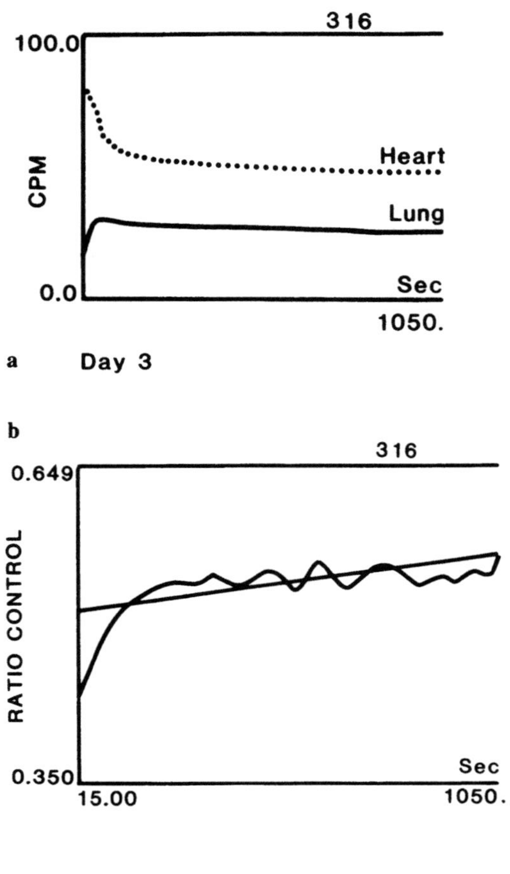

Fig. 1a,b. Extravasation study in patients on the third day of the study to show the degree of activity in the lungs and the heart. **a** Curves of the regions of interest in the heart (*dotted line*) and the lungs (*unbroken line*). *CPM*, counts per minute. **b** Curve of the changes in the lung/heart ratio.

20 min. The ratio of the degree of activity in the lungs to the degree of activity in the heart was made for each 10-s time period and plotted against time. A linear regression analysis of this plot for the time interval 5–15 min after injection was done by the method of least squares. The slope (or slope index, SI) of the resultant regression line was determined. This slope, reported as units per time interval is an indicator of the degree of permeability in the lungs (see Fig. 1). Figure 1a shows the curves for the cardiac and pulmonary regions of interest. In Fig. 1b, the curve of the change in the lung/heart ratio with time is shown. The linear regression of this curve is also shown. As can be seen, higher SI are indicative of increased levels of permeability.

Our use of the time interval 5–15 min after injections represents a modification of the method used by Sugerman et al. (1981). In their studies, the first 15 min after injection are considered an equilibration period and linear regression is performed between 15 and 45 min after injection. We compared 'early slopes' obtained between 5 and 15 min after injection with 'late slopes' obtained between 15 and 45 min after injection in 22 different studies. The result is shown in Fig. 2. As can be seen, the correlation is high. It was important to minimize the time necessary for the investigation to be performed, we therefore felt justified in limiting our scanning to this 'early slope' time period.

Two control groups were also studied using albumin extravasation scintigraphy. One group (n = 7) consisted of patients without known lung pathology who were undergoing cardiac ejection fraction studies. These studies were used to determine normal values for albumin extravasation and the SI. A second group (n = 5) was made up of patients studied within 48 h of routine elective total hip replacement. None had preexisting lung disease. All of these patients had routine operative and postoperative courses and none was intubated at the time of scan.

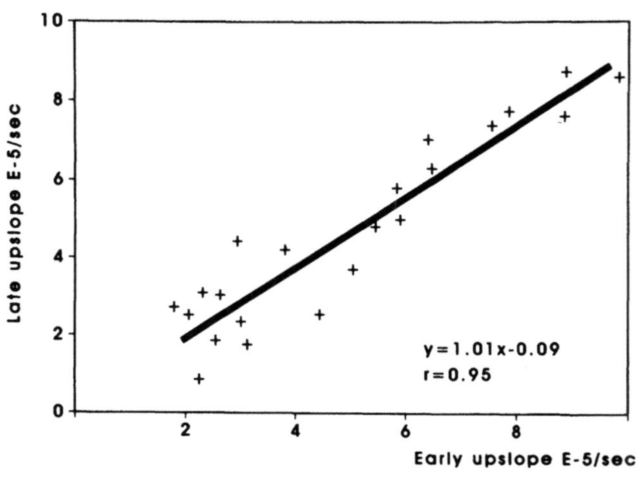

Fig. 2. Comparison of different curve fittings

Results

A total of 22 patients were studied. There were 17 men and 5 women; the average age was 38.4 years, the average PTS was 43.9 ± 12.6, and the average injury severity score (ISS) was 33.8 ± 6.6. The mortality in this study group was 54.6% (12/22). Most of these deaths (8/12) occurred at least 1 week after injury. Because of the high mortality during the 2nd week of the study, data presented as mean values are shown only for the first 7 days of the study period. Values are reported as mean ± standard error of the mean unless otherwise stated.

Data for the OQ are seen in Fig. 3. At 6 h after admission, the OQ was 385.2 ± 27.7 mmHg. The mean value for the OQ remained between 345 and

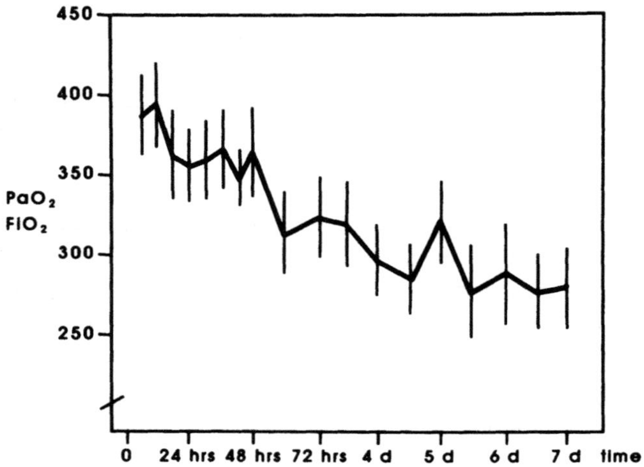

Fig. 3. Data for the oxygenation quotient

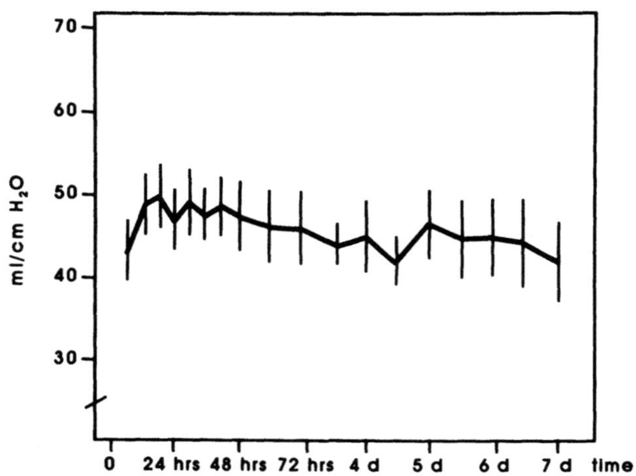

Fig. 4. Data for dynamic compliance

400 mmHg until 48 h after trauma. Between 48 and 72 h, it dropped from 365.0 ± 26.2 mmHg to 323.0 ± 18.8 mmHg and remained at or below this level for the following 4 days.

DC is shown in Fig. 4. The 6-h value was 43.6 ± 3.2 ml/cm H_2O. This increased to 50.7 ± 4.0 ml/cm H_2O by 12 h and remained between 40 and 55 ml/cm H_2O for the first 7 days after trauma, reaching a low of 41.4 ± 3.2 ml/cm H_2O on day 4. There was a steady, gradual decrease in compliance seen between 48 h and 4–5 days after trauma. Figure 5 contains data for the A-aDO_2. As with the OQ and the DC, this parameter deteriorated between 48 and 72 h (88.7 ± 13.3 mm Hg vs 118.6 ± 25.4 mm Hg) The A-aDO_2 continued to increase over days 4–7.

Q_S/Q_T (Fig. 6) revealed a somewhat different course, with an increase seen as early as 12 h after trauma. The 6-h value was 7.0 ± 1.4%, compared with 48- and 72-h values of 11.7 ± 2.1% and 13.5 ± 2.1%, respectively. By

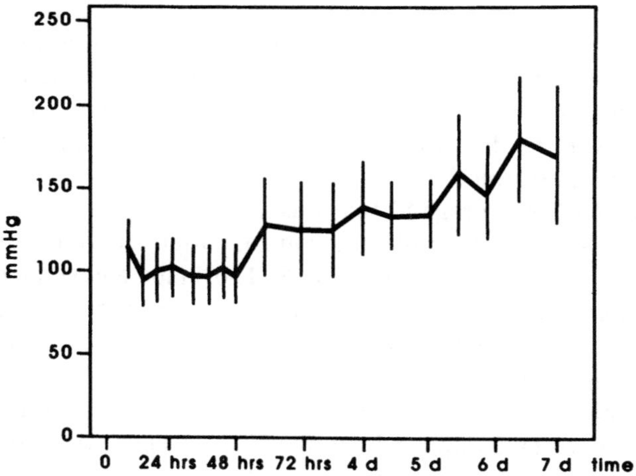

Fig. 5. Data for the arterial-alveolar difference in partial pressure of oxygen

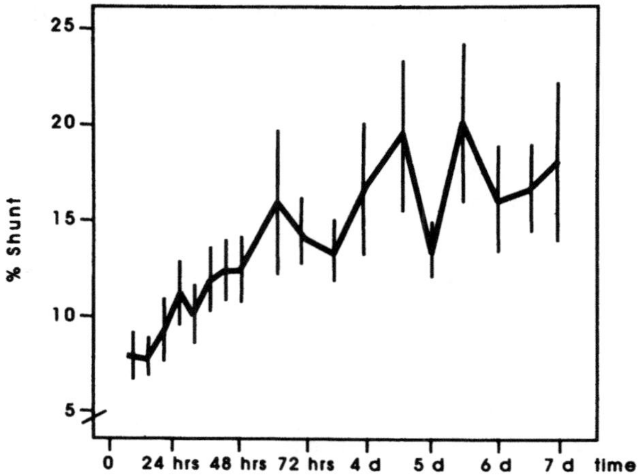

Fig. 6. Data for the shunt fraction

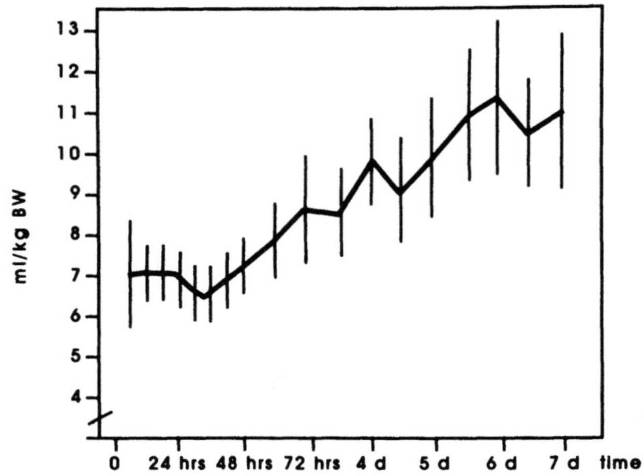

Fig. 7. Data for extravascular lung water

4.5 days after trauma, the mean value for Q_S/Q_T had reached $19.5 \pm 3.5\%$.

EVLW data are seen in Fig. 7. The 6-h value for this parameter was 6.9 ± 1.03 ml/kg and had risen only to a value of 7.11 ± 0.49 ml/kg within the first 48 h. By 72 h EVLW had risen substantially to 8.46 ± 1.00 ml/kg and it continued to increase over the following 4 days. A total of 82 albumin extravasation studies were performed.

The control patients had an average SI that was actually negative: $(-0.1 \pm 0.7) \times 10^{-5}$ s (mean ± SD). An example of a control patient curve for the change in lung/heart ratio with time is seen in Fig. 8. The shape and slope of this curve can be compared with the example from a study patient seen in Fig. 16. The range of SI values between -2 SD and $+2$ SD from the control patient mean of -0.1×10^{-5} s was between -1.5×10^{-5} s and 1.3×10^{-5} s. The upper limit of normal for the SI was thus set at 1.3×10^{-5} s. Using a range of ± 2 SD should encompass approximately 95% of expected normal values for the SI if it is assumed to be normally distributed.

The average value for patients studied after hip replacement was $(1.6 \pm 0.9) \times 10^{-5}$ s (mean ± SD). Patients in this group had significantly higher SI

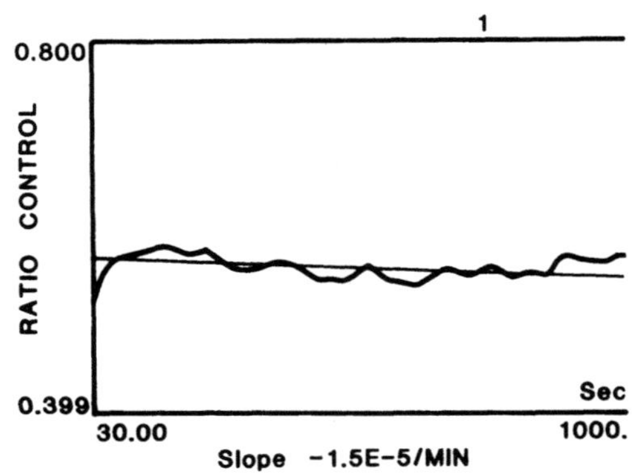

Fig. 8. Curve of the changes in the lung/heart ratio in control patients

than controls ($p < 0.05$, two-tailed t-test for unpaired data). In the trauma study patients, there was a great deal of variation both in different individuals and in different time periods in the same individual. The values for SI performed within 24 h of trauma, for example, ranged between 0.8×10^{-5} s and 83.0×10^{-5} s. What was striking in spite of this variation was the regularity with which the SI was above the upper limit of normal; 87.5% of the studies done within 24 h of trauma were above 1.3×10^{-5} s, as were 75% of the studies done on the 2nd day. Over the entire 2-week period of the study, 88.6% of the investigations done were above this normal upper limit. These data are summarized in Fig. 9.

Also of interest were five studies done in three different patients at 3 weeks (three studies) and 4 weeks (two studies) after trauma. The SI values for the studies done at 3 weeks were 0.5, 4.35, and $4.5 \times 10 \times {}^{-5}$ s. Values for the studies done at 4 weeks were -0.35 and 3.8×10^{-5} s.

The time courses of the SI compared with that of EVLW for two different patients are shown in Fig. 10. Figure 10a shows the time course for the SI and EVLW in a patient who survived. Values for the SI were generally above the normal range. However, this was not reflected by increased EVLW. In Figure 10b, the course for a nonsurvivor who died on the 12th day after trauma is shown. The SI was elevated throughout this patient's early course, but

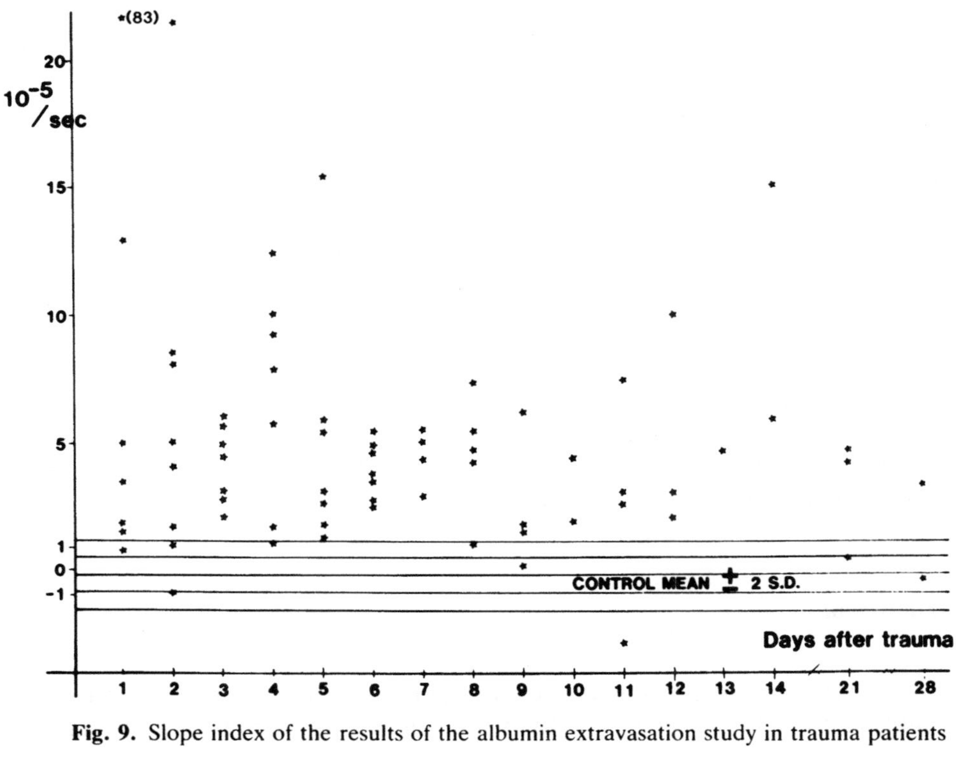

Fig. 9. Slope index of the results of the albumin extravasation study in trauma patients

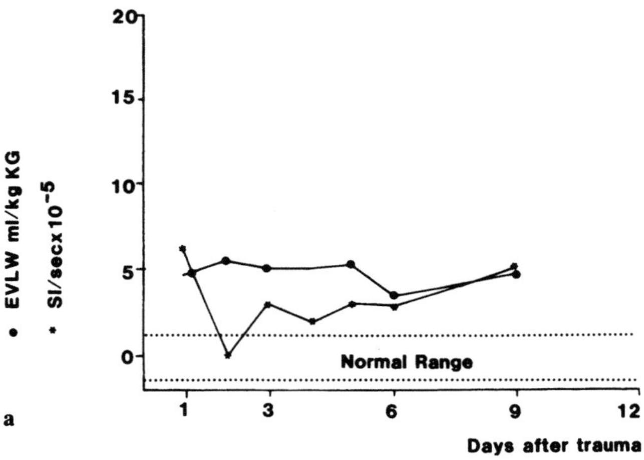

a

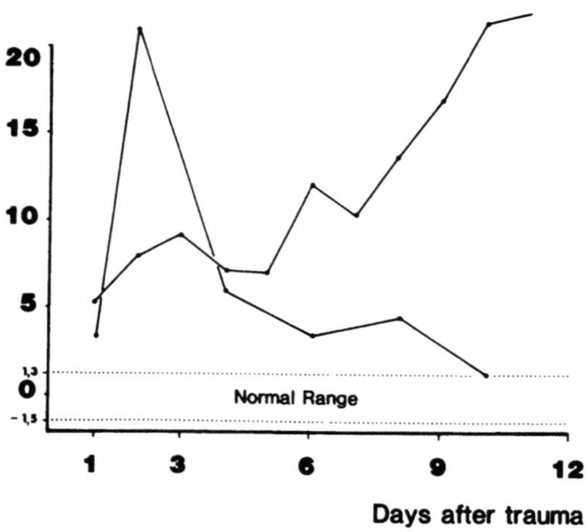

b

Fig. 10a,b. Comparison of the time courses for extravascular lung water (*EVLW*) and slope index (*SI*) in a patients who survived (**a**) and in a patient who died (**b**)

decreased during his later course simultaneous with a marked increase in the EVLW. This pattern of a decrease in the SI to normal or near normal values in the presence of markedly increased EVLW was repeatedly seen in nonsurvivors shortly before death.

Discussion

The assessment of pulmonary capillary permeability in vivo is extremely difficult. In addition to the commonly used clinical parameters of pulmonary function, a variety of different methods have been tried. In animals, draining of lung and lung lymph can be used as a quantitative reflection of fluid and solute flux across the pulmonary capillary membrane. Using radioactively labeled substances with different volumes of distribution, a number of different techniques have been developed to measure capillary permeability in the lung. Due to practical considerations associated with using several different radioactive substances and external counting of multiple blood samples, the clinical use of these techniques is limited. Also, there are concerns about the accuracy of some of these methods in clinical settings.

For example, it has been proposed that radiolabeled markers should be injected intravenously and radioactivity should be subsequently measured in tracheal suction samples. However, frequent suctioning has to be performed, and blood sampling as well as precise quantification of the relative volumes of tracheal fluid are necessary. The determination of clearance times after inhalation has also been suggested. This is a method which involves the use of radioactive aerosols and which cannot discriminate between increases in alveolar and in endothelial permeability.

Sugerman et al. (1984) developed a method by which scintigraphy is used to measure albumin extravasation. This method offers several advantages in a clinical setting:

1. It is easily repeatable on a daily or even more frequent basis and is relatively easy to perform
2. Doses of radioactivity are small, and only one radiolabel is used so that counting is simplified
3. The method has been extensively evaluated in animal experiments and the level of albumin extravasation has been shown to correlate well with the different levels of pulmonary damage produced by varying doses of oleic acid.

In a previous clinical study, a group of patients identified as suffering from respiratory failure were studied using this method. They were found to have increased SI compared with patients recovering from congestive heart failure and head injury and with controls. It was also noted that the SI could remain elevated for an extended period. The patient population in this study already had established pulmonary dysfunction. They suffered from a variety of underlying illnesses including wound infections, peritonitis, and mediastinitis. Only a few patients had suffered moderate to severe trauma. No conclusions about the onset or time course of changes in albumin extravasation after trauma could therefore be made.

The patients in our study were measured as soon as possible after trauma; all of them were studied on a prospective basis. By limiting our study to multiple trauma victims, we investigated only patients whose initial insult could be precisely defined temporarily. We were thus better able to follow the subsequent changes in various tests of pulmonary function and permeability. We found that the commonly used clinical measures of pulmonary function did not generally show marked deterioration until at least 48 h after trauma. The OQ, DC, and A-aDO_2 were all relatively stable between 12 and 48 h after trauma. Between 48 and 72 h, all three deteriorated. Although beginning to rise somewhat sooner, Q_S/Q_T also showed substantial increases between 48 and 72 h, and the lowest values for this parameter were found in the first 24 h after trauma. These findings appear to indicate either an acute change in permeability occurring between 48 and 72 h or that the reflection of permeability change with an earlier time of onset is not seen immediately in these parameters.

EVLW was also remarkedly stable for up to 48 h, at which point it began to increase markedly. Previous studies have shown a good correlation between the level of EVLW and survival. The time course of EVLW in our patients again suggests either a marked increase in pulmonary capillary permeability beginning several days after trauma, or the delayed reflection of earlier and possibly compensated permeability increases. Endotoxemia and the onset of the beginning stages of sepsis are one etiologic possibility for the change in clinical parameters and EVLW often seen after several days.

We found a strikingly different time course in our results of albumin extravasation. The frequent finding of markedly elevated SI as early as 24 h after trauma indicates an increase in permeability occurring much earlier than detected by currently used measures. A number of events known to be associated with severe trauma could cause this early permeability increase. Complement activation, microemboli of fat, platelets, and fibrin, and the activation of granulocytes are possible factors. The reason why methods other than albumin extravasation scintigraphy are unable to demonstrate this early increase in permeability may be a lag time between the onset of increased permeability and its subsequent detection. It is also possible that the increase in permeability must reach a certain level in order to create measurable interstitial edema. EVLW, for example, can detect only accumulations of fluid in the lung. The extensive lymph drainage capacity of the lung may be able to temporarily compensate for a permeability increase and increase in transendothelial fluid flux into the interstitial space. It is only when this compensatory mechanism is overwhelmed, that the EVLW begins to rise. This may be due to further increases in permeability or gradual accumulation. Changes in the OQ, DC, A-aDo_2, and Q_S/Q_T only indirectly reflect changes in lung water and are, therefore, even less sensitive to the earliest changes in pulmonary capillary permeability.

We did not see consistent correlations between the SI and other parameters. Many of our patients had elevated SI throughout their entire 2-week study course and the small number of scintigraphic investigations done at 3 and 4 weeks after trauma revealed that persistent elevations in the SI are possible even late in a patient's course and are not necessarily correlated with progressive deterioration in the clinical status.

The typical course of EVLW in patients who die with post-traumatic ARDS can be seen in the example in Fig. 10b. While often stable at normal or only modestly elevated levels during the early post-trauma period, the EVLW shows progressive and marked elevation during this patient's later course. The increase in EVLW is associated with a worsening of pulmonary function and is often seen in conjunction with sepsis and multiple organ failure.

Surprisingly, a number of our patients had a normal or only midly elevated SI, coincident with very high preterminal values for EVLW. If the pulmonary capillary permeability increase associated with ARDS was due to a progressive lesion, parallel increases in the SI and EVLW would be expected. The finding of decreasing SI in a setting of marked increases in EVLW and impairment of pulmonary function may indicate that, at some point, the permeability damage becomes so severe that back-diffusion and slowed equilibration of albumin across the endothelium results in abnormally low values for the SI. Another explanation, however, is more likely: Swenger et al. (1988, 1989) found in our group of severely injured patients that in the late phase fewer cells can be found within the lavage fluid. They concluded that a repair mechanism must be activated which subsequently leads to closure of the capillary leak. These observations agree with those found in electron-microscopical investigations in patients dying in the late phase from ARDS (Bartels et al., this volume).

It could also be discussed that patients with high EVLW and impaired pulmonary function were being ventilated with high levels of PEEP and that the SI was reduced as a result. Work with experimental animals, however, has indicated that PEEP has minimal effects on the SI. A linear regression of SI as a function of the level of PEEP for all of the studies done in our patients with, moreover, no correlation ($y = 6.28 - 0.0182x$; $r = -0.0058$), argues against a simple relationship between these parameters.

Thus, elevated SI seen after trauma cannot be explained simply by the fact that our study patients were ventilated and that the control patients were not. Previous clinical studies have shown that patients intubated and receiving positive pressure ventilation can have consistently normal SI. Furthermore, the finding of a significantly increased SI after elective total hip replacement indicates that a smaller degree of trauma can also induce changes in pulmonary capillary permeability and that these are detectable in patients who are breathing spontaneously.

We were able to show that severe trauma can induce an early increase in pulmonary capillary permeability. This is not reflected by EVLW or clinical measures of pulmonary function until 48–72 h after the traumatic event. We did not find a relationship between increases in pulmonary capillary permeability leading to clinically evident ARDS and the onset of sepsis. These findings must be kept in mind when further investigations in this respect are planned. The time course of permeability changes associated with severe illness other than multiple trauma and with lesser forms of injury require further investigation.

References

1. Horovitz JH, Carrico CJ, Shires GT (1974) Pulmonary response to major injury. Arch Surg 108:349–355
2. Lewis FR, Sturm JA (1979) Bedside measurement of lung water. J Surg Res 27:250–261
3. Dwenger A, Regel G, Joka T, Sturm JA, Tscherne H, Schmit-Neuerburg KP (1988) Loss of protein size selectivity of the alveolar epithelium after polytrauma. Clin Chem Clin Biochem 26
4. Dwenger A, Regel G, Joka T, Sturm JA, Tscherne H, Schmit-Neuerburg KP (1989) Verlust der Molekülgrößen-Selektivität des Alveolarepithels für Plasmaproteine bei Patienten nach Polytrauma. Chir Forum 8:109–113
5. Sturm JA, Lewis RF, Elings VJ (1979), Bettseitige Bestimmung des extravasculären Lungenswassers. Langenbecks Arch [Suppl.] Chir Forum 8:73–77
6. Sugerman HJ, Hirsch JI, Strash AM (1980) Preliminary report: Gamma camera detection of oleic acid alveolar-capillary albumin leak. J Surg Res 29:93–99
7. Sugerman HJ, Tatum JL, Strash AM (1981) Effects of pulmonary vascular recruitment on gamma scintigraphy and pulmonary capillary protein leak. Surgery 90:388–395
8. Sugerman HJ, Tatum JL, Burke TS (1984) Gamma scintigraphic analysis of albumin flux in patients with acute respiratory distress syndrome. Surgery 95:674–681

Alveolar Surfactant Function in Severely Injured Patients

W. Seeger[1], U. Pison[1], Th. Joka[2], and H. Neuhof[1]

Introduction

Lack of surfactant material is the underlying abnormality of the respiratory distress syndrome in preterm infants [1–3]. Surfactant abnormalities have also been implicated in the development of adult respiratory distress in adults (ARDS) [4]. This view is supported by similarities in pulmonary failure between patients with ARDS and preterm babies with respiratory distress syndrome, as well as diffuse alveolar collapse suggesting altered surfactant properties in ARDS. Mechanisms of surfactant alteration in the course of ARDS could not only include absolute lack of surface-active compounds, but also alterations in its phospholipid or protein composition [5, 6]. There are several lines of evidence that increased lung endothelial and epithelial permeability is the decisive step in the development of ARDS or different etiology [7–11]. Subsequent leakage of protein-rich edema fluid into the interstitial and the alveolar space has been implicated in alterations of surfactant properties due to protein surfactant interaction [12–16].

There are, however, only very few data on surfactant properties of patients suffering from ARDS and being artifically ventilated. Von Wichert and Kohl [17] described a decreased dipalmitoyl-phosphatidylcholine content in lung specimens from patients dying with ARDS. Petty et al. [18] observed abnormalities in lung elastic properties and in surface tension behavior of alveolar surfactant, obtained by postmortal lung washing in patients who succumbed from this syndrome. Hallman et al. [19], who studied the lavage phospholipid profile in patients with respiratory failure of different etiology, noted a marked decrease in phosphatidylcholine as well as phosphatidylglycerol, accompanied by a relative increase in the other phospholipid species in the lavage material. Moreover, he found some decrease in the minimal

[1] Department of Trauma Surgery, University Medical School, Hufelandstr. 55, W-4300 Essen, FRG
[2] Division of Clinical Pathophysiology, Department of Internal Medicine, Justus-Liebig-University, Klinikstr. 36, W-6300 Giessen, FRG

J.A. Sturm (Ed.)
Adult Respiratory Distress Syndrome

surface tension of surfactant material isolated from lavage fluid of three of these patients.

We evaluated surfactant abnormalities in severely injured patients during the course of posttraumatic pulmonary dysfunction. Trauma patients were selected because of the homogeneity of the primary event (underlying disease of ARDS) as well as the consistency in time relationship between the insult and the development of respiratory failure in several of these patients. The study was part of the research program *Grundmechanismen des posttraumatischen progressiven Lungenversagens*, supported by the Deutsche Forschungsgemeinschaft. It was the aim of the study to describe the time course of surfactant abnormalities after onset of the initial event, to find correlations between biophysical (surface tension behavior) and biochemical (phospholipids, protein extravasation) alterations of the surfactant material, and to correlate changes in surfactant properties with the severity of respiratory failure developing in these patients. The results have been published previously [20].

Materials and Methods

The alveolar phospholipid composition, surface tension characteristics, and protein and neutrophil content were determined in serially obtained bronchoalveolar lavage fluids. For this purpose, fiberoptic bronchoscopy was carried out every 2nd day, beginning within the first 24 h after trauma and ending on the 14th day after the insult (lavage volume, 100 ml 0.15 *M* sodium chloride with an overall recovery of 60%–70% by volume). After spinning, the supernatant was analyzed for protein content (staining with Coomassy brilliant blue) [21], organic phospholipids after extraction by the Folch procedure [22, 23], and hemoglobin by standard techniques. High-performance liquid chromatography was used to separate different surfactant phospholipids including phosphatidylcholine (PC), phosphatidylglycerol (PG), phosphatidylethanolamine (PE), phosphatidylinositol (PI), phosphatitic acid (PA), sphingomyelin (SPH), phosphatidyl serine (PS), and lysophosphatidylcholine (LPC) [24]. Surface tension was measured in a modified Langmuir-Wilhelmy surface balance [25, 26], using techniques previously described in detail [16]. As the lavage material obtained from these severely injured patients was highly diluted, it was concentrated approximately fivefold by positive pressure ultrafiltration [27, 28]. Fifty micrograms surfactant phospholipids in a maximum volume of 500 μl was then applied to the Wilhelmy balance by using Trurnit's method for surface spreading [29, 30]. The reproducibility of this technique was found to be very high for all surface tension parameters (standard deviation less than 5%). The coordinates of the sixth surface tension area diagram were evaluated for hysteresis area, minimal surface tension, and stability index (example given in Fig. 1).

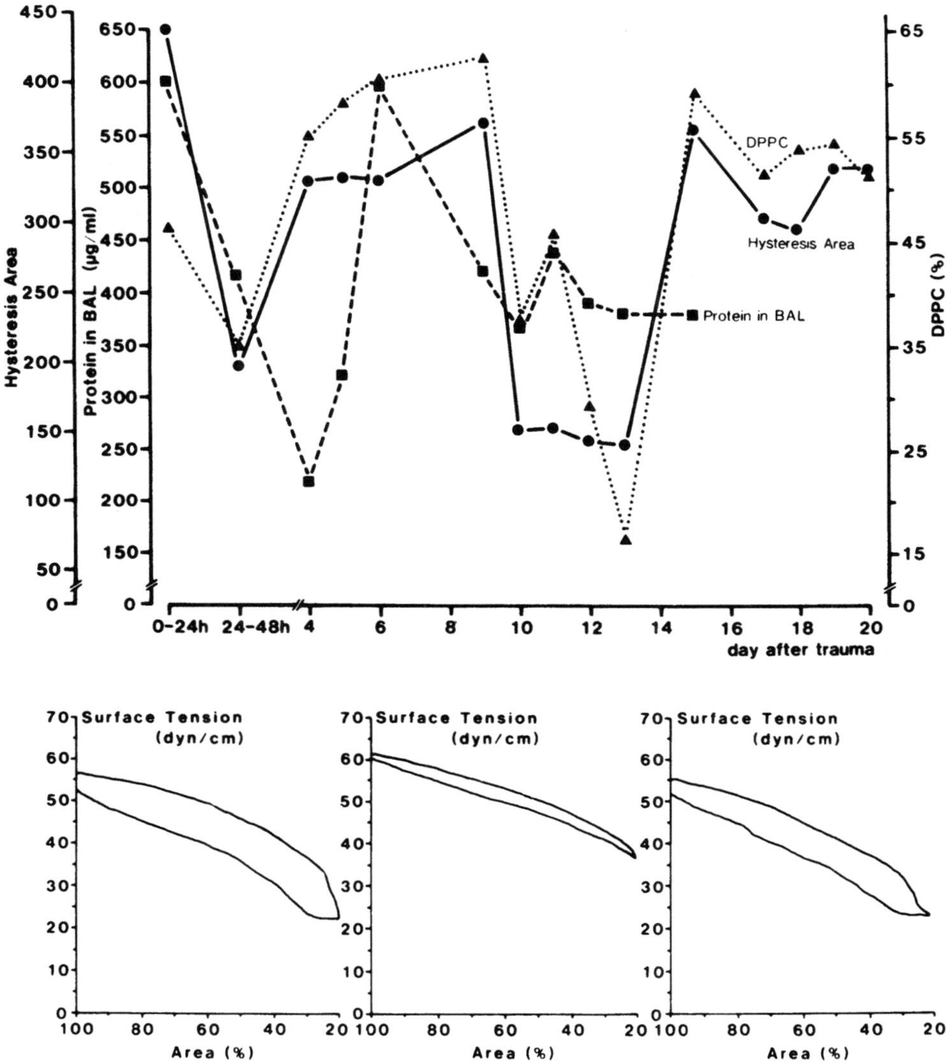

Fig. 1. *Upper*, Time course of hysteresis area, lavage protein content, and percentage of dipalmitoyl-phosphatidylcholine in lavage phospholipids (%DPPC) of a patient with a high overall ARDS score. *Lower*, Examples of surface tension isotherms (sixth cycle) obtained from lavage samples of this patient taken on day 1 (*left*), day 11 (*middle*), and day 16 (*right*) after trauma

The assessment of respiratory failure was based on a composite scoring system that combined separate evaluation of chest radiographs (range 0–4), oxygenation index ($p(Aa)O_2/pAO_2$), mean pulmonary aterial pressure, and respiratory system compliance [31, 32]. The variables of this composite respiratory failure score are weighted by using different multipliers. Patients were scored for respiratory failure every 6 h within the first 48 h after trauma

Table 1. Variables of respiratory failure, phospholipid lung profile, and in vitro surfactant function

Variables	Low ARDS score			High ARDS score			All injured patients			Healthy volunteers		
	Mean	SE	*n*	Mean	SE	*n*	Mean	SE	*n*	Mean	SE	*n*
ARDS score	0.40	0.03	267	0.78	0.04	267	0.61	0.01	534			
Mean PAP (mmHg)	19.43	0.42	334	28.18	0.50	293	23.52	0.37	627			
Compliance (ml/cm H_2O)	54.68	0.86	298	44.51	0.80	291	49.65	0.62	589			
$p(A\text{-}a)O_2/pAO_2$	0.276	0.010	369	0.533	0.013	310	0.393	0.009	679			
Shunt (QS/QT) (%)	3.10	0.23	369	7.49	0.38	310	5.10	0.23	679			
Protein (μg/ml)	143.4	12.6	75	320.8	27.3	58	220.8	15.8	133	117.9	8.4	29
Hemoglobin (mg/ml)	<0.1	–	74	<0.1	–	58	<0.1	–	132	<0.1	–	29
Total phospholipids (μg/ml)	65.7	7.4	77	65.1	5.8	58	65.4	4.8	135	84.1	5.9	29
PC[a](%)	56.3	1.0	77	48.1	1.4	58	52.8	0.9	135	62.8	1.2	29
PG(%)	1.60	0.25	77	1.88	0.26	58	1.71	0.18	135	10.02	0.67	29
SPH(%)	12.28	0.52	77	14.21	0.72	58	13.11	0.43	135	7.37	0.51	29
PI(%)	13.54	0.49	77	13.95	0.86	58	13.72	0.46	135	8.32	0.41	29
PE(%)	13.65	0.76	77	18.68	1.48	58	15.8	0.80	135	4.82	0.94	29
PA(%)	0.90	0.07	77	2.10	0.26	58	1.40	0.13	135	0.85	0.20	29
Hysteresis area[b]	313.6	12.0	75	252.0	14.9	58	286.7	9.7	133	405.7	13.1	29
Stability index	0.693	0.018	75	0.685	0.023	58	0.690	0.014	133	0.619	0.037	29
Minimum surface tension	30.86	0.82	75	28.58	0.73	58	29.87	0.57	133	34.90	1.47	29
PMN in lavage[c] ($\times 10^3$/ml)	237.4	93.3	75	136.3	32.9	47	198.4	58.7	122	13.4	3.4	28
PMN in lavage (%)	34.5	2.1	74	39.4	2.0	58	37.0	1.1	132	5.3	0.9	29

The table gives mean values averaged over the entire observation period (14 days) of 17 traumatized patients (10 with low ARDS score, 7 with high ARDS score), as well as mean values of 29 lavages obtained from 10 healthy volunteers

[a] All classes of phospholipids are given as a percentage of the total amount of phospholipids in the bronchoalveolar lavage fluid. The abbreviations are: PC, dipalmitoylphosphatidylcholine; PG, phosphatidylglycerol; SPH, sphingomyelin; PI, phosphatidylinositol; PE, phosphatidylethanolamine; PA, phosphatidic acid; PAP, pulmonary artery pressure; The difference from 100% results from the amount of phosphatidylserine and lysophosphatidylcholine

[b] Dimensions of the different surface tension parameters are given under "Methods"

[c] Total number of neutrophils (PMNs)/ml recovered lavage fluid as well as the percentage of this cell type in total lavage cell is given. [20]

and subsequently every 24 h. Based on these sequential respiratory failure scores, a mean score was calculated for the whole observation period. Using a computerized regression model the whole group of patients were thus divided into two subgroups, one with a high overall ARDS score, and one with a low overall ARDS score (mild pulmonary dysfunction) (see Table 1). The groups did not differ significantly in age or sex, and the overall survival rate was 40% in the patients with a low ARDS score and 28% in the patients with a high ARDS score (in total 17 traumatized patients were analyzed for surfactant function).

As a control group, ten healthy volunteers (all engaged in the study) underwent three bronchoalveolar lavages each by the corresponding procedure.

Results

The lavage protein content was markedly increased in the patients with a high overall ARDS score, compared with traumatized patients with a low ARDS score and compared with healthy volunteers (Table 1, Fig. 2). Analysis of the time course showed that the significantly higher alveolar protein load could

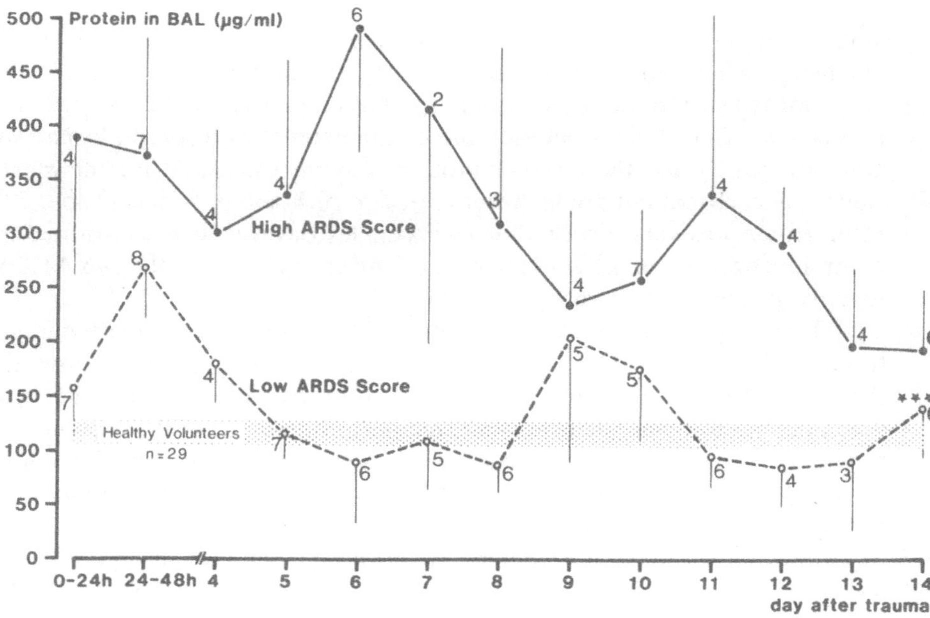

Fig. 2. Time course of the lavage protein content of patients belonging to the group with a high and with a low ARDS score. The number of observations on each day after trauma are given. *Shaded area* indicates mean ± SE of protein detected in 29 lavage fluids of healthy volunteers. The groups with high and low ARDS scores differ highly significantly (***, $p < 0.001$). [20]

Table 2. Pearson correlation coefficients – selected variables[a]

	ARDS score	Protein content	Hysteresis area	Stability index	PMN content	IgG content
Protein	0.62 $p < 0.05$ $n = 17$					
Hysteresis area	−0.57 $p < 0.05$ $n = 17$	−0.47 NS $n = 17$			−0.45 NS $n = 11$	−0.56 $p < 0.05$ $n = 17$
%PC	−0.77 $p < 0.05$ 17	−0.57 $p < 0.05$ 17	0.62 $p < 0.05$ 17	0.56 $p < 0.05$ 11	−0.36 NS	
%PE	0.65 $p < 0.05$ 17		−0.40 NS 17	−0.34 NS 17		

[a] Pearson correlation coefficients for mean values (one value for each patient and each variable) were calculated. Each cell gives correlation coefficient, statistical significance, and number of patients. The data used to calculate the Pearson product moment and the abbreviations are as for Table 1. NS, not significant. [20]

also be demonstrated within the first 24 h after trauma, often already in the first lavage taken within 6 h. In many patients, this protein leakage anteceded alterations in surfactant biophysical properties and phospholipid composition (see below). Correlations between these parameters (for instance, hysteresis area and %PC) and the alveolar protein content, calculated for the mean values of each patient, ranged between $r = 0.4$ and $r = 0.6$ (Table 2). Hemoglobin was very low in all lavage samples (lavages were performed in nontraumatized areas) and did not differ significantly between the two ARDS severity groups or the healthy controls.

There was a marked influx of granulocytes into the alveolar space in all traumatized patients ($198 \pm 58 \times 10^3$ polymorphonuclear neutrophils (PMNs)/ml in all injured patients vs. $13.4 \pm 3.4 \times 10^3$ PMNs/ml in the healthy volunteers). However, there was no significant difference in the absolute or relative alveolar PMN content between the patients with high and low ARDS, and there was no significant correlation between PMN efflux and alterations in surfactant properties.

The total phospholipid content in the lavage samples displayed quite large variability, but no significant difference between the two ARDS severity groups or the whole group of multiply injured patients and the control subjects was noted. The phospholipid profile in the lavage fluid was, however, markedly altered (Fig. 3, Table 1). There was a marked decrease in %PC in all injured patients, significantly more pronounced in patients with a high overall ARDS score than those with mild pulmonary dysfunction. Studies of

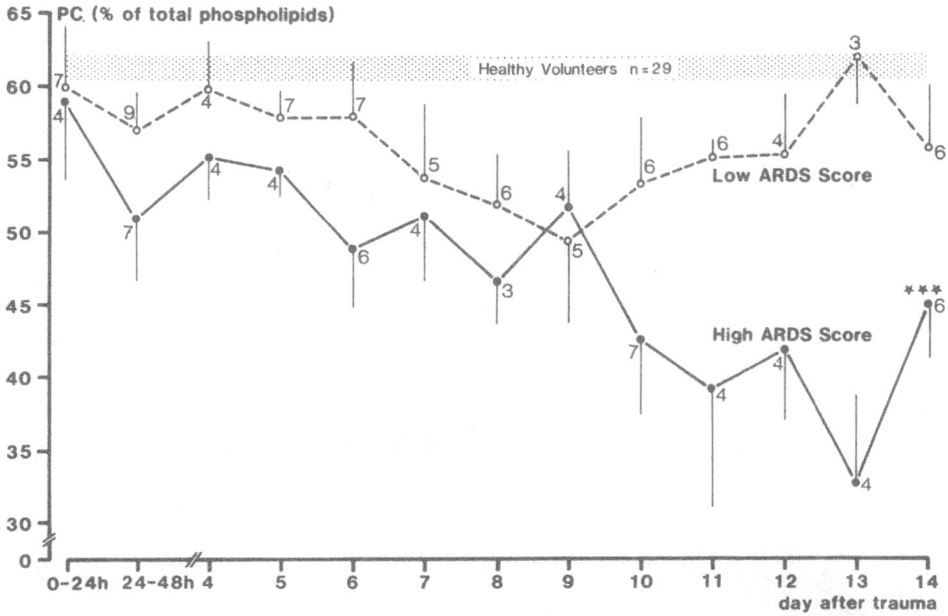

Fig. 3. Time course of the percentage of dipalmitoyl-phosphatidylcholine (PC) of the total lavage-phospholipid content in patients with a high and with a low ARDS score. The numbers of observations on each day after trauma are given. *Shaded area* indicates mean ± SE of %PC in the surfactant material of healthy volunteers. The groups with high and with low ARDS scores differ highly significantly (***, $p < 0.001$). [20]

the time course revealed that this decrease occurred progressively, with a minimum after 10–14 days in the patients who developed severe ARDS. PG was very low in all traumatized subjects (with similar progressive decrease), but no significant difference between the two ARDS severity groups was observed. In contrast, %SPH, %PI, %PE, and %PA were increased in all multiply injured patients. When calculated for all patients, there was a significant correlation between these alterations in phospholipid profile and ARDS severity score ($r = 0.77$, calculated for the decreasing PC, Table 2).

Among the parameters of surfactant function in vitro, the hysteresis area was markedly altered in all traumatized patients compared with healthy volunteers, and it efficiently discriminated between the patients with a low and high ARDS score (Table 1, Fig. 4). In most patients with severe respiratory failure, there was an initial drop in hysteresis area, followed by a more progressive decline with a minimum after 10–14 days. There was a significant correlation between the decrease in hysteresis area and the lavage phospholipid profile ($r = 0.62$ for %PC; Fig. 5). Stability index and minimal surface tension revealed marked alterations in magnitude within single patients; however, the mean values showed no significant difference between the multiply injured patients and healthy controls.

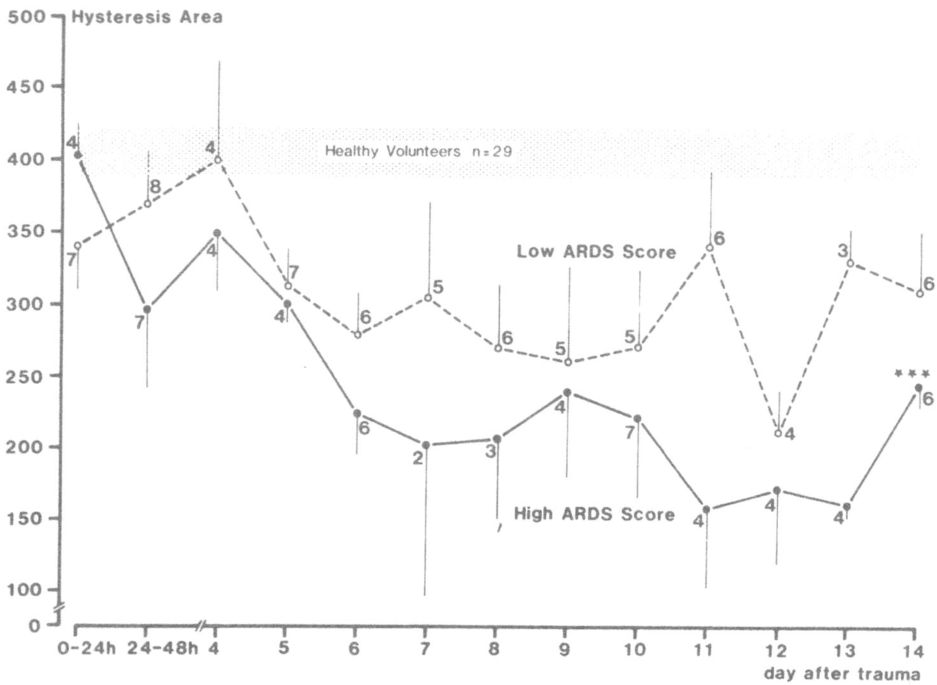

Fig. 4. Time course of surface tension hysteresis area determined in surfactant material from patients with a high and with a low ARDS score. The number of observations each day after trauma are given. *Shaded area* indicates mean ± SE of the hysteresis area determined in surfactant material from healthy volunteers. The groups with high and with low ARDS scores differ highly significantly (***, $p < 0.001$). [20]

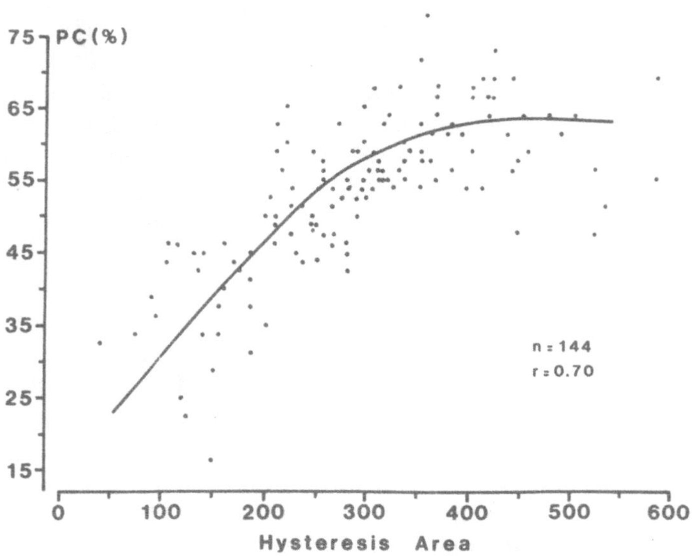

Fig. 5. Correlation of single data between %PC of total phospholipids and the hysteresis area of the surface tension diagram of all multiply injured patients. The number of observations and the Pearson correlation coefficient are given. (In total 12 lavages were obtained later than 14 days after trauma, with a maximum of 21 days.) [20]

Discussion

The data of the present study show that the alveolar surfactant system is disturbed during the course of posttraumatic ARDS.

Changes in the phospholipid lung profile were characterized by a progressive decrease in %PC and %PG and an increase in the percentages of PE, PI, and SPH. These changes are similar to the alterations reported in a heterogenous group of patients with pulmonary dysfunction of different etiology [19] and in a model of acute alveolar injury induced with *N*-nitroso-*N*-methylurethane in dogs [33]. The decrease in %PC and the increase in %PE were markedly more pronounced in patients with a high ARDS score than in those with mild pulmonary dysfunction. In contrast, the percentage of PG was low in all traumatized patients and did not discriminate between the two ARDS severity groups. This finding thus differs from the behavior of PG in preterm infants with hyaline membrane disease, in whom PG is used as a marker of fetal lung maturity. The changes in the alveolar phospholipid composition of the severely injured patients might be caused by contamination with plasma phospholipids as well as phospholipids from migrated inflammatory cells. However, the progressive time course more likely suggests that these alterations reflect alveolar type II cell injury in the course of posttraumatic pulmonary insufficiency.

A consistent finding of the surface tension-area isotherms of surfactant material recovered from traumatized patients was the reduction in hysteresis area. It was significantly more pronounced in the group of patients with a high ARDS score than those with mild pulmonary dysfunction. Hysteresis reflects the stability of the film during compression and the efficiency of reentry during expansion. These properties have recently been characterized in a variety of well-defined films, and dynamic respreading after film compression is assumed to be an important variable for physiological function in vivo. The marked decrease in hysteresis area thus reflects a severe disturbance of alveolar surfactant function in the patients with a high ARDS score.

Why was the surface tension behavior altered in these patients? The total amount of phospholipid, recovered by the standardized lavage technique, showed no significant difference between the two ARDS severity groups and the normal controls. By contrast, the alterations in the phospholipid lung profile nearly paralleled the decrease in hysteresis area in many patients (example given in Fig. 1), and there was a strong correlation between %PC and hysteresis area. These results suggested that the alterations in the phospholipid lung profile, particularly the decrease in %PC, are an important factor for the noted changes in surfactant biophysical activity. The relative amount of PG was low in all multiply injured patients, irrespective of the magnitude of hysteresis area and of ARDS severity. However, this decrease in PG was balanced by an increase in the relative amounts of PI in most of our patients. This finding seems to support the experimental observation that there is no detectable change in surfactant function in vivo when PG is replaced by PI. In addition to the changes in phospholipid lung profile, protein leakage may be an important pathophysiological event causing alterations in surfactant function. In several patients an increase in the lavage protein content preceded the decrease in hysteresis area. The impact of a high alveolar protein load on surfactant function has previously been demonstrated in many experimental studies [12–16]. Neutrophil invasion into the alveolar space was observed in all multiply injured patients. This influx, however, did not correlate significantly with parameters of surfactant function or phospholipid lung profile. Alterations in the surfactant apoproteins, which might be particularly relevant for changes in dynamic surface properties, were not addressed in the present study.

Conclusion

Surfactant abnormalities can be demonstrated in severely traumatized patients and they are significantly correlated with the development of respiratory failure. The main features are a rapidly occurring alveolar protein load (demonstrated within the first 48 h) and a progressive alteration in the alveolar phospholipid composition. The latter includes a decrease in phosphatidylcholine and phosphatidylglycerol, accompanied by a relative increase in the other phospholipid species. Alterations in the surfactant biophysical activity are noted, which are correlated with these two events (protein leakage and progressive PC decline) and which are correlated with the development of respiratory failure.

References

1. Farrell PM, Avery ME (1975) Hyaline membrane disease. Am Rev Respir Dis 111:657–688
2. Avery ME, Mead J (1959) Surface properties in relation to atelectasis and hyaline membrane disease. Am J Dis Child 97:517–523
3. Notter RH, Shapiro DL (1981) Lung surfactant in an era of replacement therapy. Pediatrics 68:781–789
4. Ashbaugh DG, Bigelow DB, Petty TL, Levine BE (1967) Acute respiratory distress in adults. Lancet 2:319–323
5. Kulovich MV, Gluck L (1979) The lung profile. II. Complicated pregnancy. Am J Ostet Gynecol 135:64–70
6. Jackson JC, Palmer S, Truog WE, Standaert TA, Murphy JH, Hodson WA (1986) Surfactant quantity and composition during recovery from hyaline membrane disease. Pediatr Res 20:1243–1247
7. Brigham KL (1985) Metabolites of arachidonic acid in experimental lung vascular injury. Fed Proc 44:43–45

8. Traber DL (1985) Pulmonary microvascular dysfunction during shock. In: Janssen HF, Barnes GD (eds) Circulatory shock: basic and clinical implications. Academic, New York, pp 23–46
9. Brigham KL, Meyrick B (1984) Interactions of granulocytes with the lungs. Circ Res 54:623–634
10. Repine JE, Tate RM (1983) Oxygen radicals and lung edema. Physiologist 26:171–181
11. Seeger W, Suttorp N (1987) Role of membrane lipids in the pulmonary vascular abnormalities caused by bacterial toxins. Am Rev Respir Dis 136:462–466
12. Taylor FB Jr, Abrams ME (1966) Effect of surface active lipoprotein on clotting and fibrinolysis, and of fibrinogen on surface tension of surface active lipoprotein. Am J Med 40:346–350
13. Tierney DF, Johnson RP (1965) Altered surface tension of lung extracts and lung mechanics. J Appl Physiol 20:1253–1260
14. Jobe A, Ikegami M, Jacobs H, Jones S, Conaway D (1983) Permeability of premature lamb lungs to protein and the effect of surfactant on that permeability. J Appl Physiol 55:169–176
15. Ikegami M, Jobe A, Jacobs H, Lam R (1984) A protein from airways of premature lambs that inhibits surfactant function. J Appl Physiol 57:1134–1142
16. Seeger W, Stöhr G, Wolf HRD, Neuhof H (1985) Alteration of surfactant function due to protein leakage: special interaction with fibrin monomer. J Appl Physiol 58:326–338
17. Von Wichert P, Kohl FV (1977) Decreased dipalmitoyl lecithin content found in lung specimens from patients with so-called shock-lung. Intensive Care Med 3:27–30
18. Petty TL, Silvers GW, Paul GW, Stanford RE (1979) Abnormalities in lung elastic properties and surfactant function in adult respiratory distress syndrome. Chest 75: 571–574
19. Hallman M, Spragg R, Harrell JH, Moser KM, Gluck L (1982) Evidence of lung surfactant abnormality in respiratory failure. Study of bronchoalveolar lavage phospholipids, surface activity, phospholipase activity, and plasma myoinositol. J Clin Invest 70:673–683
20. Pison U, Seeger W, Buchhorn R, Joka T, Brand M, Obertacke U, Neuhof H, Schmit-Neuerburg K-P (1989) Surfactant abnormalities in patients with respiratory failure following multiple trauma. Am Rev Respir Dis 140:1033
21. Bradford MM (1976) A rapid and sensitive method for the quantitation of microgram quantities of protein utilizing the principle of protein-dye binding. Anal Biochem 72:248–254
22. Folch J, Lees M, Stanley GHS (1957) A simple method for the isolation and purification of total lipids from animal tissue. J Biol Chem 226:497–509
23. Henry RJ (1964) J Clinical Chemistry. Harper and Row, New York
24. Pison U, Gono E, Joka T, Obladen M (1986) High performance liquid chromatography of adult human bronchoalveolar lavage: assay for phospholipid lung profile. J Chromatogr 377:79–89
25. Clements JA, Hustead RF, Johnson RP, Gribetz I (1961) Pulmonary surface tension and alveolar stability. J Appl Physiol 16:444–450
26. Hildebran JN, Goerke J, Clements JA (1979) Pulmonary surface film stability and composition. J Appl Physiol 47:604–611
27. Parsons PE, Fowler AA, Hyers TM, Henson PM (1985) Chemotactic activity in bronchoalveolar lavage fluid from patients with adult respiratory distress syndrome. Am Rev Respir Dis 132:490–493
28. Afford SC, Stockley RA, Kramps JA, Dijkman JH, Burnett D (1985) Concentration of bronchoalveolar lavage fluid by ultrafiltration: evidence of differential protein loss and functional inactivation of proteinase inhibitors. Anal Biochem 151:125–130
29. Trurnit HJ (1960) A theory and method for the spreading of protein monolayers. J Colloid Sci 15:1–13
30. Abrams ME (1966) Isolation and quantitative estimation of pulmonary surface-active lipoprotein. J Appl Physiol 21:718–720
31. Baker SP, O'Neill B, Haddon W, Long WB (1984) The injury severity score: a method for describing patients with multiple injuries and evaluating emergency care. J Trauma 14:187–196

32. Obertacke U, Kalotai J, Coenen T, Joka T, Schmit-Neuerburg KP (1989) Ein linearer ARDS-Schweregradscore (0–1). (submitted)
33. Liau DF, Barrett CR, Bell ALL, Ryan SF (1987) Functional abnormalities of lung surfactant in experimental acute alveolar injury in the dog. Am Rev Respir Dis 136: 395–401

Adult Respiratory Distress Syndrome As a Manifestation of a General Permeability Defect

E. Kreuzfelder[1], U. Obertacke[2], B. Neumann[1], and O. Thraenhart[1]

Introduction

Current operational definitions rely for the most part on three features of the adult respiratory distress syndrome (ARDS): hypoxia, decreased pulmonary compliance, and diffuse roentgenographic lung infiltration [5]. Diffuse roentgenographic lung infiltration is an expression of pulmonary edema and, therefore, increased lung tissue permeability. The assumption of Fleck et al. [2] that increased microvascular permeability seen after trauma occurs throughout the whole body led us to test whether systemic increases in protein permeability occur in trauma patients who develop ARDS. In probing permeability mechanisms, it is important to recognize biologic actions common to glomerular and alveolar basement membrane [1]. In order to characterize the type of permeability defect, we determined proteins with different molecular weight (MW) in urine, bronchoalveolar lavage fluid (BALF), and serum.

Methods

All proteins in serum and urine were measured every 6 h for up to 48 h after admission (early post-traumatic phase), and thereafter (late phase) once a day for up to 14 days after admission. BALF protein concentrations were estimated once a day. β_2-Microglobulin (MW 11 800, Pharmacia, Freiburg, FRG) and myoglobin (MW 17 800, CIS, Dreieich, FRG) concentrations were determined by radioimmunoassay. Concentrations of α_1-antitrypsin (MW 54 000), immunoglobulin (Ig) G (MW 150 000), and α_2-macroglobulin (MW

[1] Institute for Medical Virology and Immunology, University Hospital Essen, Hufelandstr. 55, W-4300 Essen, FRG

[2] Department of Trauma Surgery, University Hospital Essen, Hufelandstr. 55, W-4300 Essen, FRG

J.A. Sturm (Ed.)
Adult Respiratory Distress Syndrome

Table 1. Blood, bronchoalveolar lavage fluid, and urine concentrations of β_2-microglobulin, myoglobin, α_1-antitrypsin, immunoglobulin G, and α_2-macroglobulin of trauma patients with and without adult respiratory distress syndrome during a 14-day time course after hospital admission

Time after admission	Protein	Blood			Bronchoalveolar lavage fluid			Urine		
		+ARDS median (*n*)	−ARDS median (*n*)	*p* value	+ARDS median (*n*)	−ARDS median (*n*)	*p* value	+ARDS median (*n*)	−ARDS median (*n*)	*p* value
0–48 h	B2MG (mg/l)	1.4 (9)	1.4 (13)	NS	0.3 (2)	0 (3)	NS	6.2 (9)	3.0 (13)	NS
	MG [μg/l]	4,075 (9)	2,079 (13)	0.0178	40 (2)	9 (3)	NS	2,077 (9)	553 (13)	0.0123
	A1AT [mg/dl]	212 (9)	273 (13)	0.0323	0.5 (7)	0.6 (11)	NS	ND	ND	ND
	IgG [mg/dl]	518 (9)	559 (13)	NS	3.4 (7)	2.6 (11)	NS	0.5 (8)	0.9 (12)	NS
	A2MG [mg/dl]	140 (9)	174 (13)	NS	0.3 (7)	0.2 (11)	NS	ND	ND	ND
4–14 days	B2MG [mg/l]	4.1 (10)	1.7 (13)	0.0002	0.2 (3)	0 (3)	NS	67.0 (9)	6.4 (13)	0.0002
	MG [μg/l]	648 (10)	189 (13)	0.0184	0 (3)	0 (3)	NS	2,537 (9)	23 (13)	0.0009
	A1AT [mg/dl]	577 (10)	502 (13)	NS	1.8 (9)	0.2 (12)	0.0225	ND	ND	ND
	IgG [mg/dl]	612 (10)	684 (13)	NS	2.7 (10)	0 (12)	0.0318	1.7 (8)	1.5 (12)	NS
	A2MG [mg/dl]	168 (10)	211 (13)	NS	0.4 (9)	0 (12)	0.0063	ND	ND	ND

+*ARDS*, trauma patients with adult respiratory distress syndrome; −*ARDS*, trauma patients without ARDS; *A1AT*, α_1-antitrypsin; *A2MG*, α_2-macroglobulin; *B2MG*, β_2-microglobulin; *IgG*, immunoglobulin G; *MG*, myoglobin; *ND*, not done; *NS*, not significant ($p > 0.05$)

820000) in BALF and serum were measured by immunonephelometry (Beckman, Munich, FRG). IgG concentrations in urine were measured using the radial immunodiffusion technique (Behring, Marburg, FRG) after concentration (Amicon, Witten, FRG).

To ascertain differences between the ARDS and nonARDS groups of patients, Wilcoxon's two-sample tests were performed. If time intervals were analyzed, the median over time of each individual patient was calculated at first, and then distributions of medians in both groups were compared. Level of significance was designated at $\alpha = 0.05$ (two-tailed tests).

Results

Whereas β_2-microglobulin concentrations in serum and urine were significantly higher in the ARDS group than in the nonARDS group during the late post-traumatic phase only (Table 1, Figs. 1, 2), serum and urine concentrations of myoglobin were significantly increased in both the early and the late phases (Table 1, Figs. 3, 4). α_1-Antitrypsin concentrations in serum were significantly lower in ARDS group than in nonARDS group in serum during the early phase (Table 1, Fig. 5), but significantly higher in BALF during the late phase (Table 1, Fig. 6).

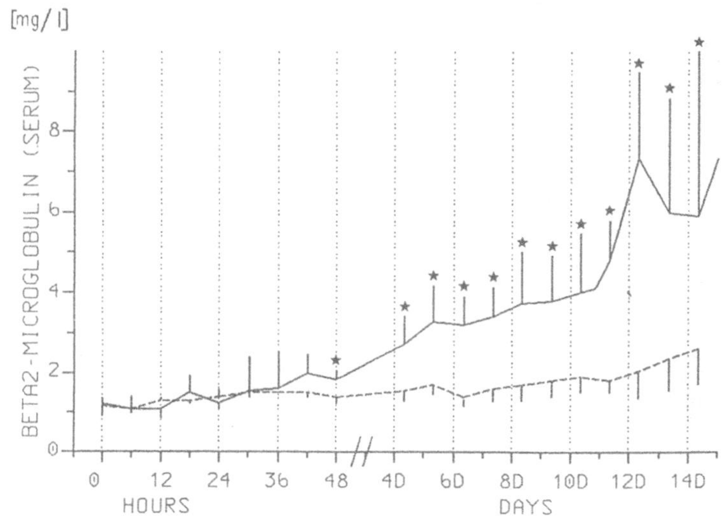

Fig. 1. Serum β_2-microglobulin concentrations of trauma patients with and without adult respiratory distress syndrome (ARDS) during a 14-day time course after hospital admission. Median values and standard deviations are presented. *Continuous line* indicates trauma patients with ARDS ($n \leq 9$); *broken line* indicates trauma patients without ARDS ($n \leq 13$); *, $p < 0.05$

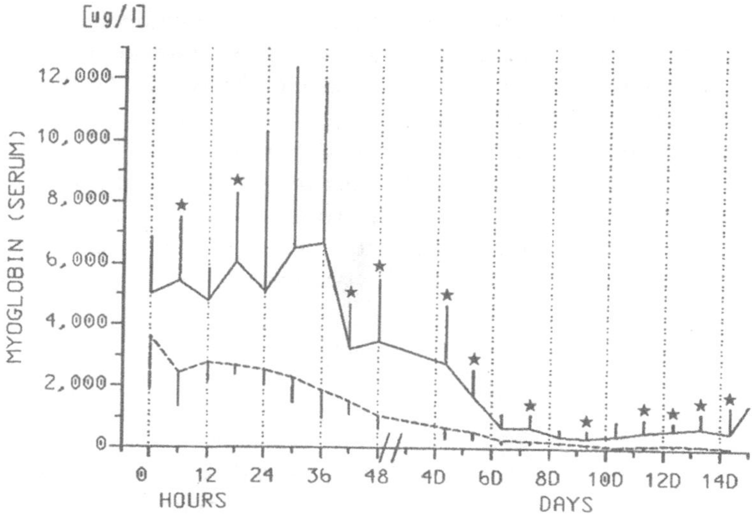

Fig. 2. Urine β_2-microglobulin concentrations of trauma patients with and without adult respiratory distress syndrome (ARDS) during a 14-day time course after hospital admission. Median values and standard deviations are presented. *Continuous line* indicates trauma patients with ARDS ($n \leq 9$); *broken line* indicates trauma patients without ARDS ($n \leq 13$); *, $p < 0.05$

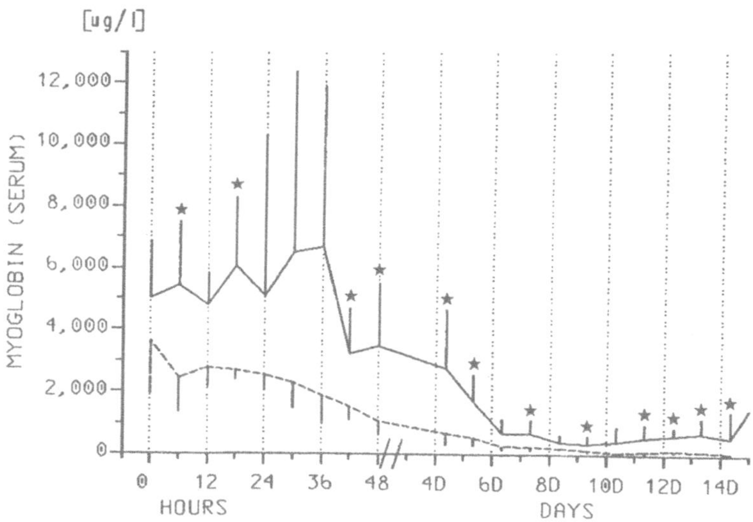

Fig. 3. Serum myoglobin concentrations of trauma patients with and without adult respiratory distress syndrome (ARDS) during a 14-day time course after hospital admission. Median values and standard deviations are presented. *Continuous line* indicates trauma patients with ARDS ($n \leq 10$); *broken line* indicates trauma patients without ARDS ($n \leq 13$) *, $p < 0.05$

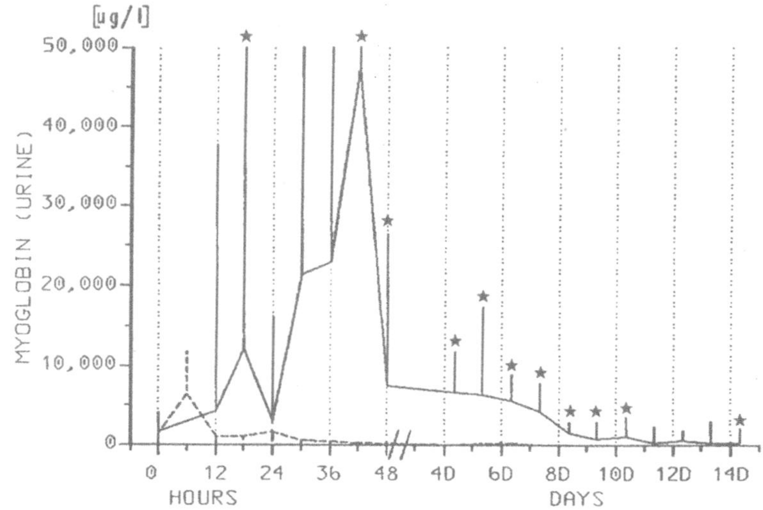

Fig. 4. Urine myoglobin concentrations of trauma patients with and without adult respiratory distress syndrome (ARDS) during a 14-day time course after hospital admission. Median values and standard deviations are presented. *Continuous line* indicates trauma patients with ARDS ($n \leq 9$); *broken line* indicates trauma patients without ARDS ($n \leq 13$); *, $p < 0.05$

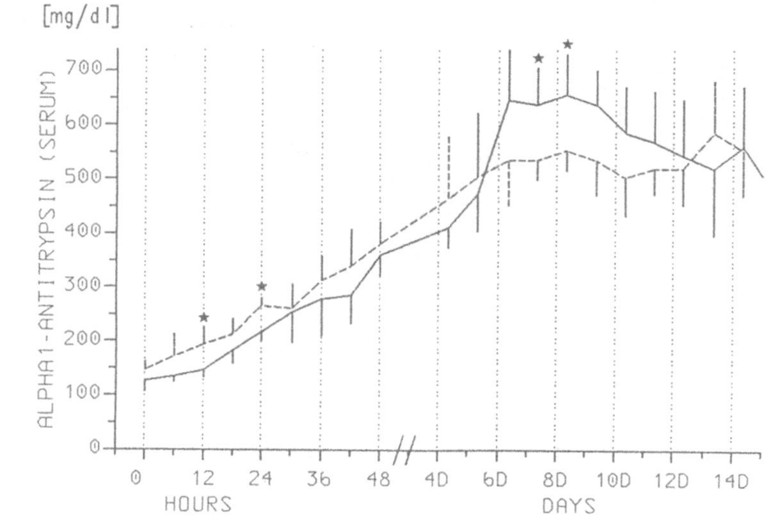

Fig. 5. Serum α_1-antitrypsin concentrations of trauma patients with and without adult respiratory distress syndrome (ARDS) during a 14-day time course after hospital admission. Median values and standard deviations are presented. *Continuous line* indicates trauma patients with ARDS ($n \leq 10$); *broken line* indicates trauma patients without ARDS ($n \leq 13$); *, $p < 0.05$

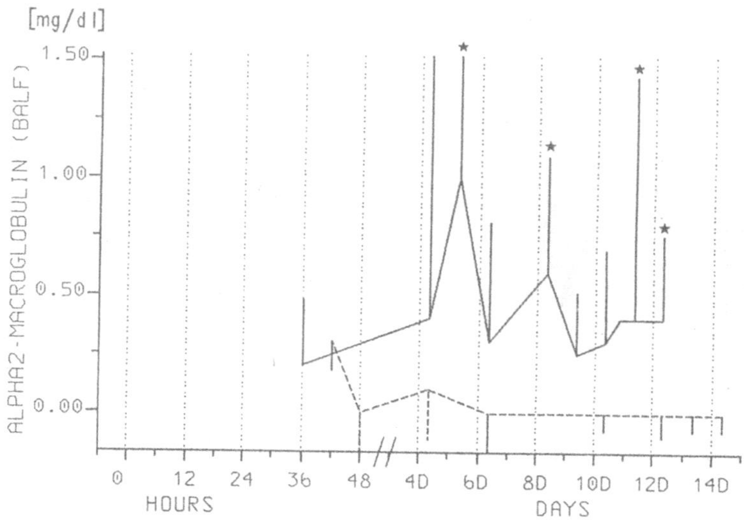

Fig. 6. Bronchoalveolar lavage fluid α_1-antitrypsin concentrations of trauma patients with and without adult respiratory distress syndrome (ARDS) during a 14-day time course after hospital admission. Median values and standard deviations are presented. *Continuous line* indicates trauma patients with ARDS ($n \leq 9$); *broken line* indicates trauma patients without ARDS ($n \leq 11$); *BALF*, bronchoalveolar lavage fluid; *, $p < 0.05$

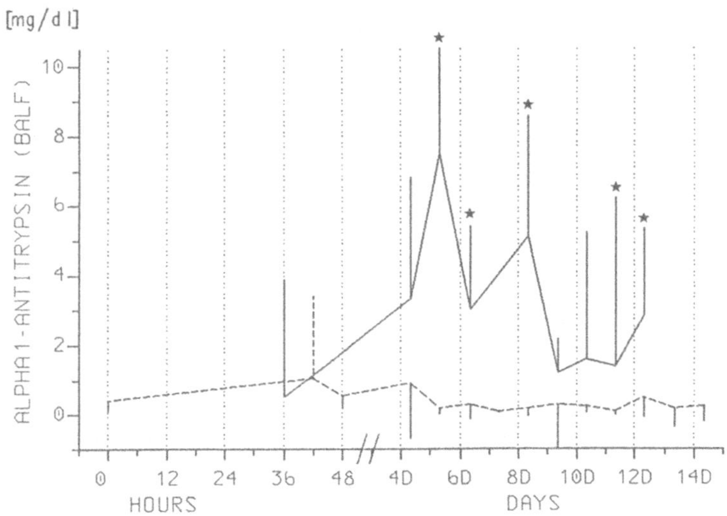

Fig. 7. Bronchoalveolar lavage fluid α_2-macroglobulin concentrations of trauma patients with and without adult respiratory distress syndrome (ARDS) during a 14-day time course after hospital admission. Median values and standard deviations are presented. *Continuous line* indicates trauma patients with ARDS ($n \leq 9$); *broken line* indicates trauma patients without ARDS ($n \leq 11$); *BALF*, bronchoalveolar lavage fluid; *, $p < 0.05$

IgG concentrations were significantly different (increased) in the two groups only in the BALF during the late post-traumatic phase (Table 1); serum and urine concentrations did not show any difference between the two groups over the entire period. α_2-Macroglobulin concentrations were significantly different (increased) in the two groups only in the BALF during the late post-traumatic phase (Table 1, Fig. 7), whereas serum concentrations did not show any difference between the two groups over the entire period.

Discussion

One of the hallmarks of ARDS is pulmonary edema. Using extravascular lung water content (EVLW) as a parameter for the development of edema and, therefore, increased, endothelial permeability, we could establish a positive correlation between increases in EVLW and β_2-microglobulin concentrations in the urine of all patients with ARDS, indicating systemically increased permeability [4].

Systemically increased permeability was also found in this study when the previous results were reevaluated using a score system to characterize ARDS and increasing the numbers of patients. This conclusion is based on the temporal relationship between increases in protein permeability in kidney and lung, as measured by increased concentrations of β_2-microglobulin in serum and urine as well as concentrations of α_1-antitrypsin and α_2-macroglobulin in the BALF of ARDS patients. Recognizing biologic actions common to glomerular and alveolar basement membrane [1] and the relationship between glomerular function and serum β_2-microglobulin concentration [7], increased protein concentrations in BALF, serum, and urine at the same time interval seem to be an expression of systemically increased protein permeability.

Whereas BALF protein concentrations (with the exception of IgG) in ARDS patients rise over time, BALF protein concentrations in nonARDS patients decrease. The downward trend in BALF protein concentrations (BALF/plasma ratio) with time in ARDS was first observed by Holter et al. [3] and explained by alveolar protein clearance in the face of a restored endothelial barrier. The conclusion drawn by Holter et al. [3] concerning the disturbed structure of the endothelial/alveolar barrier was based primarily on the measurement of concentrations of molecules with high MW such as α_2-macroglobulin. Since we found increased and different concentrations in the ARDS and nonARDS groups of patients also when the low MW protein α_1-antitrypsin was measured, and, furthermore, since concentrations of both proteins, α_2-macroglobulin and α_1-antitrypsin, were not different between groups in the early post-traumatic phase, it seems unlikely that the conclusion drawn by Holter et al. [3] was correct. On the other hand are our results in agreement with the conclusion drawn by Holter et al. [3] that normal size selectivity is destroyed by the alveolar-capillary injury caused by ARDS, since low and high MW protein BALF concentrations are increased and different between both groups.

Evidence of damage to the endothelial/alveolar barrier is seen in the elevated BALF protein concentrations during the late phase about 5 days after injury. Since serum and urine concentrations of β_2-microglobulin show a similar time pattern to the BALF proteins, and since β_2-microglobulin concentrations are related to glomerular function, increased permeability in kidney and lung seems primarily to reflect disturbed mechanisms related to the glomerular barrier. In contrast to this, proteinuria measured by urine myoglobin concentrations becomes manifest during the first 48 h, reflecting primarily disturbed tubular function. Disturbed tubular function preceded disturbed glomerular function and, therefore, measurement of serum and urine myoglobin concentrations may be used as a "... biochemical marker in either the blood or urine, which can herald the onset of ARDS with a reasonable degree of specificity and sensitivity." as PETTY [6] wrote.

Conclusion

ARDS in trauma patients is characterized by a systemically increased protein permeability in kidney and lung tissue. An increase in urine myoglobin protein concentrations reflecting tubular kidney function disturbance precedes an increase in BALF protein concentrations and may be used as early indicator of the development of ARDS.

References

1. Barrowcliffe MP, Jones JG (1987) Solute permeability of the alveolar capillary barrier. Thorax 42:1
2. Fleck A, Colley CM, Myers MA (1985) Liver export proteins and trauma. Br Med Bull 41:265
3. Holter JF, Weiland JE, Pacht ER, Gadek JE, Davis WB (1986) Protein permeability in the adult respiratory distress syndrome. Loss of size selectivity of the alveolar epithelium. J Clin Invest 78:1513
4. Kreuzfelder E, Joka T, Keinecke HO, Obertacke U, Schmit-Neuerburg KP, Nakhosteen JA, Paar D, Scheiermann N (1988) Adult respiratory distress syndrome as a specific manifestation of a general permeability defect in trauma patients. Am Rev Respir Dis 137:95
5. Murray JF, Matthay MA, Luce JM, Flick MR (1988) An expanded definition on the adult respiratory distress syndrome. Am Rev Respir Dis 138:720
6. Petty TL, (1988) ARDS: refinement of concept and redefinition. Am Rev Respir Dis 138:724
7. Vree TB, Guelen, PJM, Jongman-Nix B, Walenkamp GHIM. (1981) The relationship between the renal clearance of creatinine and the apparent renal clearance of beta-2-microglobulin in patients with normal and impaired kidney function. Clin Chim Acta 114:93

Early and Late Ultrastructural Changes in the Lungs of Patients Suffering from Severe Polytrauma

H. BARTELS and E. REALE

Introduction

The adult respiratory distress syndrome (ARDS) is a complication of a wide variety of insults which affect directly (aspiration of gastric content, viral pneumonia) or indirectly (multiple body trauma including major long bone and/or pelvic fractures, hemorrhagic shock, sepsis, pancreatitis) the lungs [10]. ARDS defines an acute respiratory failure due to noncardiogenic (permeability) pulmonary edema and is associated with diffuse alveolar damage which finally leads to pulmonary fibrosis [4].

In the present study we investigated lung biopsies from patients who died at different intervals (1 h–4 weeks) after a severe polytrauma in order to describe the initial lesions in the lung alveoli and the time course of the ultrastructural changes leading to the structural remodeling of the lung parenchyma after diffuse alveolar damage.

Material and Methods

Lung biopsies were obtained from four patients who died during the first 24 h after severe polytrauma and from 27 patients who suffered from ARDS as a complication of polytrauma. In these latter patients the time lapse between the accident and death was 1–4 weeks. All biopsies were taken as transcutaneous fine-needle biopsies from the right and left lung immediately after the patient's death in the intensive care unit.

The biopsies were fixed in phosphate-buffered (0.1 M) glutaraldehyde (3%), postfixed in OsO_4 (2% in the same buffer), dehydrated in ethanol, and embedded in Agar-Araldite (epoxy resin) CY 212. Sections 1–2 µm thick were stained with toluidine blue and thin sections, cut on an LKB 4800–III

Department of Cell Biology and Electron Microscopy, Hannover Medical School, Konstanty-Gutschow-Str. 8, W-3000 Hannover 61, FRG

J.A. Sturm (Ed.)
Adult Respiratory Distress Syndrome

Ultrotome, were stained with uranyl acetate and lead citrate. In addition, freeze-fracture replicas were made from eight biopsies obtained from patients suffering from ARDS according to the standard protocol (cryoprotection: 30% glycerol in Ringer's solution; freezing in Freon 22, fracturing and shadowing the fracture face at 2×10^{-6} Torr and $-100°C$ in a Balzers BA 360 M freeze fracture device). Electron microscope: Siemens Elmiskop IA, 80kV).

Results

In biopsies obtained during the first 24 h after trauma, the general architecture of the interalveolar septa was always present: capillary endothelium and alveolar epithelium were separated from each other by a single basal lamina at the minimal barrier, while the interstitial space on the thick side of the septum was frequently markedly dilated, indicating the presence of interstitial edema (Fig. 1). Flocculent material and various amounts of red

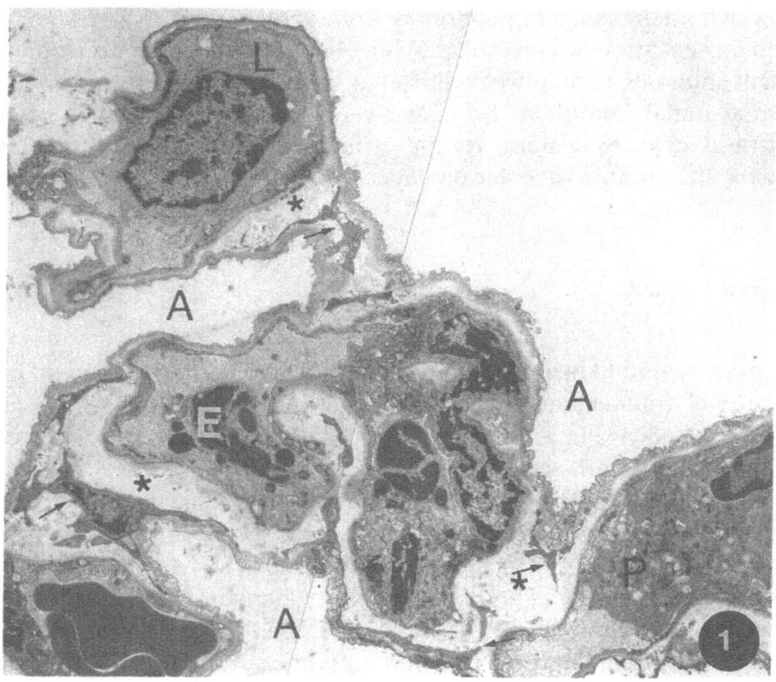

Figs. 1–3. Lung biopsies from patients who died during the first 24 h after polytrauma

Fig. 1. Survey micrograph of an interalveolar septum showing a dilated interstitial space (*asterisks*) and various leukocytes in the lumen of capillaries. *E*, eosinophil granulocyte; *L*, lymphocyte; *P*, polymorphonuclear leukocyte. *Arrows* indicate contractile interstitial cells, extending between the epithelial basal laminae. *A*, alveolar lumen, × 3500

blood cells in the alveolar lumen indicated a proteinaceous alveolar edema and bleeding. Macrophages were particularly abundant in alveoli filled with edema fluid and red blood cells. In some septa, the capillaries were collapsed. White blood cells, among which polymorphonuclear leukocytes (PMNs) were predominant, occurred in capillaries (Figs. 1, 2) and occasionally in the

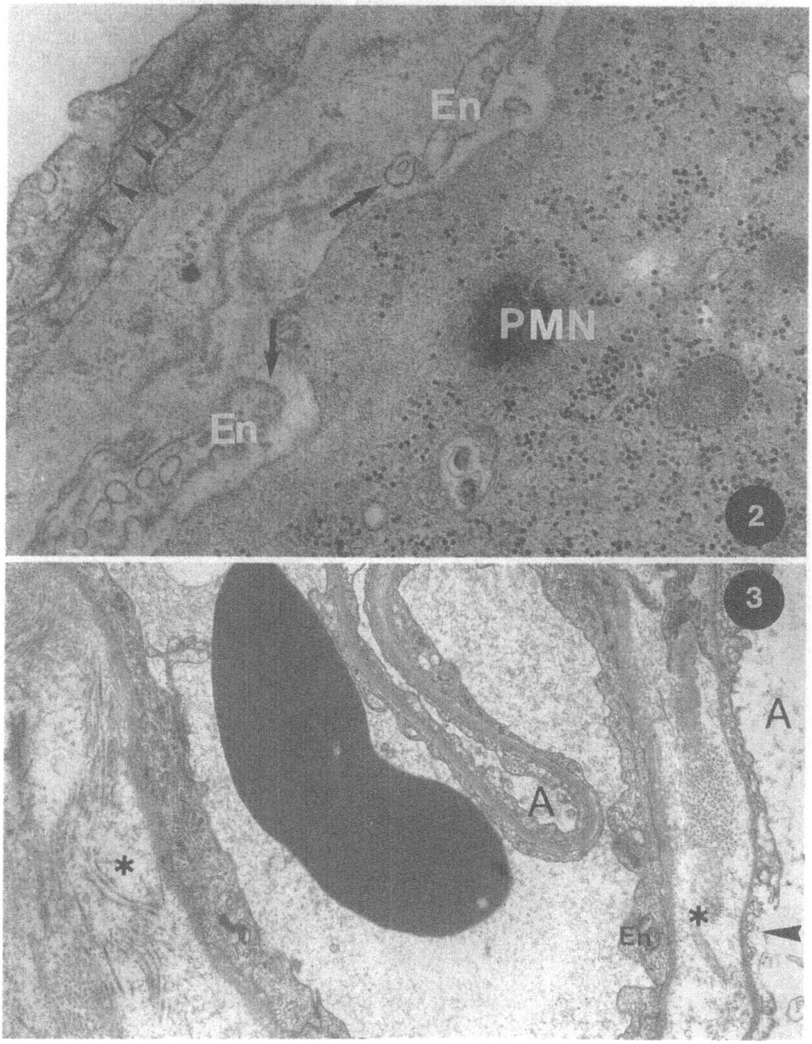

Fig. 2. A polymorphonuclear leukocyte (*PMN*) moving through a gap (*between arrows*) in the capillary endothelium (*En*). *Arrowheads* indicate a zonula occludens in the alveolar epithelium (1 h after trauma), × 32 000

Fig. 3. Cellular damage of a type I pneumocyte (*arrowhead*) in a biopsy taken 18 h after trauma. The interstitial space is dilated (*asterisks*). *A*, alveolar lumen; *En*, endothelium, × 9000

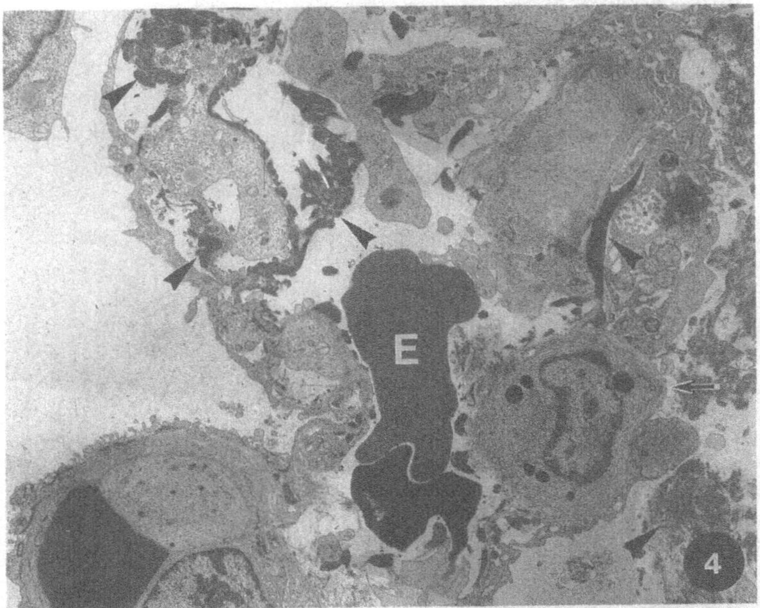

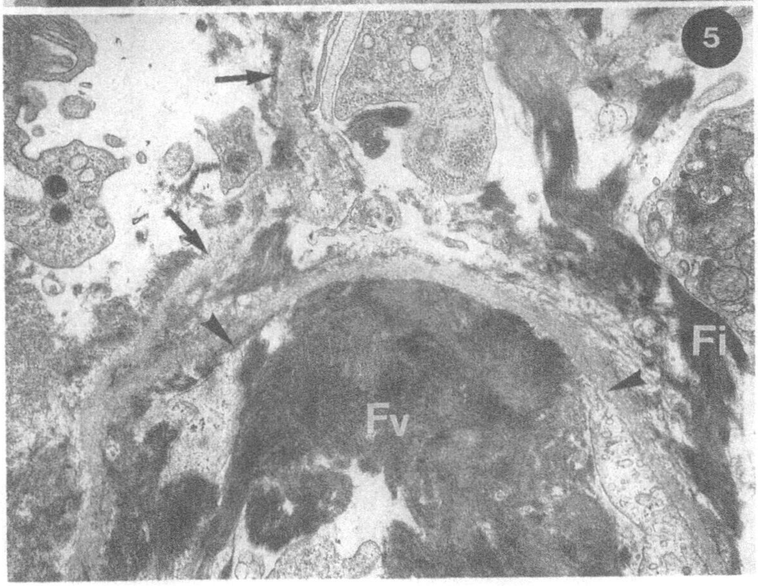

Figs. 4, 5. Acute stage of ARDS characterized by diffuse alveolar damage. One week after trauma

Fig. 4. Survey micrograph showing fibrin (*arrowheads*) in the interstitial space and alveolar lumen. *Arrow* indicates a denuded epithelial basal lamina. *E*, erythrocyte in the interstitial space, × 4000

Fig. 5. Intravascular (*Fv*) and interstitial (*Fi*)fibrin at higher magnification. Note denuded endothelial (*between arrowheads*) and epithelial (*arrows*) basal laminae × 13 000

interstitial space of the interalveolar septa. The distance between the plasma membranes of the PMN and endothelial cells was often only 15–20 nm. A cellular edema and fragmentation of endothelial cells to which PMN adhered was observed in a biopsy taken 1 h after trauma (Fig. 2). Swelling and damage of thin processes of type I epithelial cells were present in a biopsy taken 18 h after trauma (Fig. 3). The intercellular junctions in the capillary endothelium and alveolar epithelium appeared to be intact with thin-section electron microscopy. Fat droplets were present in small arteries and in septal capillaries, occluding the lumen of the latter.

Biopsies from patients who survived the polytrauma for more than 1 week and had developed ARDS by clinical definition (Neumann, this volume) showed a less uniform pattern of structural changes. An exudative (acute) stage could be distinguished from a proliferative and fibrotic stage as described by Fukuda et al. [4].

The *acute stage* of ARDS was investigated in biopsies of patients who died about 1 week after the trauma. This stage was characterized by diffuse alveolar damage [6], as a notably dilated interstitial space, and as severe damage of epithelial and endothelial cells (Figs. 4, 5). The epithelial basal lamina was widely denuded due to the loss of the thin processes of type I pneumocytes and it was occasionally discontinuous. Denudation of the endothelial basal lamina was less frequently observed (Fig. 5). Where type I pneumocytes and endothelial cells were still present, they showed marked swelling, indicating cellular edema. Fibrin thrombi, red blood cells, and PMNs were present in all compartments: intravascular, interstitial, and intraalveolar (Figs. 4, 5). Small fibrin thrombi were also interposed between the basal surface of pneumocytes and the epithelial basal lamina. Cellular debris was conspicuous in the alveolar lumen.

The most prominent changes in more progressive stages of ARDS took place in the alveolar lumen. In the *proliferative stage* the alveoli were usually filled by numerous macrophages, plasma cells, fibrin thrombi, and cellular debris (Fig. 6). In addition, fibroblasts which passed the epithelial basal lamina moved into the alveolar lumen. They showed typical features of protein-secreting cells as abundant cisternae of the rough endoplasmic reticulum and a prominent Golgi complex. Bundles of 5-nm (actin) filaments were present in the peripheral cytoplasm directly underneath the plasma membrane (Fig. 7). Intraalveolar fibroblasts, fibrin thrombi, and blood-borne cells were incompletely covered by a single layer of epithelial cells which detached themselves from their basal lamina (Fig. 8). These cells were mainly cuboidal and retained their polarity, as they showed short microvilli on their "apical" surface. They were joined to each other by zonulae occludentes, and often contained multilamellar bodies, thereby resembling type II pneumocytes.

In regions where the septal architecture was still present the interalveolar septa were extremely widened (up to 35 μm) by a vast dilatation of the interstitial space due to excessive amounts of edema fluid (Fig. 9). There was a marked reduction in capillary profiles within the septa and many of the

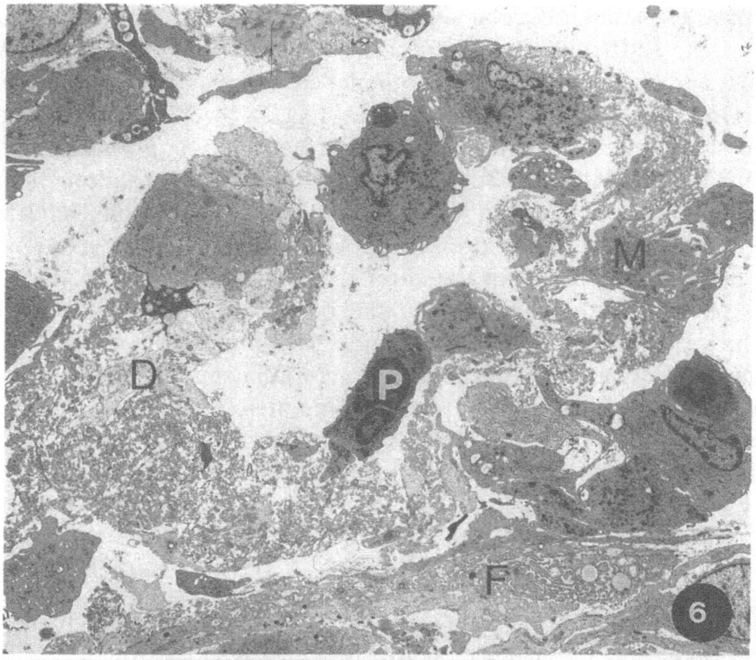

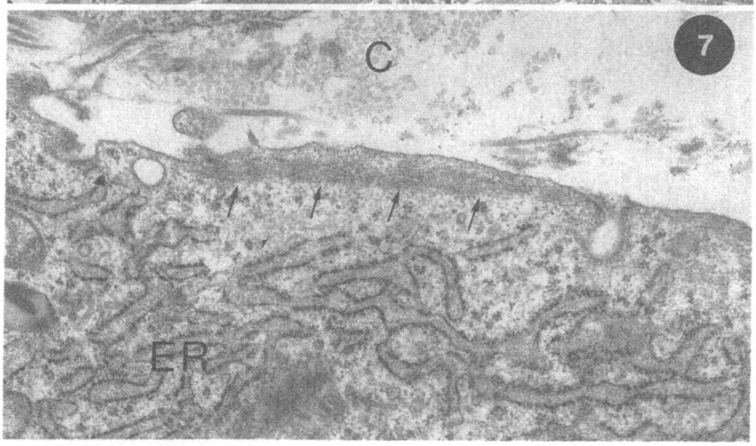

Figs. 6–10. Proliferative stage of ARDS

Fig. 6. Various blood-borne cells, mainly polymorphonuclear leukocytes (*P*) and macrophages (*M*), fibroblasts (*F*), and cellular debris (*D*) in the alveolar lumen, × 1300
Fig. 7. Bundles of 5-nm filaments (*arrows*) directly underneath the plasma membrane of a fibroblast. *C*, collagen fibrils; *ER*, cisternae of rough endoplasmic reticulum, × 10000

endothelial cells were swollen. Fibroblasts, PMNs, and bundles of collagen fibrils occurred at various frequencies in these septa. Occasionally, contractile interstitial cells [5], which are characterized by bundles of 5-nm (actin) filaments, were attached to the epithelial basal lamina by focal contacts. The

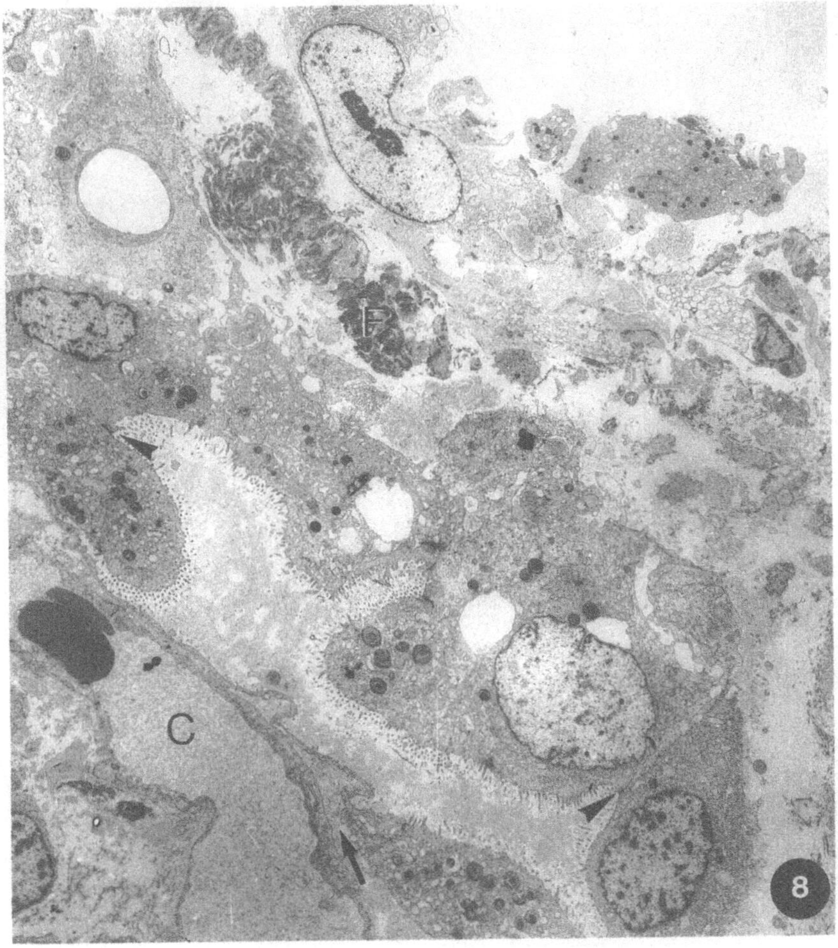

Fig. 8. Epithelial cells detach themselves from their basal lamina (*arrow*) and direct their basal surface toward intraalveolar fibrin (*F*). *Arrowheads* point to zonulae occludentes between the detached epithelial cells. *C*, capillary lumen, × 2400

existing epithelial basal lamina was reepithelialized by a single layer of mainly cuboidal cells, resembling type II cells by the presence of multilamellar bodies. They were linked by zonulae occludentes (Fig. 10) and the apical surface of many cells was increased by numerous short microvilli each containing a bundle of 5 nm (actin) filaments (Fig. 9). Alternatively, in some regions a squamous epithelium, resembling type I pneumocytes, was present (Fig. 9).

In the *fibrotic stage* the alveolar lumen appeared cleft-like, lined by a few flattened cells resembling type I pneumocytes and by numerous cuboidal epithelial cells resembling type II pneumocytes by the presence of numerous

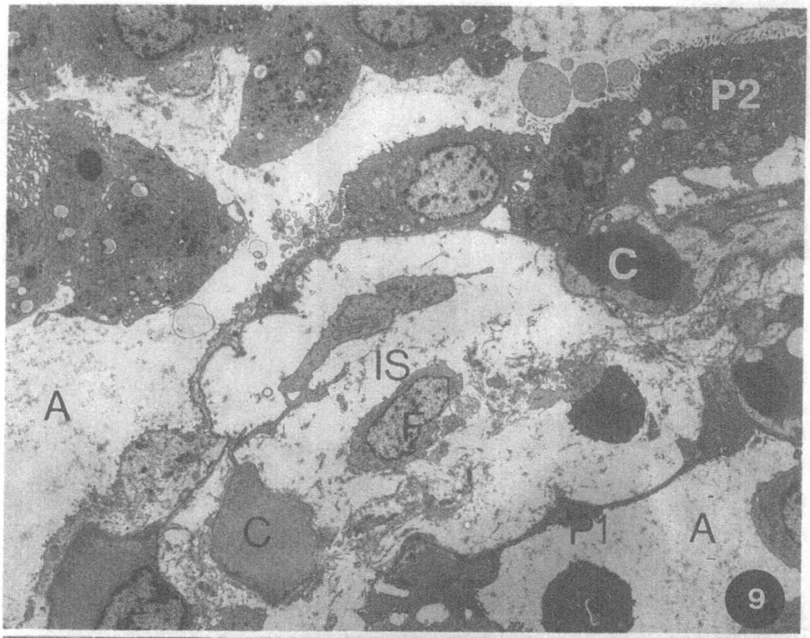

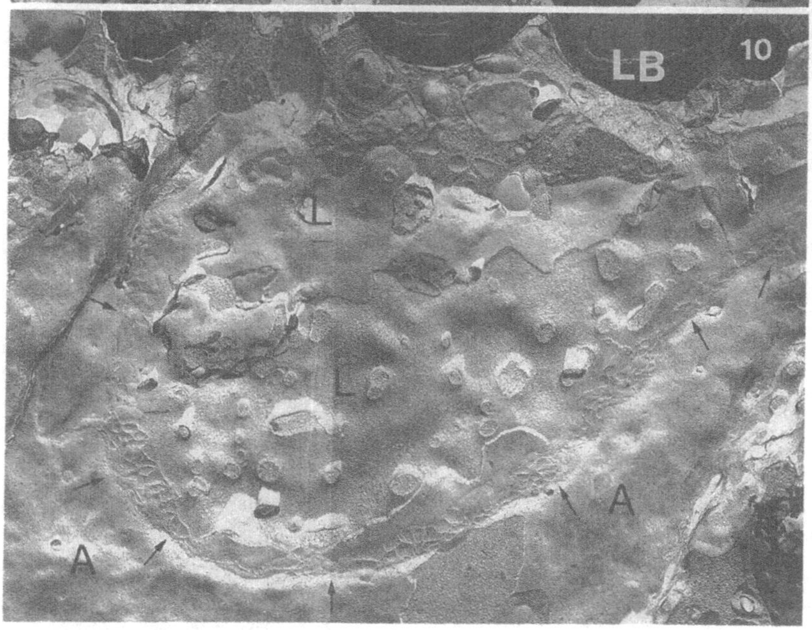

Fig. 9. Vastly dilated interalveolar septum (*IS*) covered by type I-like (*P1*) and type II-like (*P2*) pneumocytes. Note reduction of capillaries (*C*). *A*, alveolar lumen; *F*, fibroblast, × 1300

Fig. 10. Freeze-fracture replica of regenerating alveolar epithelium. *Arrows* indicate zonula occludens. *A*, apical membrane; *L*, lateral membrane; *LB*, lamellar body, × 13000

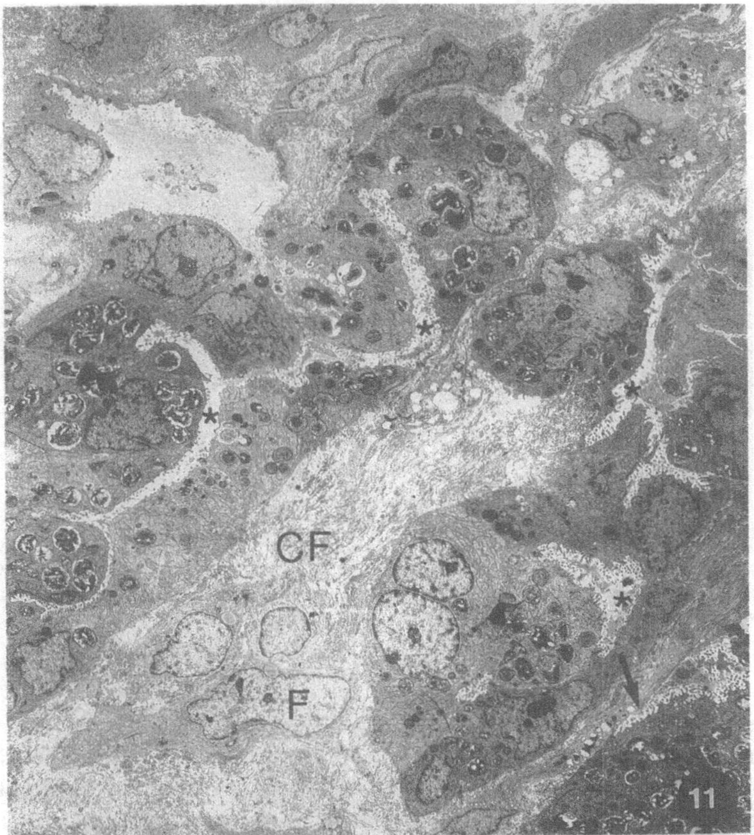

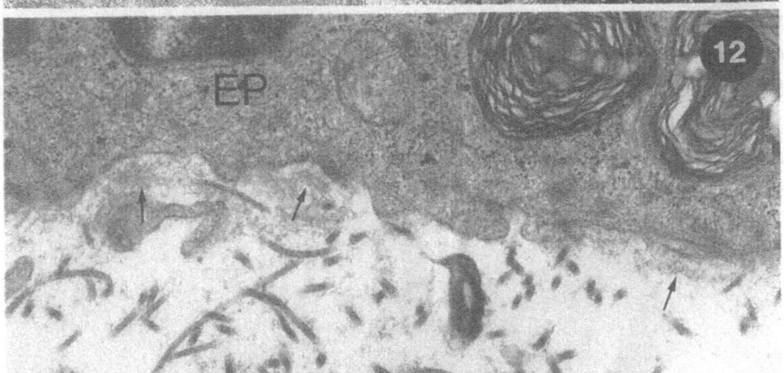

Figs. 11–13. Fibrotic stage of ARDS

Fig. 11. Intraalveolar fibrosis. Air spaces are cleft-like (*asterisks*) and lined by cuboidal epithelium showing lamellar bodies. Occasionally the apical membrane of the epithelial cells faces interstitial fibroblasts (*F*) and collagen fibrils (*CF*) (*arrow*), × 1300

Fig. 12. Basal surface of an epithelial cell (*EP*), *Arrows* indicate basal lamina-like material produced by the cell, × 18000

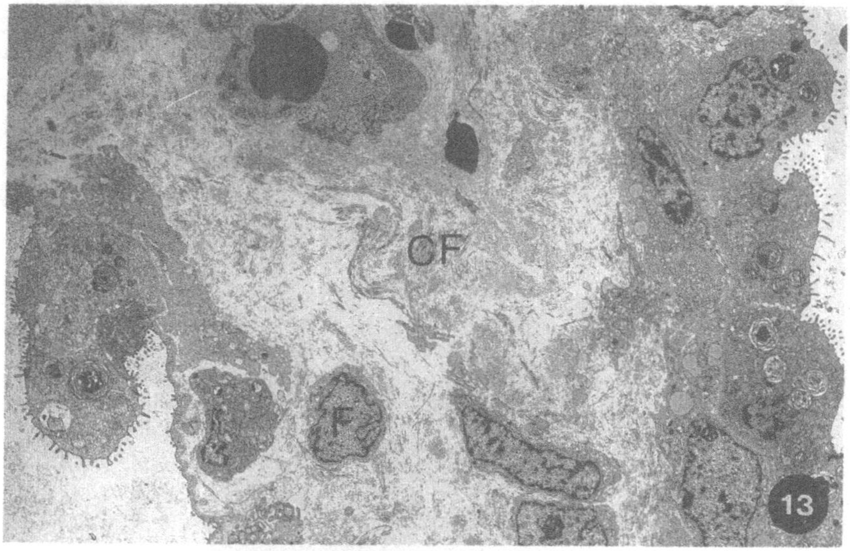

Fig. 13. Interstitial fibrosis. The interalveolar septum is lined by a cuboidal epithelium, the thickened interstitial space is filled with fibroblasts (*F*) and collagen fibrils (*CF*), and capillaries are markedly reduced, × 2000

lamellar bodies. The epithelial cells rested on either a preexisting or a newly produced basal lamina (Figs. 11, 12). The interstitial space, i.e., the space between the basal surfaces of the epithelial cells and bordered by the basal laminae, was filled with bundles of collagen fibrils and fibroblasts. Occasionally, however, the microvilli of these epithelial cells were in direct contact with interstitial collagen or fibroblasts (Fig. 11). Blood-borne cells were scarce in the interstitial space at this stage of ARDS. While most of the fibrotic regions appeared intraalveolar, interstitial fibrosis was only occasionally observed. In the latter case the thickened septa (up to 50 μm) contained scanty capillaries and the interstitial space was filled with fibroblast, bundles of collagen fibrils, and edema fluid (Fig. 13).

Discussion

In this study we demonstrated that (a) after a severe polytrauma initial lesions of the air-blood barrier are ultrastructurally present within the 1st h after the event; (b) an acute stage can be distinguished from progressive stages during ARDS; and (c) intra-alveolar fibrosis appears more prominently than interstitial fibrosis in structurally remodeled lung alveoli.

Initial Lesions

The results of the present study confirm previous reports that adherence of PMNs to the capillary endothelium, intravascular fat droplets, and interstitial and intraalveolar edema are the predominant ultrastructural changes in the lung alveoli which occur in the initial phase after polytrauma [8, 11] or sepsis [1], i.e., conditions known to lead to ARDS. In contrast to these previous reports, edema of endothelial and epithelial cells was less prominent in our material. These findings may be due to an earlier and more effective therapy during the initial phase of shock.

Although ARDS can develop in neutropenic patients [7], a causal relationship between the adherence of PMN to endothelial cells and the development of interstitial edema has been proposed for several years [10, 13]. In the present study a fragmentation of endothelial cells close to adherent PMNs has been shown, suggesting that oxygen metabolites and/or proteolytic enzymes released from the PMNs have injured the adjacent endothelial cell and thereby created "pores" in the endothelial lining. At these pores, the capillary lumen and the interstitial space (endothelial basal lamina) are in direct contact, presumably allowing the unrestricted and unselective leakage of serum proteins and fluid into the interstitial compartment. In addition, functional changes of the interendothelial occluding junctions not detectable by routine thin-section electron microscopy may also contribute to an increased endothelial permeability to serum proteins [12].

In contrast, the pathway by which proteins enter the alveolar lumen immediately (1st h) after trauma remains obscure. A fragmentation of alveolar epithelial type I cells similar to capillary endothelial cells has not been found as yet in the initial phase, but only several hours after polytrauma, and the tight junctions between the pneumocytes appeared to be intact. Since alveolar edema was usually found to be associated with intraalveolar erythrocytes, microhemorrhage from small intra- and/or extraacinar arteries and veins could be the cause of serum proteins in the alveolar lumen.

Acute ARDS

In contrast to the minute and focal structural lesions of the air-blood barrier in the initial phase after polytrauma, the lung biopsies from patients who died about 1 week after the trauma show diffuse alveolar damage, characterized by a destruction of the septal architecture and numerous PMNs and macrophages in the alveolar lumen. This massive increase of both PMNs and macrophages resembles the situation found in the inflammatory stage ("alveolitis") of idiopathic pulmonary fibrosis [3]. The extended loss of endothelial and epithelial cells and the discontinuity particularly of the epithelial basal lamina implicates the breakdown of any barrier in the alveoli which may be caused by an interdependent and uncontrolled activity of the PMN and alveolar macrophages.

The presence of fibrin in all three compartments of the lung parenchyma is a further indication of the loss of the air-blood barrier and the presence of so-called hyaline membranes in which albumin, immunoglobulins (IgG, IgM, IgA), and fibronectin have been detected immunochemically [4].

Vracko [14] has demonstrated that an intact epithelial basal lamina is a necessary condition for the organotypic repair of the injured lung. It is conceivable that, in contrast to the initial lesions of the air-blood barrier after polytrauma which probably heal without defect, the destruction of both cellular barriers associated with multiple disruptions of the epithelial basal lamina leads to structural remodeling of the lung alveoli similar to those of various interstitial lung disease [2, 3], characterized by severe alveolitis.

Structural Remodeling of the Alveoli

The purpose of the repair processes is to eliminate the various materials which accumulate in the alveoli in the acute phase of ARDS and to restore air spaces for gas exchange. However, these repair processes finally lead to deleterious pulmonary fibrosis. Two stages can be distinguished in the course of remodeling, an earlier proliferative and a successive fibrotic stage [4].

In the proliferative stage, the denuded epithelial basal lamina is reepithelialized by cuboidal cells and fibroblasts migrate into the alveolar lumen, possibly attracted by fibronectin secreted by alveolar macrophages [9], where both cell types are present on the surface of the intraalveolar material. In a second step, epithelial cells which have lost contact with their basal lamina migrate over the fibroblasts and also uncovered "hyaline membranes" and intraalveolar collagen, secreted by the fibroblasts. The epithelial cells frequently retain polarity as they show a rather smooth basal, but microvillous, apical surface and are furthermore linked by zonulae occludentes. The epithelial cells thus create cleft-like or even cyst-like new "alveoli." It remains questionable whether these prospective air spaces are always connected to conductive airways. They are by no means capable of gas exchange as contacts to capillaries are rare and angiogenesis has never been observed. Finally the space between the newly formed small "alveoli" is rapidly filled by fibroblasts and collagen fibrils, while the macrophages and also the hyaline membranes gradually disappear.

Although intraalveolar fibrosis, as described above, prevails, interstitial fibrosis occasionally occurs in the biopsies. Interstitial fibrosis is characterized by broad septa lined by a cuboidal epithelium, a marked reduction of capillary profiles, and an interstitial space filled with fibroblasts and collagen fibrils. It is speculated that interstitial fibrosis occurs in interalveolar septa which are less severely injured during the acute phase of ARDS and which largely retain a scaffold of septal structure throughout the disease.

Acknowledgments. This study was supported by the Deutsche Forschungsgemeinschaft Re 657/6. The expert technical assistance of M. Ramspott, K. Scheiber, and S. Krämer is gratefully acknowledged.

References

1. Bachofen M, Weibel ER (1977) Alterations of the gas exchange apparatus in adult respiratory insufficiency with septicemia. Am Rev Respir Dis 116:589–615
2. Basset F, Ferrans VJ, Soler P, Takemura T, Fukuda Y, Crystal RG (1986) Intraluminal fibrosis in interstitial lung disorders. Am J Pathol 122:443–461
3. Crystal RG, Bitterman PB, Rennard SI, Hance AJ, Keogh BA (1984) Interstitial lung diseases of unknown cause. Disorders characterized by chronic inflammation of the lower respiratory tract. N Engl J Med 310:154–166, 235–244
4. Fukuda Y, Ishizaki M, Masuda Y, Kimura G, Kawanami O, Masugi Y (1987) The role of intraalveolar fibrosis in the process of pulmonary structural remodeling in patients with diffuse alveolar damage. Am J Pathol 126:171–182
5. Kapanci Y, Assimacopoulos A, Irle C, Zwahlen A, Gabbiani G (1974) "Contractile interstitial cells" in pulmonary alveolar septa: a possible regulator of ventilation/perfusion ratio? J Cell Biol 60:375–392
6. Katzenstein AL, Bloor CM, Leibow AA (1976) Diffuse alveolar damage – the role of oxygen, shock, and related factors. Am J Pathol 85:210–228
7. Ognibene FP, Martin SE, Parker MM, Schlesinger T, Roach P, Burch C, Shelhamer JH, Parrillo JE (1986) Adult respiratory distress syndrome in patients with severe neutropenia. N Engl J Med 315:547–551
8. Pietra GG, Rüttner JR, Wüst W, Glinz W (1981) The lung after trauma and shock – fine structure of the alveolar-capillary barrier in 23 autopsies. J Trauma 21:454–462
9. Rennard SI, Hunninghake GW, Bittermann PB, Crystal RG (1981) Production of fibronectin by the human alveolar macrophages: mechanisms for recruitment of fibroblasts to sites of tissue injury in interstitial lung diseases. Proc Natl Acad Sci USA 78:7147–7157
10. Rinaldo JE, Rogers RM (1982) Adult respiratory distress syndrome. Changing concepts of lung injury and repair. N Engl J Med 306:900–909
11. Schlag G, Voigt WH, Schnells G, Glatzl A (1976) Die Ultrastruktur der menschlichen Lunge im Schock. Anaesthesist 25:512–521
12. Schneeberger EE (1983) Proteins and vesicular transport in capillary endothelium. Fed Proc 42:2419–2424
13. Tate RM, Repine JE (1983) Neutrophils and the adult respiratory distress syndrome. Am Rev Respir Dis 128:522–559
14. Vracko R (1974) Basal lamina scaffold-anatomy and significance for maintenance of orderly tissue structure. Am J Pathol 77:314–346

VI Experimental Studies

Simultaneous Measurement of Endothelial Cell Damage, Elastase Release, and Chemiluminescence Response During Interaction Between Polymorphonuclear Leukocytes and Endothelial Cells

E. Jonas[1], A. Dwenger[1], B. Lueken[1], and U. Böhme[2]

Introduction

The polymorphonuclear leukocyte (PMNL, neutrophil) has been suggested to play a central role in the pathogenesis of lung injury in adult respiratory distress syndrome (ARDS) [18]. A causal relationship between neutrophil accumulation at sites of inflammation and subsequent endothelial cell (EC) changes has been proposed. Under some circumstances, e.g., endotoxemia, neutrophils adhere to the vessel wall and release toxic products that might alter endothelial structure and function [20] and may therefore precede the development of ARDS. Using cultured human umbilical cord vein ECs and human blood neutrophils, the in vitro interaction between neutrophils and has been studied [11]. Nylon fiber as a model for certain endothelial reactions ECs has shown a respiratory burst stimulation of neutrophils during adherence of neutrophils to nylon fiber [5]. Furthermore, amplification of oxygen-derived metabolite production during adherence to nylon fiber by lipopolysaccharide (LPS) priming of neutrophils has been shown [5]. LPS is able to stimulate neutrophil secretion of enzymes and oxygen-derived metabolites [7].

The aim of this study was to examine whether a respiratory burst stimulation would also be observed by EC/PMNL interaction and whether the respiratory burst stimulation of neutrophils by ECs could be enhanced by LPS stimulation of neutrophils. The second goal of the study was to examine whether oxygen-derived metabolites could explain EC damage in vitro, or whether EC damage could be shown to be mainly mediated by elastase released by LPS-stimulated neutrophils. Low concentrations of LPS similar to those detectable in blood of patients with gram-negative bacteremia were used [12]. In the present study, chemiluminescence (CL) as an indicator of oxygen-derived metabolites produced by neutrophils, elastase release by

[1] Department of Clinical Biochemistry, Hannover Medical School, Konstanty-Gutschow-Str. 8, W-3000 Hannover 61, FRG
[2] Department of Gynecology, Friederikenstift, Humboldtstr. 5, W-3000 Hannover 1, FRG

J.A. Sturm (Ed.)
Adult Respiratory Distress Syndrome

neutrophils, and EC damage based on [^{111}In] oxine release from labeled ECs was measured simultaneously.

For experimental use a technique was set up whereby ECs were established as suspensions, monolayers, or ECs grown on microcarrier beads.

Methods

Preparation of Endothelial Cells

Human umbilical cord vein ECs were harvested by collagenase digestion [6, 10]. Briefly, the cord was severed from the placenta soon after birth, placed in a sterile container filled with "cord buffer" (0.14 *M* NaCl, 0.004 *M* KCl, 0.001 *M* phosphate buffer, pH 7.4), and stored for no longer than 6 h until further processing. The vein was infused with cord buffer containing 0.01% collagenase (Gibco BRL, Eggenstein, FRG), clamped shut, and incubated at 37°C for 30 min. The collagenase solution containing ECs was flushed from the umbilical cord with cord buffer. The cells were sedimented, washed, and resuspended in culture medium (mixture of M199 and RPMI 1640 medium, Flow Laboratories, Meckenheim, FRG), which contained 12% human AB serum and is a selective medium for ECs. The cells were transferred to 75-cm^2 culture flasks (Corning, New York) and grown to confluence, when the typical cobblestone morphology was identified by phase contrast microscopy. In addition, the cells expressed Factor VIII antigen as detected by fluorescein-conjugated rabbit antihuman Factor VIII antibody (Behringwerke, Marburg, FRG). Transmission electron microscopy revealed a normal ultrastructure [9].

Experimental Design

The assays were performed with EC suspensions, ECs grown on Thermanox coverslips (Lux Scientific Corporation, Naperville, IL, USA), or ECs grown on microcarrier beads (Cytodex 3, Pharmacia Fine Chemicals, Sweden).

Endothelial Cell Suspensions

When experiments were performed with EC suspensions, they were trypsinized [trypsin, 0.05%/ethylenediaminetetraacetic acid (EDTA), 0.02% in phosphate-buffered saline solution, Boehringer] and resuspended in minimum essential medium (MEM) Dulbecco buffer solution (Boehringer). Primary passage ECs were used at 1×10^4 cells/vial.

Endothelial Cell Monolayer

For monolayer experiments, ECs were plated on sterilized coverslips which were cut to 8 mm in diameter. The final plating density was 1×10^4 cells/coverslip counted by hemocytometry, providing a visually confluent monolayer after overnight incubation in culture medium. Adherent cell counts after 18 h were approximately 10000 cells with 5%–10% variation between replicates.

Endothelial Cells Grown on Microcarrier Beads

The microcarrier technique allowed for the generation of large numbers of ECs in suspension, but growing as monolayers [19]. Experiments with ECs grown on microcarrier beads were conducted using a microcarrier system of negatively charged spherical dextran beads. The diameter range was 133–215 μm. The setup was a modification of a technique described elsewhere [3]. Cells were allowed to attach to the beads in the absence of flow after incubating the beads with RM 12% medium. The unattached cells and beads were then gently mixed with a siliconized glass rod and left undisturbed. After cells had become attached (within 3 h), they were agitated gently (30 rpm) by a microcarrier stirrer system (Techne, Cambridge, UK).

To determine cell numbers, small aliquots of beads were sampled from the culture and transferred to a siliconized test tube. The medium was removed, the microcarrier system rinsed twice with PBS, without Ca and Mg, then incubated briefly with a solution of EDTA: trypsin. The detached cells and denuded beads were suspended by pipetting and aliquots were removed for cell counting by hemocytometry.

Neutrophils, suspended in MEM Dulbecco buffer solution, were added to ECs at a final concentration of 7×10^4 cells/vial (7 neutrophils/EC). [^{111}In]Oxine (Amersham Buchler, Braunschweig, FRG) -labeled target ECs (either as suspensions or monolayers) were mixed with stimulated or unstimulated neutrophils and agitated gently. After the addition of neutrophils, CL measurement was started and recorded continuously. After a 60-min incubation time, one-third of the supernatant was removed to determine [^{111}In]oxine release by ECs and elastase release by neutrophils.

Priming and Preparation of Human Polymorphonuclear Leukocytes

Blood from healthy donors was preincubated for 20 min at 37°C without and with different concentrations of LPS (*E. coli* serotype 0.55:B5, extracted with phenol from *E. coli*, Sigma, Deisenhofen, FRG). Small amounts of LPS were used (5, 10, and 20 ng LPS/ml blood). The lyophilized LPS was dissolved in MEM buffer solution at 250 μg/100 μl. Frozen aliquots were thawed and diluted to the appropriate concentration prior to use. Neutrophils were prepared using Percoll density gradient centrifugation [4], and were resuspended in MEM buffer solution.

Chemiluminescence

Chemiluminescence was measured by luminol-enhanced chemiluminescence, using a six-channel Biolumat (LB 9505, Berthold, FRG) for simultaneous measurement. Chemiluminescence measurements of non-stimulated and LPS-stimulated PMNLs were performed in both the absence and presence of ECs. The chemiluminescence parameters were calculated from the peak maximum counts/min values. When experiments were performed with EC suspensions, the reaction mixture consisted of 415 μl MEM buffer solution, 10 μl luminol (22.6 mmol/l), 20 μl human plasma, 100 μl EC suspension, and 25 μl PMNL suspension. When experiments were performed with EC monolayers and ECs grown on microcarrier beads, the reaction mixtures were identical. Release of oxygen-derived metabolites was determined in duplicate or triplicate reaction mixtures.

Endothelial Cell Damage

The evaluation of EC damage was based on [^{111}In]oxine release from labeled ECs. The assay used was a modification of a previously described monolayer injury assay [1]. [^{111}In]Oxine can label ECs in vitro both in monolayers and suspensions with low spontaneous leakage. [^{111}In]Oxine has the advantage, as a cell label, of high labeling and high counting efficiency. It has been shown that labeling of ECs with [^{111}In]oxine does not affect the ability of ECs to attach to or spread out on tissue culture petridishes [15]. On the day of assay ECs were washed three times with phosphate-buffered saline. To label the EC suspensions, [^{111}In]oxine was added to the cells to achieve a final concentration of 1 μCi [^{111}In]oxine/10^4 cells. The cells were incubated for 20 min at room temperature. After labeling, the ECs were washed three times with buffer and were resuspended in MEM buffer solution. When experiments were performed using endothelial monolayers or ECs grown on microcarrier beads, the cells were treated in an identical manner.

Injury to ECs was quantified in terms of percentage specific ^{111}In release which was calculated to be: A/A + B, where A is the counts/min value in the supernatant of samples containing neutrophils and target cells and B is the counts/min value of the pellet of the same sample. In addition, control values for [^{111}In]oxine release were determined using samples containing target cells alone. Controls for spontaneous release consisted of labeled cells which were derived from the same umbilical cord and which were identically treated.

Elastase

The immunologic determination of elastase concentration in the samples was performed using the enzyme immunoassay test combination kit "PMN Elastase" (E. Merck, FRG).

Calculations

Chemiluminescence values, measured using neutrophils alone, were subtracted from values obtained after interaction between neutrophils and ECs. EC damage was expressed as percentage specific [^{111}In]oxine release. The value for percentage specific [^{111}In]oxine release was obtained by subtracting the control value. Results are shown as $\bar{x} \pm$ SEM. For statistical analysis, Student's *t* test for nonpaired data was applied.

Results

Chemiluminescence Measurements

Neutrophils treated with different concentrations of LPS released increased amounts of oxygen-derived metabolites in comparison to unstimulated neutrophils (data not shown). A significant increase in photon emission was observed during interaction between unstimulated neutrophils and ECs, as suspensions ($p < 0.01$), ECs grown on coverslips ($p < 0.025$), and ECs grown on microcarrier beads ($p < 0.02$). Data are shown in Table 1.

Table 1. Photon emission (peak maximum counts/min) during interaction between unstimulated neutrophils and ECs (70000 PMNLs: 10000 ECs), both as suspensions and as ECs grown on coverslips and on microcarrier beads

	PMNLs	PMNLs + ECs
EC suspension (cpm × 10^3)	265.5 ± 24.6 $n = 25$	411.9 ± 43.1*
ECs grown on coverslips (cpm × 10^3)	195.5 ± 31.1 $n = 15$	326.7 ± 41.8**
ECs grown on microcarrier beads (cpm × 10^3)	207.7 ± 28.6 $n = 13$	348.7 ± 48.8***

*$p < 0.01$ vs. value for PMNLs alone; **$p < 0.025$ vs. value for PMNLs alone; ***$p < 0.02$ vs. value for PMNLs alone
Values are shown as $\bar{x} \pm$ SEM

In Figs. 1–3, the dose response relationship between blood pretreatment with varying LPS concentrations and CL response of neutrophils exposed to endothelial cells is shown.

When experiments were performed with EC suspensions, CL increases following LPS stimulation were significantly different ($p < 0.01$) at 10 ng/ml blood compared with unstimulated neutrophils (Fig. 1). This effect could not be further increased by an LPS concentration of up to 20 ng LPS/ml blood. Even stimulation of blood with 100 ng LPS/ml blood did not further increase the CL response (data not shown). When experiments were performed with ECs grown on coverslips or microcarrier beads, CL increases following LPS stimulation of neutrophils were already significantly different ($p < 0.005$ for ECs grown on coverslips or $p < 0.001$ for ECs grown on microcarrier beads)

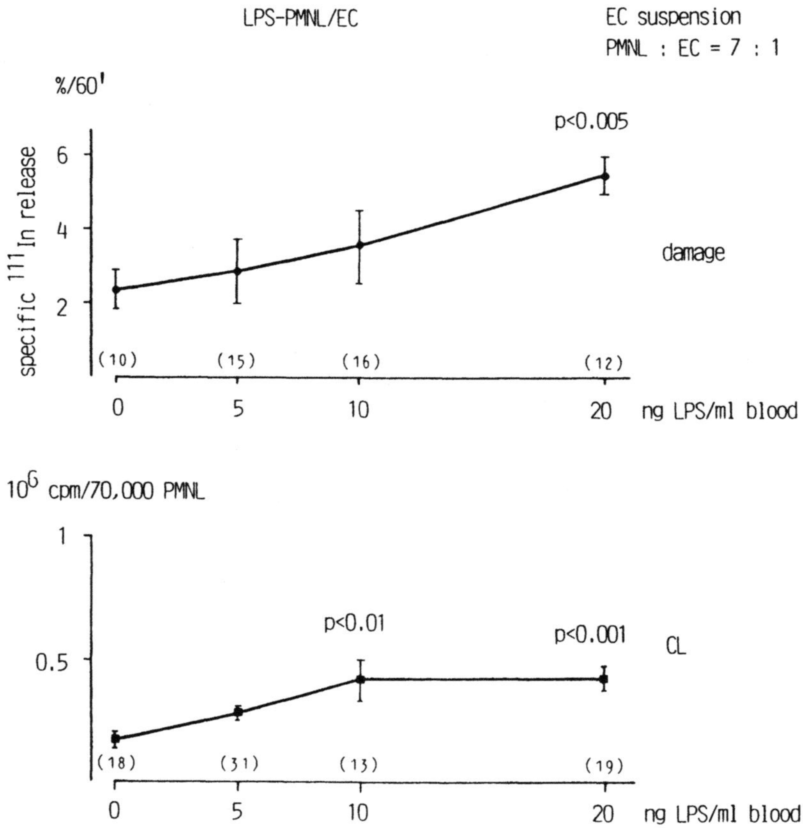

Fig. 1. *Upper*, effect of neutrophils stimulated with different concentrations of LPS on [^{111}In]oxine release from EC suspensions. *Lower*, chemiluminescence response (counts/min of peak maximum) of neutrophils in contact with EC suspensions. The incubation time was 1 h. Data are shown as $\bar{x} \pm$ SEM; significance versus value for unstimulated PMNLs

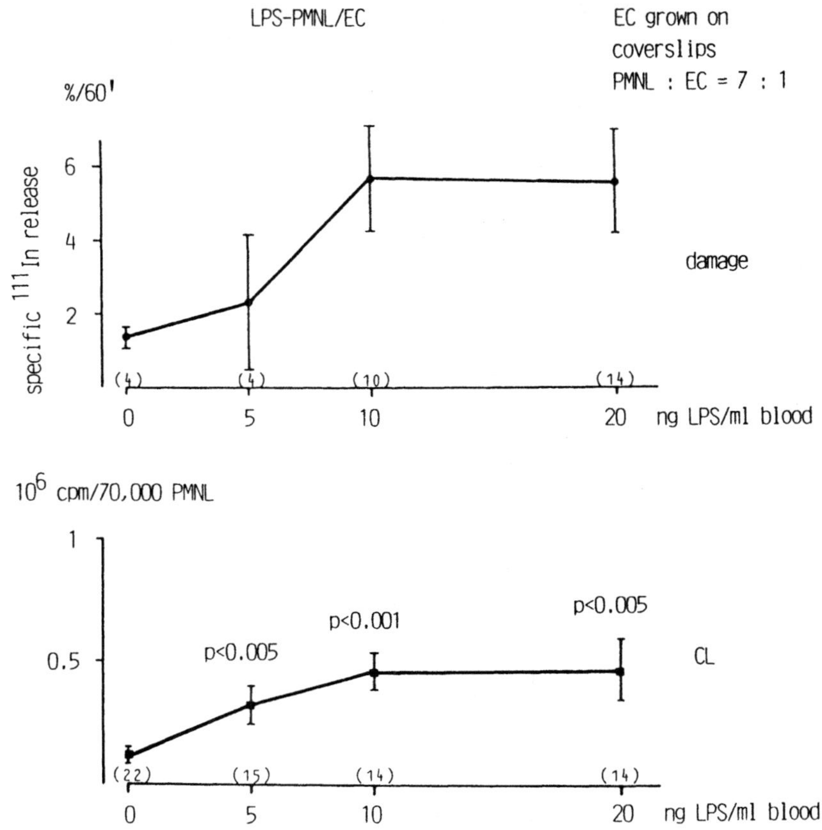

Fig. 2. *Upper*, effect of neutrophils stimulated with different concentrations of LPS on [^{111}In]oxine release from ECs grown on coverslips. *Lower*, chemiluminescence response counts/min of peak maximum) of neutrophils in contact with ECs grown on coverslips. Data are shown as $\bar{x} \pm$ SEM; significance versus value for unstimulated PMNLs

at 5 ng LPS/ml blood (Figs. 2, 3). This effect could not be further increased by an LPS concentration of 20 ng LPS/ml blood or 100 ng LPS/ml blood, respectively.

Endothelial Cell Damage

Unstimulated neutrophils did not elicit significant release of [^{111}In]oxine from endothelial cell suspensions after 1 h incubation. Yet, neutrophils stimulated with 20 ng LPS/ml blood caused significant damage ($p < 0.005$) after 1 h incubation in comparison to controls (Fig. 1). LPS alone did not mediate significant cytotoxicity ($p < 0.30$; $n = 4$). Neutrophils stimulated with different LPS concentrations caused a slight, but not significant, release of [^{111}In]oxine from labeled endothelial cells grown on coverslips (Fig. 2). A

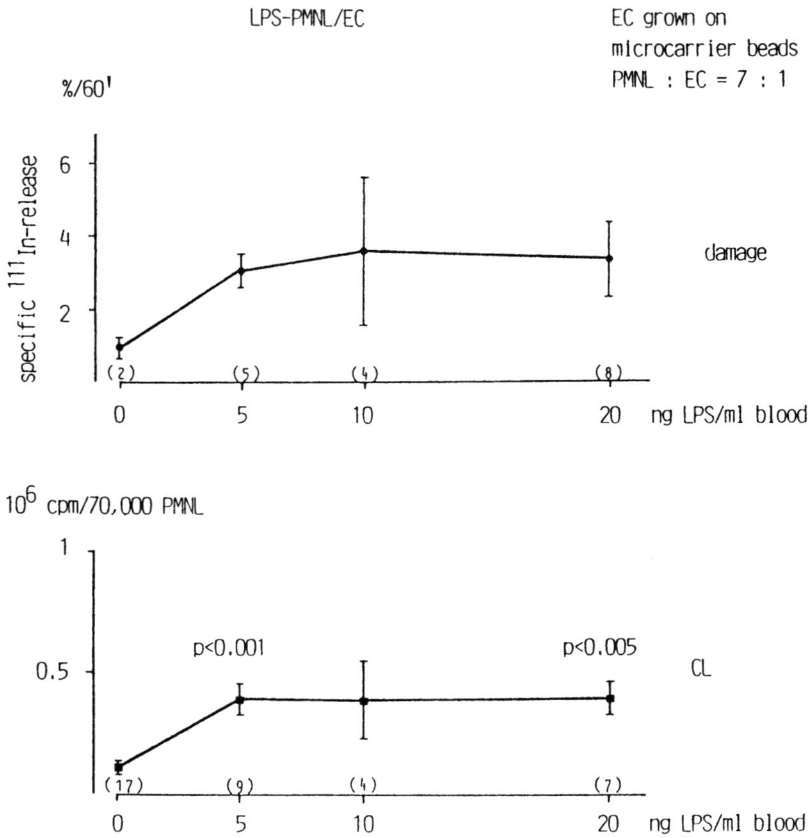

Fig. 3. *Upper*, effect of neutrophils stimulated with different concentrations of LPS on [^{111}In]oxine release from ECs grown on microcarrier beads. *Lower*, chemiluminescence response (counts per minute of peak maximum) of neutrophils in contact with ECs grown on microcarrier beads. Data are shown as $\bar{x} \pm$ SEM; significance versus value for unstimulated PMNLs

slight but not significant [^{111}In]oxine release was also obtained with ECs grown on microcarrier beads exposed to PMNLs stimulated with different concentrations of LPS (Fig. 3).

Elastase Release

Elastase release by PMNLs is shown in Tables 2 and 3. Elastase release by PMNLs, stimulated with varying LPS concentrations, increased significantly ($p < 0.0005$) in comparison with unstimulated PMNLs (Tables 2, 3). Table 2

Table 2. Elastase release by PMNLs stimulated with different concentrations of LPS during interaction with EC suspensions

EC suspension	Elastase (µg/l in 60 min) 70000 PMNLs			
	0	5	10	20 ng LPS/ml blood
PMNLs	70.8 ± 7.2 ($n = 8$)	89.0 ± 10.0* ($n = 7$)	109.2 ± 7.7** ($n = 7$)	107.4 ± 5.3*** ($n = 9$)
PMNLs + ECs	85.6 ± 16.8 ($n = 7$)	118.3 ± 18.8 ($n = 8$)	113.9 ± 18.2 ($n = 6$)	110.6 ± 6.8 ($n = 9$)

*$p < 0.01$ vs. value for unstimulated PMNLs; **$p < 0.0025$ vs. value for unstimulated PMNLs; ***$p < 0.0005$ vs. value for unstimulated PMNLs
Data are shown as $\bar{x}$ ± SEM

Table 3. Elastase release by PMNLs stimulated with different concentrations of LPS during interaction with ECs grown on coverslips

EC monolayer	Elastase (µg/l in 60 min) 70000 PMNLs			
	0	5	10	20 ng LPS/ml blood
PMNLs	65.3 ± 6.0 ($n = 5$)	98.9 ± 27.2* ($n = 5$)	105.0 ± 3.0** ($n = 2$)	141.9 ± 7.0*** ($n = 6$)
PMNLs + blank coverslips	62.7 ± 3.4 ($n = 5$)	87.1 ± 6.5 ($n = 7$)	136.4 ± 27.7 ($n = 4$)	130.8 ± 13.5 ($n = 10$)
PMNLs × ECs	66.7 ± 6.8 ($n = 6$)	81.2 ± 10.8 ($n = 12$)	129.0 ± 21.4 ($n = 5$)	141.0 ± 14.0 ($n = 10$)

*$p < 0.15$ vs. value for unstimulated PMNLs; **$p < 0.01$ vs. value for unstimulated PMNLs; ***$p < 0.0005$ vs. value for unstimulated PMNLs
Data are shown as $\bar{x}$ ± SEM

shows the results for endothelial cell suspensions. The difference in elastase release by PMNL and by PMNL during interaction with EC suspensions was not significant at any LPS concentration. When experiments were performed with endothelial cell monolayers, elastase release did not significantly increase during interaction between PMNLs and blank coverslips or PMNLs and ECs grown on coverslips in comparison to PMNL alone (Table 3), even when neutrophils were treated with different concentrations of LPS. Similar results were obtained when experiments were performed with ECs grown on microcarrier beads (Table 4). There was no significant difference between PMNLs in contact with blank microcarrier beads and PMNLs in contact with endothelial cells grown on microcarrier beads in comparison to PMNLs alone.

Table 4. Elastase release by PMNLs stimulated with different LPS concentrations in contact with ECs grown on microcarrier beads. Data are shown as $\bar{x} \pm$ SEM

EC microcarrier	Elastase (μg/l in 60 min) 70 000 PMNLs			
	0	5	10	20 ng LPS/ml blood
PMNLs + blank microcarrier	114.2 ± 11.5 (*n* = 5)	104.8 ± 2.3 (*n* = 2)	131.6 ± 9.6 (*n* = 3)	166.3 ± 11.8 (*n* = 5)
PMNLs + ECs	130.5 ± 33.8 (*n* = 7)	121.1 ± 6.4 (*n* = 2)	158.9 ± 35.5 (*n* = 3)	157.2 ± 9.5 (*n* = 5)

Discussion

The current investigation utilizing cultured ECs and granulocytes provides the data base for a model to study the mechanisms by which unstimulated and LPS-stimulated PMNLs interact with ECs. The data presented suggest that neutrophils can be directly stimulated by ECs, as demonstrated by increased oxygen-derived metabolite production during interaction between ECs and unstimulated PMNLs. These observations, made by experiments performed with EC suspensions, EC monolayer, and ECs grown on microcarrier beads, indicate that human ECs may have the potential to influence PMNL functions. Therefore, our findings support previous observations indicating that ECs and EC products can modify PMNL chemotaxis and adherence [21] and PMNL aggregation [22].

In addition, it could be shown that methods which increased the contact of PMNLs to ECs, e.g., centrifugation, were associated with increases in CL (data not shown), suggesting that contact is an important step during interaction between PMNLs and ECs.

Oxygen-derived metabolites could be shown to be increased under conditions of LPS stimulation, an observation that has already been described [5]. Furthermore, it has been shown in the present study that respiratory burst stimulation of PMNLs by ECs could be enhanced by LPS stimulation of PMNLs even with low doses of LPS. Because previous investigations performed with nylon fiber have shown a similar effect [5], a similarity between PMNL adherence to nylon fiber as an artificial model and ECs can be supposed, an effect that has been assumed by other investigators [2, 13].

In the present study, culture methods were divided into two groups, one group using enzymes and one group avoiding exposure of ECs to enzymes during subculture. The similar dose response pattern regarding photon emission by PMNLs of all three EC models suggests that the morphologic state of the ECs has no influence on EC-PMNL interaction regarding photon emission by PMNL. Even when ECs are trypsinized, there is no significant difference in comparison to EC monolayer cells and ECs grown on microcarrier beads, although trypsinization causes the monolayer cells to lose their flattened appearance and become round. The investigation has been extended by demonstrating a technique whereby oxygen radical production, [^{111}In]oxine release, and elastase production could be measured simultaneously. The aim was to study a possible injurious potential of LPS alone, unstimulated, and LPS-stimulated PMNLs. For this reason, ECs were labeled with [^{111}In]oxine. By using phase contrast microscopy and electron microscopy it could be confirmed that labeling of ECs with [^{111}In]oxine did not affect the ability of ECs to attach to culture flasks or coverslips [15]. LPS alone had no measurable injurious effect on EC damage, suggesting the essential participation of the PMNL in the genesis of EC damage in this system. Even unstimulated PMNLs did not cause [^{111}In]oxine release from labeled ECs, thus indicating that stimulation of neutrophils played a necessary role in this system. A significant [^{111}In]oxine release in comparison with controls occurred following neutrophil stimulation between 10 and 20 ng LPS/ml blood in the trypsin-treated EC group. This effect could be explained as a consequence of previous possible EC-membrane damage by trypsinization followed by damage caused by PMNLs. In contrast, experiments performed with ECs grown on coverslips or microcarrier beads indicate slight, but not significant, EC damage. This suggests that there is no indication of extensive EC-membrane damage. This observation is supported by trypan blue exclusion and by the observation that phase contrast microscopy showed focal disruption of the monolayer by stimulated PMNLs but no clear lytic effect.

Contradictory results have been reported on effects of stimulated neutrophils on ECs [14]. However, there are several important differences between the assays that may account for at least some of the differences. Apparently, the selection of stimulus [LPS vs. pyridylmercuric acetate (PMA), (FMLP)] plays an important role in the determination of the mechanisms of cytotoxicity. The fact that in the present study ECs cultured from human umbilical vein are nearly unaffected by a dose of LPS that causes extensive lysis and detachment of bovine pulmonary artery ECs [8] further points to the possibility that ECs from different species or perhaps different tissue beds can lead to different responses. Therefore, it should be pointed out that no clear conclusions from data based on cells obtained from different species can be drawn. The amount of elastase release by PMNLs was shown to be increased under conditions of LPS stimulation, but not by the EC itself. Additionally, it is interesting to note CL increases but no elastase increases when PMNLs are in contact with blank coverslips or microcarrier beads. The failure to detect increased amounts of elastase during interaction between ECs and neutrophils supports the hypothesis that in this system proteases, such as elastase, are not primarily responsible for the observed increase in [^{111}In]oxine release, although it is possible that other (unmeasured) lysosomal enzymes, e.g., cathepsin G, could contribute to the observed increase in [^{111}In]oxine release.

Contradictory results have been reported by other investigators [17], who found the elastase to be mainly responsible for EC damage in the model of adipose tissue ECs. Our observations are similar to those reported by other investigators, who have reported that oxygen radicals were the causative agent of neutrophil-mediated injury [14], even when these work groups have used large doses of LPS. Again, this discrepancy also seems to be based on the type of EC chosen. The type of EC probably determines, in part, the mechanism by which they are injured. Our results are partly supported by other investigators [17], who compared studies performed with human umbilical vein ECs and adipose tissue ECs and reported that ECs were ten times more sensitive to H_2O_2-induced injury than human microvascular cells. An explanation for this observation was provided by a recent study suggesting that umbilical vein ECs lack catalase [16].

Conclusion

In conclusion, the present investigation demonstrates that neutrophils can be directly stimulated by ECs. A further amplification of this process following LPS priming up to 10 ng/ml blood could be demonstrated. A slight EC damage occurs following neutrophil stimulation, although elastase secretion does not increase during interaction between neutrophils and ECs. These results raise the possibility that oxygen-derived metabolites rather than elastase contribute to EC damage which might occur in conditions such as endotoxin-induced ARDS.

Acknowledgment. The authors thank the staff members and nurses of the "Friederikenstift" Delivery Room and "Oststadtkrankenhaus" Delivery Room, Hannover, for their invaluable help in collecting umbilical cords.

References

1. Chopra J, Joist JH, Webster RO (1987) Loss of 51 chromium, lactate dehydrogenase, and ^{111}indium as indicators of endothelial injury. Lab Invest 57:578
2. Clifford DP, Rasp FL, Repine JE (1984) Simultaneous measurement of adherence and chemiluminescence by polymorphonuclear leukocytes. Inflammation 8:101
3. Davies PF (1981) Microcarrier culture of vascular endothelial cells on solid plastic beads. Exp Cell Res 134:367
4. Dwenger A, Schweitzer G, Regel G (1986) Bronchoalveolar lavage fluid and plasma proteins, chemiluminescense response and protein contents of polymorphonuclear leukocytes from blood and lavage fluid in traumatized patients. J Clin Chem Clin Biochem 24:73
5. Dwenger A, Schweitzer G, Funck M (1988) Lipopolysaccharide-dependent enhancement of adherence-mediated chemiluminescence response of polymorphonuclear leukocytes. J Biolum Chemilum 2:35

6. Gimbrone MA, Shefton EJ, Cruise SA (1978) Isolation and primary culture of endothelial cells from human umbilical vessels. Tissue Culture Assoc Manual 4:813
7. Guthrie LA, McPhail LC, Henson PM, Johnston RB (1984) Priming of neutrophils for enhanced release of oxygen metabolites by bacterial lipopolysaccharide. J Exp Med 160:1656
8. Harlan JM, Killen PD, Harker LA, Striker GE, Wright DG (1981) Neutrophil-mediated endothelial injury in vitro (mechanisms of cell detachment), J Clin Invest 68:1394
9. Haudenschild CC, Cotran RS, Gimbrone MA, Folkman J (1975) Fine structure of vascular endothelium in culture. J Ultrastruct Res 50:22
10. Jaffe EA, Hoyer LW, Nachman RL (1973) Synthesis of antihemophilic factor antigen by cultured human endothelial cells. J Clin Invest 52:2757
11. Jonas E, Dwenger A, Lueken B (1988) Chemiluminescence response and endothelial cell damage following lipopolysaccharide priming of polymorphonuclear leukocytes. Fresenius Z Anal Chem 333:421
12. Levin J, Poore TE, Zauber NP, Oser RS (1970) Detection of endotoxin in the blood of patients with sepsis due to gram-negative bacteria. N Engl J Med 283:1313
13. MacGregor RR, Macarak EJ, Kefalides NA (1978) Comparative adherence of granulocytes to endothelial monolayers and nylon fiber. J Clin Invest 61:697
14. Sacks T, Moldow CF, Craddock PR, Bowers TK, Jacob HS (1978) Oxygen radical mediated endothelial cell damage by complement-stimulated granulocytes. J Clin Invest 61:1161
15. Sharefkin JB, Lather C, Smith M, Rich NM (1983) Endothelial cell labeling with indium-111-oxine as a marker of cell attachment to bioprasthetic surface. J Biomed Mater Res 17:345
16. Shingu MK, Yoshioka K, Nobunaga M, Yoshida K (1985) Human vascular smooth muscle cells and endothelial cells lack catalase activity and are susceptible to hydrogen peroxide. Inflammation 9:309
17. Smedly LA, Tonnesen MG, Sandhaus RA, Haslett C, Guthrie LA, Johnston RB, Henson PM, Worthen GS (1986) Neutrophil mediated injury to endothelial cells. J Clin Invest 77:1233
18. Tate RM, Repine JE (1983) Neutrophils and the adult respiratory distress syndrome. Am Rev Respir Dis 128:552
19. Van Wezel AL (1967) Growth of cell strains and primary cells on micro-carriers in homogeneous culture. Nature 216:64
20. Worthen GS, Haslett C, Smedly LA, Rees AJ, Gumbay RS, Henson JE, Henson PM (1986) Lung vascular injury induced by chemotactic factors: enhancement by bacterial endotoxins. Fed Proc 45:7
21. Zimmerman GA, Wiseman GA, Hill HR (1985) Human endothelial cells modulate granulocyte adherence and chemotaxis. J Immunol 134:1966
22. Zimmerman GA, Klein-Knoeckel D (1986) Human endothelial cells inhibit granulocyte aggregation in vitro. J Immunol 136:3839

Influence of Short- and Long-Term Endotoxin Administration on the Phagocytic Functions of Polymorphonuclear Leukocytes and Reticuloendothelial System in a Sheep Model

G. Regel[1], A. Dwenger[2], G. Schweitzer[2], A. Seekamp[1], and J.A. Sturm[1]

Introduction

The reticuloendothelial system (RES) is thought to ensure the clearance of embolic particulate matter and blood-borne bacterial substances after trauma, burns, and sepsis [14]. It thereby helps to prevent disturbances to organ integrity, for instance, lung capillary injury, and consequently the development of adult respiratory distress syndrome (ARDS) [1, 7, 11, 25]. In cases of RES blockade, an enhanced deposition of debris and bacterial matter is seen in the lung [13]. It has been suggested that polymorphonuclear leukocytes (PMNLs) then become activated, migrate to the lung, and can take on a major phagocytic role [8, 21]. It is unclear what mechanisms lead to the activation of neutrophils [26] and their pooling in the lung [5]. This is important in that stimulated PMNLs, in addition to substituting for a blocked RES, may lead to pulmonary endothelial damage [14, 16]. The relative injury-producing role of activated PMNLs alone, as opposed to activated PMNLs that have subsequently decompensated, is unknown [15]. It is therefore questionable whether toxic degranulation is a sign of appropriately increased PMNL function or rather a sign of dysfunction. To clarify these issues we used two animal models that would cause acute and chronic lung injury [2] and examined the behavior of the PMNLs and the RES following single and multiple endotoxin bolus injection.

This study was an attempt to answer the following questions:

1. Does injection of a standardized dose of endotoxin, an insult known to cause an increase in lung permeability [3], also lead to RES blockade [3, 4, 20]?
2. By what mechanisms do PMNLs localize in the lung?

[1] Department of Trauma Surgery, Hannover Medical School, Konstanty-Gutschow-Str. 8, W-3000 Hannover 61, FRG
[2] Department of Clinical Biochemistry, Hannover Medical School, Konstanty-Gutschow-Str. 8, W-3000 Hannover 61, FRG

J.A. Sturm (Ed.)
Adult Respiratory Distress Syndrome

3. Are neutrophils activated or decompensated after endotoxin administration and with what time course?

Materials and Methods

Reticuloendothelial System Function Test

Twenty-four female sheep weighing 27–45 kg were used in the study. All animals were monitored for several days before the experiment to ensure they were in a good, healthy condition, afebrile, and with no signs of infection [normal white blood cell count (WBC)]. Twenty-four hours prior to the experiment, catheters were placed in both jugular veins of the unanesthetized animals. After injecting a bolus of 100 μCi [^{99}Tc]phytate (a biometabolizable colloid) [4, 21] into one of the venous lines, 5-ml venous blood aliquots were extracted every 2 min from the other line. This was performed to measure the blood clearance by the RES, as the phytate colloid is normally 85% phagocytized by the Kupffer cells. Blood samples were centrifuged at 3000 rpm for 10 min and the ^{99}Tc activity in 1 ml plasma subsequently measured. Radioactivity was analyzed with a scintillation counter and the reticuloendothelial function expressed by the half-life time formula: $1nA = 1nB \times X$, with $t_{1/2} = 0.6931{:}B$. Directly following RES function testing, the sheep were anesthetized with 15–20 mg/kg body wt. sodium pentobarbital. We then placed polyvinyl arterial and venous catheters via a femoral incision and a Swan-Ganz thermodilution catheter (Edwards model 93A-131-9F) via the external jugular vein. The animals were allowed to recover for 24 h and were then studied in an unanesthesized and unrestrained state.

Endotoxin Animal Models

The short-term model was studied for 24 h and the chronically instrumented sheep were studied for 5 days. Aortic (Part), pulmonary artery (Ppa), pulmonary arterial wedge (Ppaw), and central venous (CVP) pressures were recorded and cardiac output (CO) was measured by the thermodilution method. To ensure a steady state, all measurements were obtained during a 2-h baseline. The hematologic and biochemical parameters described below were also collected during the control period. Following the intravenous bolus injection of *Escherichia coli* endotoxin (serotype 055:B5, Sigma chemicals) (2 μg/kg body wt), samples were collected according to the time-table shown in Table 1. RES function was again studied by the above method from 15 to 45 min postendotoxin administration.

Hematologic samples were anticoagulated with ethylenediaminetetraacetic acid (EDTA) and biochemical aliquots with sodium citrate (10%).

Table 1. Protocol for hemodynamic measurements and sample collection

	Hemodynamics	CL	Hematology	RES function
Baseline	*	*	*	
Endotoxin	(ET)—	—	—	—
15 min pET		*	*	*
30 min	*	*	*	
1 h	*	*	*	
1 h 30 min	*			
2 h	*			
2 h 30 min	*			
3 h	*			
3 h 30 min	*			
4 h	*	*	*	
12 h	(ET)—	—	—	—
24 h/baseline	*	*	*	

CL, chemiluminescence

Polymorphonuclear Leukocyte Separation

One milliliter of venous sheep blood was mixed with 1 ml saline solution and layered on Percoll (4 ml 1.070 g/cm^2 density) and centrifuged at 350 *g* at 25°C for 20 min. The supernatant was discarded and the erythrocytes of the cell pellet were lysed with 4 ml icecold water for 30 s. Then, 2 ml 2.7% NaCl was added, the granulocytes were washed twice with phosphate-buffered saline (PBS) (530 *g*, 25°C, 5 min), resuspended with 200–500 µl PBS, and counted using a Neubauer hemocytometer after cell staining with Türk's solution (viability rate, 90%).

Polymorphonuclear Leukocyte Function

Chemiluminescence Measurement

Luminol-enhanced chemiluminescence (CL) was determined using the six-channel Bioluminat LB 9505 in combination with an Apple II plus computer and an Epson MX 82 F/T printer (Laboratory Prof. Dr. Berthold, Wildbad, FRG) in 3-ml polystyrene CL vials. For CL measurements the following reagents were prepared: luminol in minimum essential medium (MEM) Dulbecco (Boehringer, Mannheim, FRG), 22.6 mmol/l containing triethylamine, 40 mmol/l, daily fresh preparation; zymosan A, washed twice with PBS, once with MEM (centrifugation at 800 *g* for 10 min at 22°C) and resuspended in MEM, 100 mg/ml, frozen in aliquots at −70°C. CL measurements were performed at 37°C with prewarmed reagents.

For CL characterization we used the following parameters:

Whole blood (CL of 2.5×10^5 PMNLs):

1. Base activity: reaction measured after mixture of 520 µl MEM, 10 µl luminol, and 50 µl whole blood
2. Activity after stimulation: 500 µl MEM, 10 µl luminol, 20 µl zymosan (2 mg), and 50 µl whole blood

Isolated cells (CL of 25 000 isolated PMNLs):

1. Base activity: 520 µl MEM, 50 µl plasma of the baseline sample, 10 µl luminol, 50 µl cell suspension (25 000 PMNLs)
2. Activity after stimulation: 500 µl MEM, 50 µl plasma of the baseline sample, 10 µl luminol, 50 µl cell suspension, and 20 µl opsonized zymosan (2 mg)

The peak maximum CL was determined and is abbreviated as CLPM in the following text. CL measurements were started simultaneously in six channels and the photon emission was recorded continuously for at least 60 min. All measurements were corrected by subtraction of the base activity from the stimulation value.

Adherence of Isolated PMNLs (Acute Model)

A nylon fiber column was produced by filling a 1-ml syringe with 0.05 g nylon pressed to a volume of 0.25 cm^2 and moistened with 500 µl PBS. One milliliter of PMNL suspension containing approximately 10^6 PMNLs/ml was incubated together with 10% sheep serum for 10 min at 37°C and placed in the prepared syringe. The adherence was measured by determining the cell count in the suspension both before (*B*) and after (*A*) passage through the column. Percentage adherence was calculated by the following formula: $100 - (A) \times 100/(B)$.

Adherence of PMNLs in Whole Blood (Long-Term Model)

A quantity of 400 µl MEM and 100 µl citrated blood were incubated with (A) and without (B) 5 mg nylon fiber in 3-ml polystyrene vials for 20 min at 37°C. After removing the nylon fiber the nonadhered portions of granulocytes were counted in A and B, respectively, after cell staining with Türk's solution.

$$\% \text{ adherence} = \frac{(\text{PMNLs/ml}_B - \text{PMNLs/ml}_A)\ 100}{(\text{PMNLs/ml}_B)}$$

Results

Base Data

All animals were studied after a steady baseline period.

Short-Term Model

Reticuloendothelial System Function

Reticuloendothelial system function was measured at 15 min pET. Nine out of 11 animals of the short-term model showed an increase in RES clearance after endotoxin administration, as revealed by changes in the half-life times ($t_{1/2}$) ($p < 0.05$) (Fig. 1). A correlation between changes in cardiac output and changes in RES function was not seen ($p < 0.05$, two-tailed Wilcoxon test for matched pairs).

Polymorphonuclear Leukocyte Function

White Cell Count. Total white count as well as granulocytes decreased rapidly during the first 15 min pET, as seen in Table 2. Granulocytes showed the

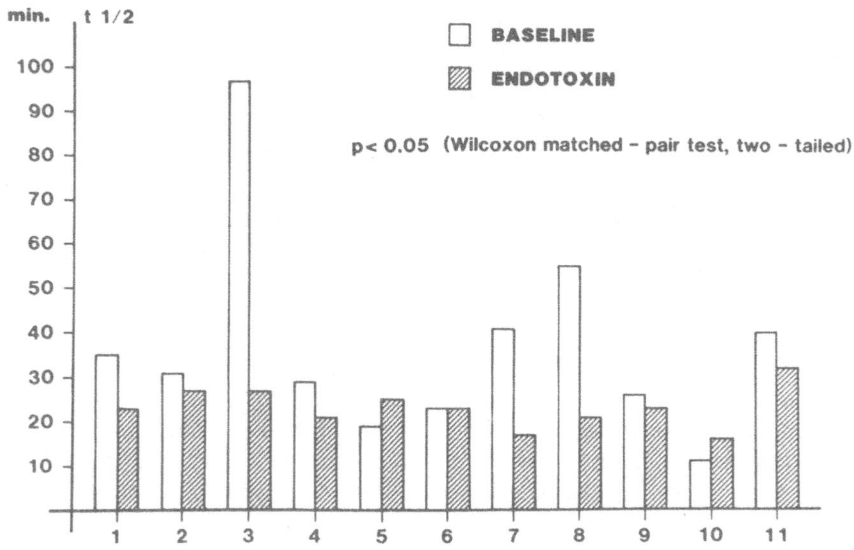

Fig. 1. Half-life of ^{99}Tc colloid: baseline versus 15 min postendotoxin in the short-term model

Table 2. White blood count before and after endotoxin administration

	Baseline			15 min			4 h			24 h		
	$\bar{x}$	SEM	*n*	$\bar{x}$	SEM	*n*	$\bar{x}$	SEM	*n*	$\bar{x}$	SEM	*n*
Leukocytes (WBC) (1/mm^3)	9519	1104.85	8	4780	958.13	8	2088	207.4	8	12014	978.36	8
Granulocytes (1/mm^3)	5121	1017.75	8	1579	335.38	7	754	55.68	6	7433	1246.44	6
As % of WBC:												
Neutrophils	64.5	3.62	4	30.5	2.21	4	43.5	9.75	4	55.7	7.13	3
Monocytes	2.3	1.03	4	5.2	1.89	4	1.5	0.96	4	3.0	0.58	3
Lymphocytes	31.0	5.20	4	63.5	13.05	4	55.0	9.81	4	41.3	7.53	3
Others (eosinophils + basophils)	2.2	1.93	4	0.8	0.50	4	0.0	0.0	4	0.0	0.0	3

lowest level, with a mean of $x = 0.75 \pm 0.06 \times 10^6$/ml 4 h after ET. Both the 15-min and 4-h measurements were significantly different from baseline values ($p < 0.05$). The lymphocyte count showed no significant changes.

Adherence

Adherence was tested at 15 min, 4 h, and 24 h pET. The results of these tests are seen in Fig. 2. A significant increase in adherence was seen only at 4 h pET (66.14% ± 3.7%).

Chemiluminescence

The peak maximum (CPLM), or the peak value of CL after stimulation with zymosan, was assessed in whole blood samples as well as isolated ovine white cell suspensions. CLPM for whole blood showed a continuous decline to a low point at 1 h after endotoxin administration ($x = 0.41 \pm 0.08 \times 10^6$ cpm) (Fig. 3) and subsequently increased steadily until the last measurement at 24 h. Baseline values were reached after 6 h. At 24 h the CLPM mean value was $1.46 \pm 0.27 \times 10^6$ cpm, which was not significantly different from the baseline value ($p < 0.2$). The CLPM for isolated cells fell to a minimum at 1 h. This minimum was significantly lower than baseline CL ($0.52 \pm 0.13 \times 10^6$ cpm, $p < 0.05$). A return to baseline values occurred after approximately 5 h ($1.64 \pm 0.38 \times 10^6$ cpm) and there was a continuous increase up to 24 h ($2.47 \pm 0.62 \times 10^6$ cpm).

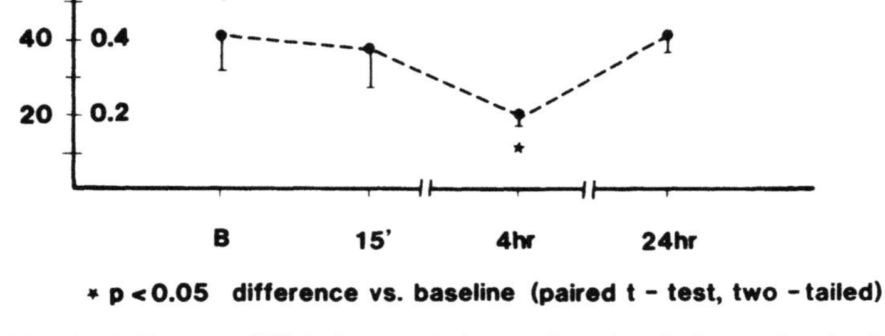

Fig. 2. Adherence (%) before and after endotoxin administration in the short-term model

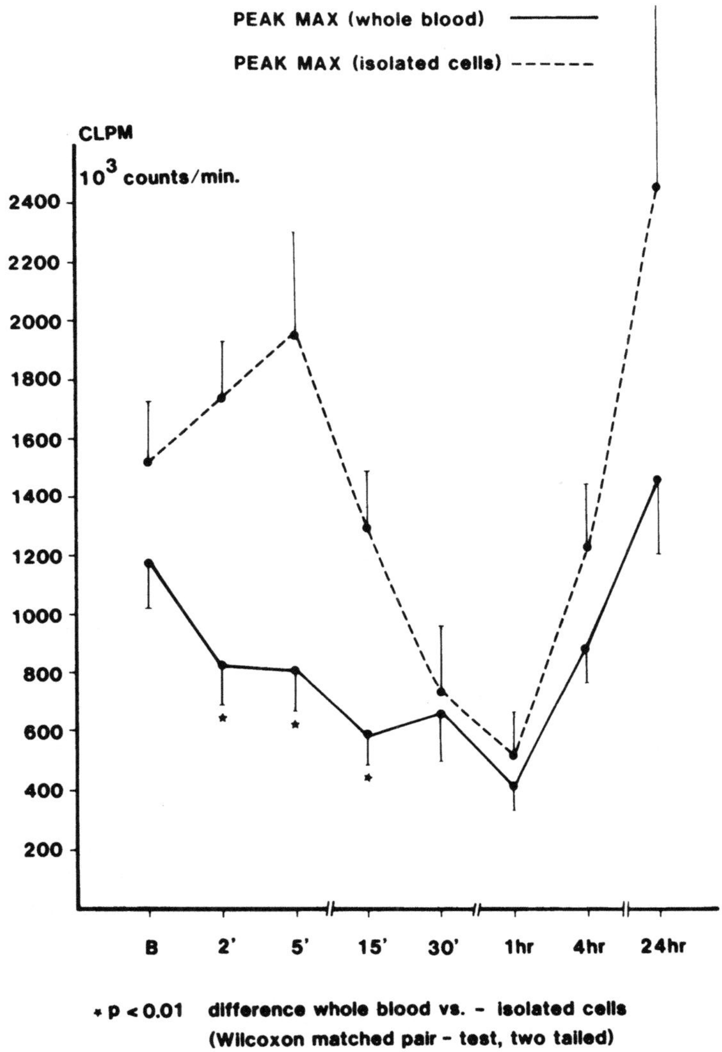

Fig. 3. Chemiluminescence peak maximum of whole blood versus isolated cell samples after endotoxin administration in the short-term model

Long-Term Model

Reticuloendothelial system function was measured at 15 min pET on 5 days in the long-term model (Fig. 4). Similar to the short-term model an increase (reduction of half-life) of clearance was seen. This was maximal on the 3rd experimental day. Baseline values were still not reached at the end of the study period (5th day).

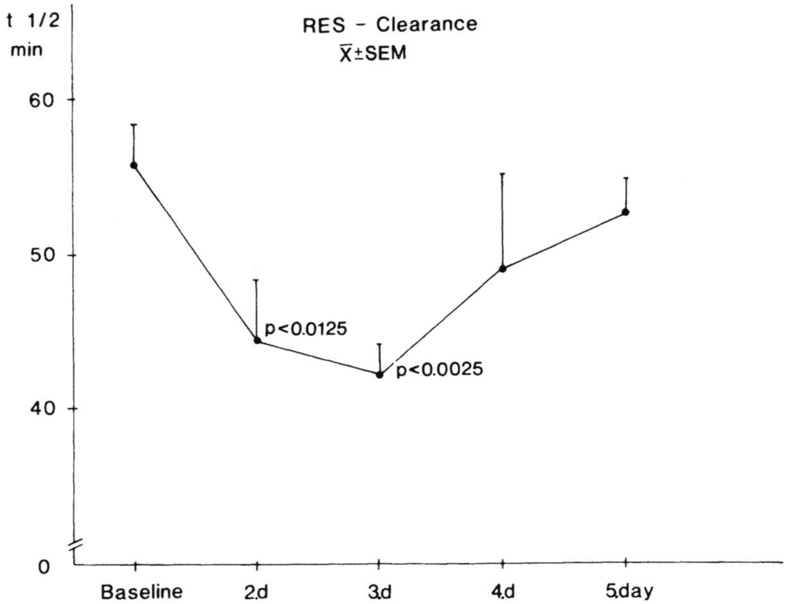

Fig. 4. Half-life of ^{99}Tc colloid: baseline versus 2nd, 3rd, 4th, and 5th day in the long-term model

White Cell Count

Recurrent endotoxin bolus injection (12-h intervals) resulted in a steady decrease of granulocytes in the peripheral blood, up to a minimum at 30 min to 1 h after administration of endotoxin. This minimum was altered during the time course from $0.45 \pm 0.02 \times 10^6$/ml on the 1st day to $1.23 \pm 0.04 \times 10^6$/ml on the 5th day (Fig. 5).

Adherence

The chronic endotoxin effect led to an increase in adherence up to a maximum of 58% ± 2% on the 3rd day. A return to baseline values could not be found during the investigation period (Fig. 5).

Chemiluminescence

A decompensation state was seen following each endotoxin bolus with a minimum at 30 min to 1 h after administration of endotoxin. Again this minimum was lowest on the 1st day with $0.51 \pm 0.01 \times 10^6$ cpm and increased up to $0.98 \pm 0.02 \times 10^6$ cpm on day 5 (Fig. 6). These results were confirmed by the whole blood measurements.

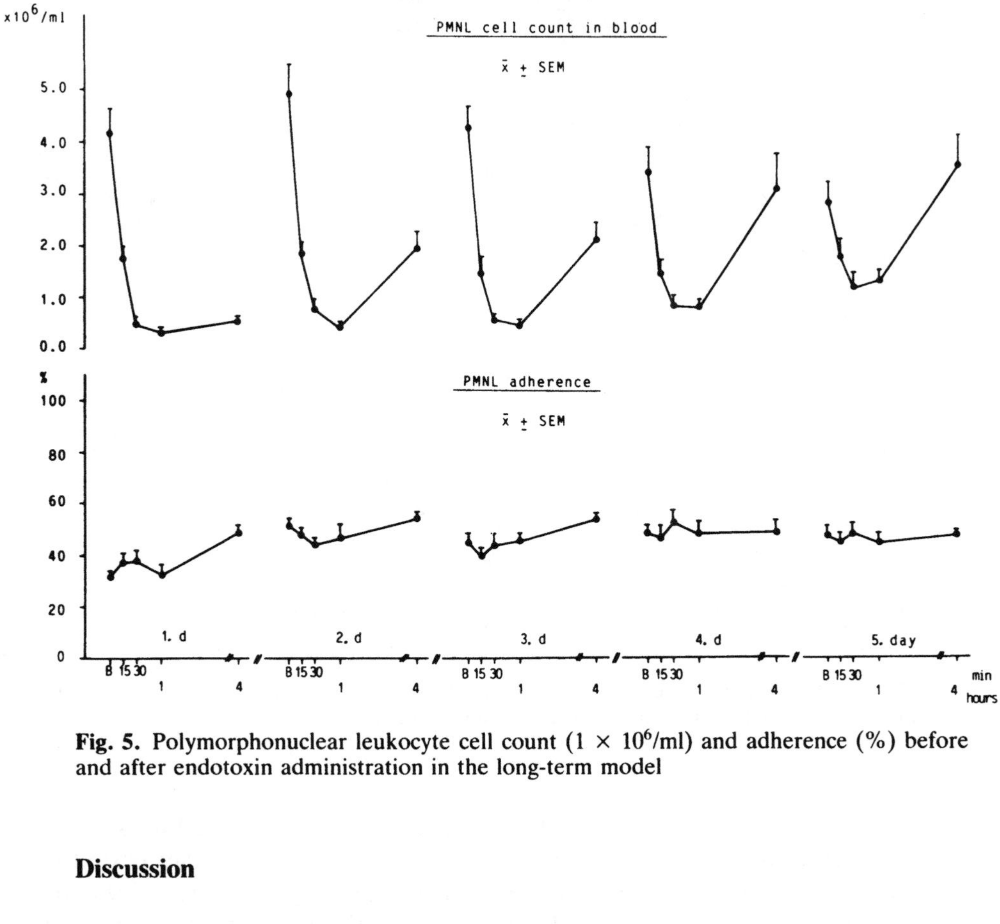

Fig. 5. Polymorphonuclear leukocyte cell count (1×10^6/ml) and adherence (%) before and after endotoxin administration in the long-term model

Discussion

Individual tests of PMNL and RES function in septic animal models have often been performed [6, 9, 10, 12, 19, 22]. Comprehensive determinations of these functions, however, are lacking. In order to clarify the questions mentioned in the introduction, we studied the changes (induced with ET) in a standardized animal model [2]. Our intention was to follow the behavior of the PMNL and RE phagocytic systems after endotoxemia in sheep, using both short- and long-term administration. This allowed us to determine the functional state of these systems at various times following the injury insult.

Reticuloendothelial System Function

Since endotoxin is normally cleared by the RES immediately after bolus injection, we tested RES function at this time point [17, 24]. The RES was not blocked early after endotoxin bolus administration. A comparison of baseline and post-endotoxin half-lives (Fig. 1) demonstrated that the RES clearance

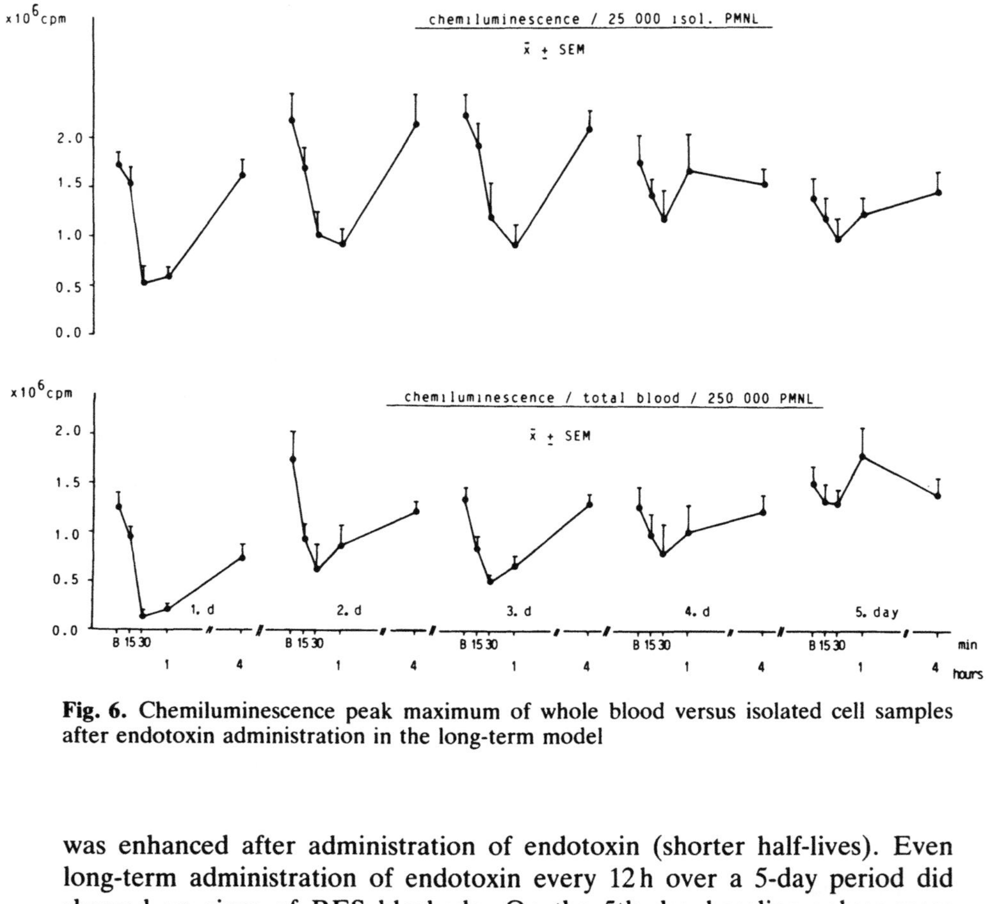

Fig. 6. Chemiluminescence peak maximum of whole blood versus isolated cell samples after endotoxin administration in the long-term model

was enhanced after administration of endotoxin (shorter half-lives). Even long-term administration of endotoxin every 12 h over a 5-day period did showed no signs of RES blockade. On the 5th day baseline values were reached, which can probably be associated with an adaptation status. The increased clearance of the RES in both models apparently has no influence on the effect of endotoxemia. Probably even the enhanced RES function is not able to clear the circulating endotoxin totally, and therefore cannot prevent the stimulation of the PMNLs and consequently the development of lung capillary damage.

Polymorphonuclear Leukocyte Function

Several responses to bolus injection of endotoxin in animal models are described [2, 3]. As others have also observed, we noted neutropenia after endotoxin administration (Table 2). The increased permeability phase (3–4 h pET) seems to coincide with the sequestration of PMNLs in the lung:

First we found an increase of PMNL adherence, correlating with the varying peripheral granulocyte count, which suggests that adherence may be important for the margination of PMNLs at the endothelial surface. Second we found a massive modulation of PMNL activity (CL) immediately after injection of the ET bolus, ending in a decompensatory state at 1 h postendotoxin. Probably the permeability damage seen 3–4 h after injection of the endotoxin bolus is directly related to this enormous stimulation of the PMNLs and liberation of O_2 radicals during the 1st h after endotoxin administration.

The changes in PMNL function in the long-term model are difficult to interpret. Probably, the PMNLs become adapted to the effect of recurrent endotoxin bolus injections. The mechanisms are still unclear, but possibly this adaption is related to the so-called desensitization theory. Long-term interaction with an endotoxin-induced chemotactic factor leads to a decrease in PMNL migration into the lung (Fig. 5) [18, 23]. On the other hand, adherence remains continuously high over the 5-day period. This is possibly related to the irreversible change of the PMNL membrane structures under ET influence. The desensitization of the PMNLs can also be demonstrated in the CL measurements: there, the endotoxin influence decreases subsequently in the 5-day period. The decompensation, phenomenon at 30 min–1 h after endotoxin administration practically disappears on the 4th day in the long-term model (Fig. 6, isolated PMNLs). This effect also means that the O_2 – radical liberation from the PMNLs similarly decreases during this period. This is even more pronounced in the CL whole blood measurement, where apparently the normalizing opsonin concentrations influence this phenomenon. Consequently the damage to the lung and the increase in capillary permeability decrease from day to day in this experiment.

In conclusion we can say that:

1. The injection of a standardized dose of endotoxin results in an activation of RES function (increase of clearance) in both the short- and long-term models. However, this stimulation obviously does not prevent the circulatory and pulmonary effect of endotoxin. Sufficient clearance cannot be achieved.

2. Therefore, PMNLs become stimulated in the circulation and migrate into the lung, as seen in both short- and long-term models. Here they adhere to the capillary membrane and possibly cause the damage to the lung capillary routinely seen after 3–4 h in the sheep model. In the long-term experiment, adherence remains increased, which is possibly an expression of an irreversible cellular membrane defect.

Adherence to the capillary endothelium and increased O_2-radical production (CLPM) immediately after injection of an endotoxin bolus are probably related to the change in capillary permeability seen after 3–4 h. This phenomenon is attenuated in the long-term model, which can possibly be explained by the desensitization of the PMNLs after recurrent injection of an endotoxin bolus.

References

1. Barie PS, Minnear FL, Malik AB (1981) Increased pulmonary vascular permeability after bone marrow injection in sheep. Am Rev Respir Dis 123:648
2. Brigham KL, Bowers RE, Heynes J (1979) Increased sheep lung vascular permeability caused by *Escherichia coli* endotoxin. Circ Res 45:292
3. Demling RH, Smith M, Gunther R, Flynn J, Gee M (1981) Pulmonary injury and prostaglandin production during endotoxemia in conscious sheep. Am J Physiol 240:348
4. George EA, Hendershott LR, Klos DJ et al. (1980) Mechanism of hepatic extraction of gelatinized 99 m technetium sulfur colloid. Eur J Nucl Med 5:241
5. Heflin JM, Brigham KL (1981) Prevention by granulocyte depletion of increased vascular permeability of sheep lung following endotoxemia. Clin. Invest. 68:1253
6. Henson PM (1971) Interaction of cells with immune complexes: adherence, release of constituents and tissue injury. J Exp Med 134:1145
7. Hinson JM, Hutchinson AA, Ogletree ML, Brigham KL, Snapper JR (1983) Effect of granulocyte depletion on altered lung mechanics after endotoxin in sheep. J Appl Physiol 55:92
8. Hollingsworth JW, Beeson PB (1955) Experimental bacteremia in normal and irradiated rats. Yale J Biol Med 28:56
9. Issekutz AC, Bhimji S (1982) Role for endotoxin in the leukocyte infiltration accompanying *Escherichia coli* inflammation. Infect Immunol 36:558
10. Johnston RB, Lehmeyer JE (1976) Elaboration of toxic oxygen byproducts by neutrophils in a model of immune complex disease. J Clin Invest 57:836
11. Jones JG, Minty BD, Beely JM, Royston D, Crow J, Grossmann RF (1982) Pulmonary epithelial permeability is immediately increased after embolization with oleic acid but not with neutral fat. Thorax 37:169
12. Kaplan JE (1981) Effect on reticuloendothelial blockade on the development of hypotension after trauma, sepsis and intravascular coagulation. Adv Shock Res 2:73
13. Lanser ME, Saba TM (1980) Opsonic glycoprotein (plasma fibronectin) enhances bacterial phagocytosis by neutrophils. J Reticuloendothel Soc 28:21a
14. Lanser ME, Saba TM (1981) Neutrophil-mediated lung localization of bacteria: a mechanism for pulmonary injury. Surgery 90:473
15. Larsen GL, Parrish DA, Henson PM (1983) Lung defense, the paradox of inflammation. Chest [Suppl] 5:18
16. Loegering DJ, Garrett LJ (1981) Reticuloendothelial system depression with hemolyzed blood and susceptibility to endotoxin shock and thermal injury. Circ Shock 8:473
17. Lucas CE, Walt AJ (1970) Critical decisions in liver trauma. Experience based on 604 cases. Arch Surg 101:277
18. Nelson RD, McCormack RT, Fiegel, VD et al. (1979) Chemotactic deactivation of human neutrophils: possible relationship to stimulation of oxidative metabolism. Infect. Immunol 23:282
19. O'Flaherty JT, Kreutzer DL, Ward PA (1978) Chemotactic influences on the aggregation, swelling and foreign surface adhesion of human leukocytes. Am J Pathol 90:537
20. Reske SN, Vyska K, Feinendegen LE (1981) In vivo assessment of phagocytic properties of Kupffer cells. J Nucl Med 22:405
21. Rimola A, Soto R, Bory F (1981) Reticuloendothelial system phagocytic activity in cirrhosis and its relation to bacterial infections and prognosis. Hepatology 4:53
22. Skarnes RC (1970) Host defense against bacterial endotoxemia, mechanism in normal animals. J Exp Med 132:300
23. Spilberg I, Mandall B, Hoffstein SA (1979) Proposed model for chemotactic deactivation: evidence for microtubule modulation of polymorphonuclear leukocyte chemotaxis. J Lab Clin Med 94:361

24. Steinberg B, Martin RA (1954) Hematopoietic responses to provocatives. Arch Pathol 57:277
25. Tahamont MV, Malik AB (1983) Granulocytes mediate the increase in pulmonary vascular permeability after thrombin embolism. J Appl Physiol 54:1489
26. Wong C, Flynn J, Demling RM (1984) Role of oxygen radicals in endotoxin-induced lung injury. Arch Surg 119:77

The Three-Compartment Model in Sheep: The Effect of Recurrent Endotoxemia on Endothelial and Epithelial Permeability in the Lung

A. SEEKAMP, A. DWENGER, G. REGEL, and J.A. STURM

Introduction

Posttraumatic sepsis syndrome is a hyperdynamic state characterized by decreased systemic vascular resistance and increased oxygen consumption. Pulmonary failure combined with a sepsis syndrome has often been diagnosed and is characterized by pulmonary hypertension, increased vascular permeability, and hypoxia [13].

The major role of polymorphonuclear leukocytes (PMNL) in this pathomechanism has been clearly defined in the recent past. In experimental protocols of acute endotoxemia, the migration of PMNL into the microvessels of the lung, their adherence to vascular endothelial cells, and the localized release of proteases and oxygen radicals have been shown to cause endothelial cell injury leading to pulmonary edema [8, 11, 16]. However, it is not yet clear in which way PMNL function is modulated under frequent stimulation by circulating endotoxin as in a sepsis syndrome. Since, in other studies, single-dose endotoxemia only resulted in transient lung injury without a hyperdynamic state, we used a model of recurrent endotoxemia designed to result in a more characteristic sepsis syndrome.

Our purpose was to investigate PMNL function in recurrent endotoxemia and to find more evidence for the relationship between damage to the endothelial barrier and PMNL. We also tried to determine whether the alveolar epithelium was also affected by PMNL. We, therefore, used the well-known chronic lung lymph fistula model in sheep for monitoring endothelial integrity and performed bronchoalveolar Lavage (BAL) to monitor epithelial integrity.

Methods

Using the method described by Staub et al. [15] a chronic lung lymph-fistula was prepared in eight sheep (mean weight 35 kg). After the efferent lymph-

Department of Trauma Surgery, Hannover Medical School, Konstanty-Gutschow-Str. 8, W-3000 Hannover 61, FRG

J.A. Sturm (Ed.)
Adult Respiratory Distress Syndrome

atic duct of the inferior mediastinal lymph node had been cannulated, the distal part of the node was cut and cauterized at the inferior pulmonary ligament in order to diminish abdominal lymph contamination. The collected lymph was clear, a steady flow was only modulated by inspiration and expiration. Polyvinyl catheters were placed in the femoral artery and vein, additionally a Swan-Ganz thermodilution catheter was placed in the pulmonary artery. The sheep were allowed to recover for at least 4 days before the study began to ensure the establishment of a steady state lymph flow (>4 ml/h, <10 ml/h), and hemodynamics (mean pulmonary artery pressure 15–20 mm Hg) for baseline values.

Measurements

Arterial, central venous, pulmonary artery, and pulmonary capillary wedge (Paw) pressure were recorded using pressure transducers which had been positioned at the level of the left atrium and were calibrated before each measurement. Cardiac output (Q) was measured by thermodilution. Lung lymph (Q_L) was collected in heparinized grade tubes for each 30-min period. Within each period, heparinized blood samples were drawn and, unless total protein was to be determined, samples were frozen at −80°C immediately. Arterial blood gases were only measured every 60 min. Samples for chemiluminescence (CL) and PMNL cell count were drawn once during the baseline period and 15 min, 30 min, 1 h, and 4 h after the administration of endotoxin. Total protein was measured using the biuret test, and albumin was determined using the bromcresol green method.

Protocol

The animals were studied in an unanesthetized state while standing in a metal cage with free access to food and water. One day prior to the first endotoxin injection, the first BAL was performed (Table 1). After a baseline period of 2 h, sheep were given 1 µg/kg body weight (BW) endotoxin (Serotype 0.55:B5, Sigma Chemicals, St. Louis, USA) as an intravenous bolus injection every 12 h over a 5-day period. Hemodynamic parameters were monitored for 6 h in the daytime, including the taking of lymph and blood samples every 30 min. On the third day, prior to the baseline measurement, the second lavage was performed, and the last one was performed at the end of the study immediately before the animals were killed by an overdose of pentobarbital. Four additional sheep, also receiving endotoxin in the same time course, were monitored over a 5-day period without undergoing BAL.

Bronchoalveolar Lavage

For bronchoscopy followed by lavage, the sheep were anesthetized with a single injection of 1.5 mg/kgBW of thiopental sodium and subsequent

Table 1. Protocol for hemodynamic measurements and sample collection

	Hemodynamics	CL	Hematology	Lymph	BAL
Baseline	*	*	*	*	*
Endotoxin	(ET) –	–	–	–	
15 min pET		*	*	*	
30 min	*	*	*		
1 hr	*	*	*	*	
1 hr 30 min	*			*	
2 hr	*			*	
2 hr 30 min	*			*	
3 hr	*			*	
3 hr 30 min	*			*	
4 hr	*	*	*	*	
12 hr	(ET) –	–	–	–	
24 hr/Baseline	*	*	*		

CL = Chemiluminescence

injection of pentobarbital of a maximum concentration of 2 mg/kgBW. The sheep were then intubated and mechanically ventilated with an inspiration oxygen concentration (FiO_2) of 30%. They did not receive any halothane or nitrogen gas. Over a vent positioned in line, the broncho-endoscope (Fuiji Optical) was inserted into the tube and pushed further down to the trachea. After the removal of secretion, the tip of the endoscope was positioned in a bronchioll. At this point 60 ml (3 × 20 ml) saline solution (0.9%) were instilled via the proximal end of the endoscope. During suctioning, the lavage fluid was collected in cylindrical grade tubes, which were positioned in line with the suction tube. The recovery was approximately 60% of the instilled amount of fluid. Each time the lavage was performed, another pulmonary segment was chosen to make sure that the appearance of PMNL in the alveolus was not caused just by mechanical irritation.

The BAL fluid was first centrifuged for 10 min at 350 *g* and 10°C. The cell sediment was washed twice with phosphate buffer solution (PBS; Dulbecco, Boehringer Mannheim, FRG) and again centrifuged for 5 min at 350 *g* and 10°C. The final sediment was resuspended in 1 ml PBS and put in a Neubauer hemocytometer for cell counting. In the upper layer, which had been taken off after the first centrifugation, the concentrations of total protein and albumin were measured. All measurements of any protein concentrations or cell count in the lavage fluid were corrected by the urea concentration of plasma and the BAL fluid, which was determined separately. According to the following formula we calculated the actual epithelial lining fluid (ELF) [12] as follows:

$$\text{ELF} = C_{\text{urea}}\ \text{BAL} \times \text{Volume BAL}/C_{\text{urea}}\ \text{Plasma}$$

and the cell count in the ELF as follows:

$$\text{cells/ml ELF} = \text{cells/ml BAL} \times \text{Volume BAL/ELF}$$

PMNL Separation

One milliliter of venous sheep's blood was mixed with 1 ml of saline solution, layered on a one-step discontinous Percoll gradient (Lot No. OB 05847, 1.130 g/cm^3, Pharmacia, Sweden; diluted to 3 ml of 1.070 g/cm^3 density), and centrifuged with 350 *g* at 22°C for 20 min. The intermediate PMNL layer was extracted and washed several times with PBS. In order to hemolysate the erythrocytes, cells were washed with 4 ml of aqua destillata for 30 s at 0°C. To restore isotonic media 2 ml of 2.7% sodium chloride solution was added immediately. Cells were then resuspended in 200–500 µl PBS and counted using a Neubauer hemocytometer after cell staining with Türk's solution (viability rate >90%).

CL Measurement

Luminol-enhanced CL [18] was determined using a six-channel Bioluminat LB 9505 in combination with an Apple II plus computer, and an Epson MX 82 F/T printer (Laboratory of Prof. Berthold, Wildbad, FRG) in 3-ml polystyrene CL vials. For CL measurement the following reagents were prepared: 22.6 mmol/liter luminol in minimal essential medium (MEM; Dulbecco, Boehringer Mannheim) also containing 40 mmol/l triethylamine, prepared freshly daily, and zymosan A (Sigma Chemicals, St. Louis) washed twice with PBS, once with MEM, centrifuged at 800 *g* for 10 min at 22°C, resuspended in 100 mg/ml MEM, and frozen in aliquots at −70°C. CL measurements were performed at 37°C with prewarmed reagents.
PMNL function was characterized by the following parameters:

CL in whole blood:

1. To measure base activity, 520 µl MEM, 10 µl luminol, and 50 µl whole blood were mixed.
2. To measure activity after stimulation, 500 µl MEM, 10 µl luminol, 50 µl whole blood, and 20 µl zymosan were mixed. Activity was expressed in CL of 5×10^6 PMNL/ml.

CL of isolated PMNL:

1. To measure base activity, 520 µl MEM, 10 µl luminol, 50 µl cell suspension, and 50 µl pooled plasma were mixed.
2. To measure activity after stimulation, 500 µl MEM, 10 µl luminol, 50 µl cell suspension, 50 µl pooled plasma, and 20 µl nonopsonized zymosan were mixed. The cell suspension should contain 25 000 PMNL.

Measurements were started simultaneously in six channels and photon emission was recorded for at least 60 min. Activity was then calculated by subtracting base activity from stimulation values. Peak maximum of CL (CLPM) was then determined.

Statistics

Within each group, paired data of the individual time periods were compared to baseline employing the two-way analysis of variance. Data between both groups were compared at the individual time periods using Student's unpaired *t*-test.

Results

All monitored animals survived the 5-day study. Data are presented in the figures as mean values ± standard deviation. We noted no significant difference either in pulmonary and systemic response or in PMNL response between those animals which were not undergoing BAL but also received the endotoxin injections in the same time course and those sheep, which were anasthetized intermittently for BAL.

Pulmonary Response

As in the model of acute endotoxemia, we noted a two-phase response after the first endotoxin injection. The initial phase lasting for about 1.5 h was characterized by pulmonary hypertension up to 44 mm Hg paralleled by a protein-poor lymph flow (lymph/plasma protein ratio of 0.53) and hypoxia (P_aO_2 70 mm Hg). About 3–4 h after the endotoxin injection, we noted a slight decrease in pulmonary artery pressure down to 30 mm Hg but a protein-rich lymph flow (lymph/plasma protein ratio of 0.74) (Figs. 1, 2).

Under subsequent endotoxin injections, the acute response became attenuated but the pulmonary artery pressure remained significantly increased at values of 24–30 mm Hg. Also lung lymph flow did not return to baseline values. After the lymph/plasma protein ratio had increased significantly within 4 h after the first endotoxin injection, values returned to baseline and were not affected very much by further endotoxin administration. The initial hypoxia was totally compensated. After the fourth to fifth endotoxin injection, arterial P_aO_2 returned to baseline and then increased constantly till the end of study.

Systemic Response

Arterial pressure and cardiac output decreased significantly after administration of the first endotoxin. Within the following 4 h values returned to

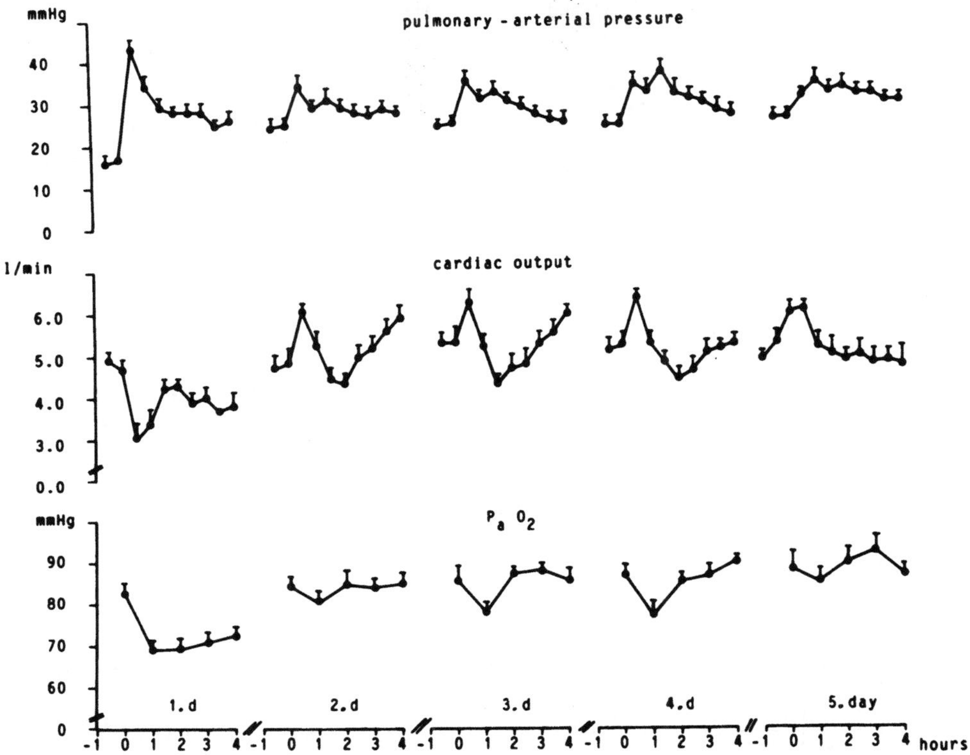

Fig. 1. Pulmonary artery pressure remained significantly increased over the whole period of time. Cardiac output decreased only after the first endotoxin injection and increased significantly after subsequent injections. P_aO_2 also increased constantly after initial hypoxia

baseline. Over the next 4 days, a significant increase in cardiac output could be noted (Fig. 1). Body temperature increased significantly right after the initial endotoxin injection and returned to baseline values within the first day. A transient increase could be noted also after any of the following endotoxin injections, an increase which was, however, no longer significantly different from baseline values.

PMNL Response

First we noted a rapid decrease in the PMNL cell count till the first hour after administration of endotoxin; after about 4 h, a slight recovery was noted. Before the third endotoxin injection was given, the PMNL cell count almost returned to baseline. After subsequent endotoxin administration, we noted an attenuation in the acute leukopenia, but also a decrease in the cell count recovery (Fig. 3).

The CL response reflected a maximal stimulation of the PMNL 1 h after the first endotoxin injection. Within the next 3 h, the CL response returned to

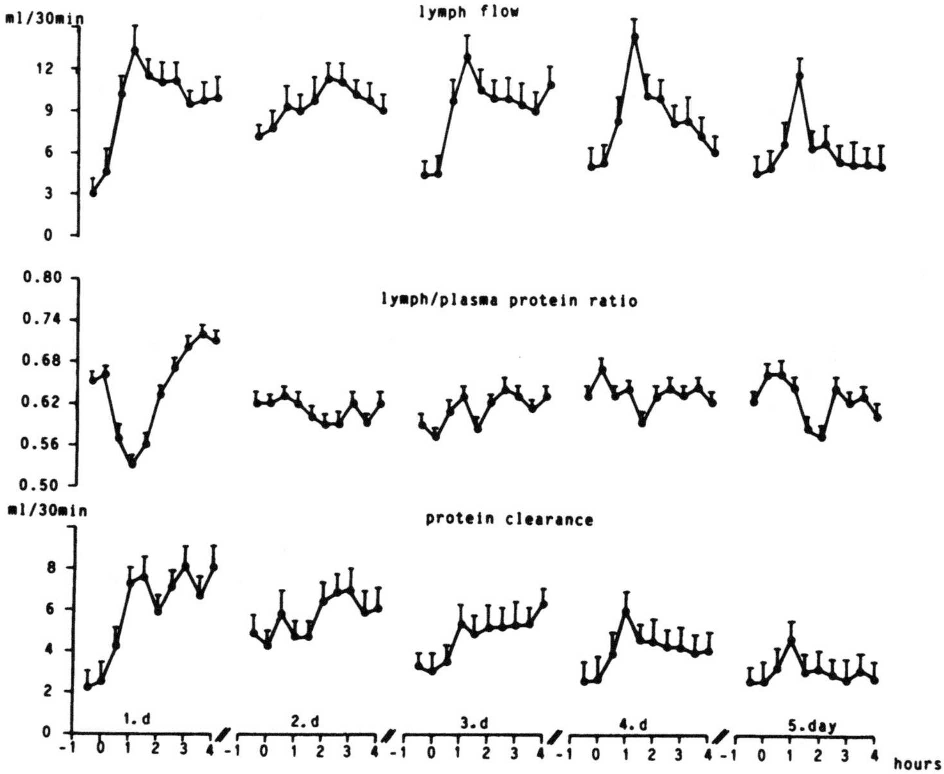

Fig. 2. By calculating the protein clearance from lymph flow and the lymph/plasma protein ratio, it became evident that the microvascular permeability tended to move down to normal values even after recurrent endotoxin injections

baseline values. From the third injection on, the acute response was less dramatic and by the tenth endotoxin injection only a transient change was measured in the CL response. In spite of the attenuation in the acute response, a decline in the overall CL response was noted. On the last day of the study the CL value prior to endotoxin administration was significantly higher than the baseline value of the first day (Fig. 4).

Bronchoalveolar Lavage

In the ELF, the total cell count increased over the 5-day period, but not significantly (Fig. 5). Considering the cell pattern in the BAL, macrophages, PMNL, and leukocytes, we noted a significant increase only in the PMNL, which had a percentage of less than 1% in the baseline lavage and increased up to 25% of the total cell count at the end of study (Fig. 6).

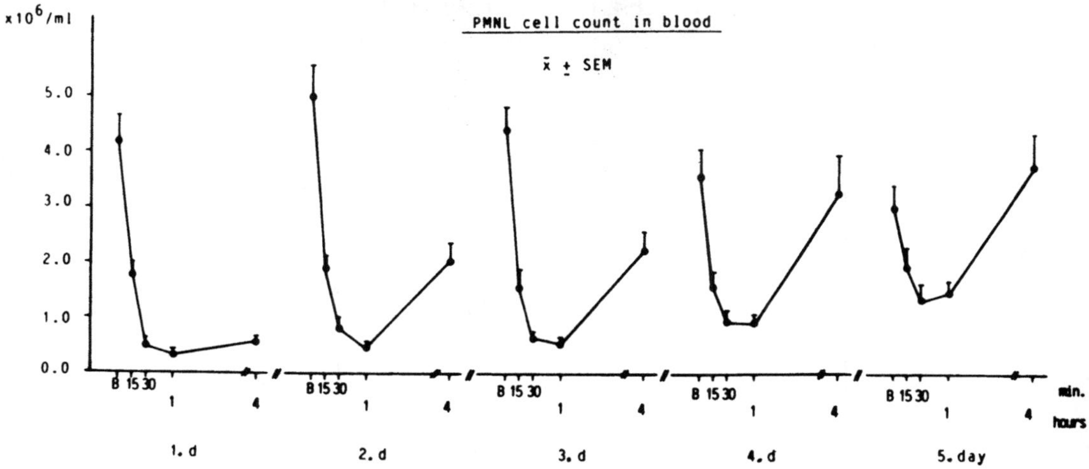

Fig. 3. The acute leukopenia after the administration of endotoxin was attenuated over the 5 days, whereas the cell count recovery decreased

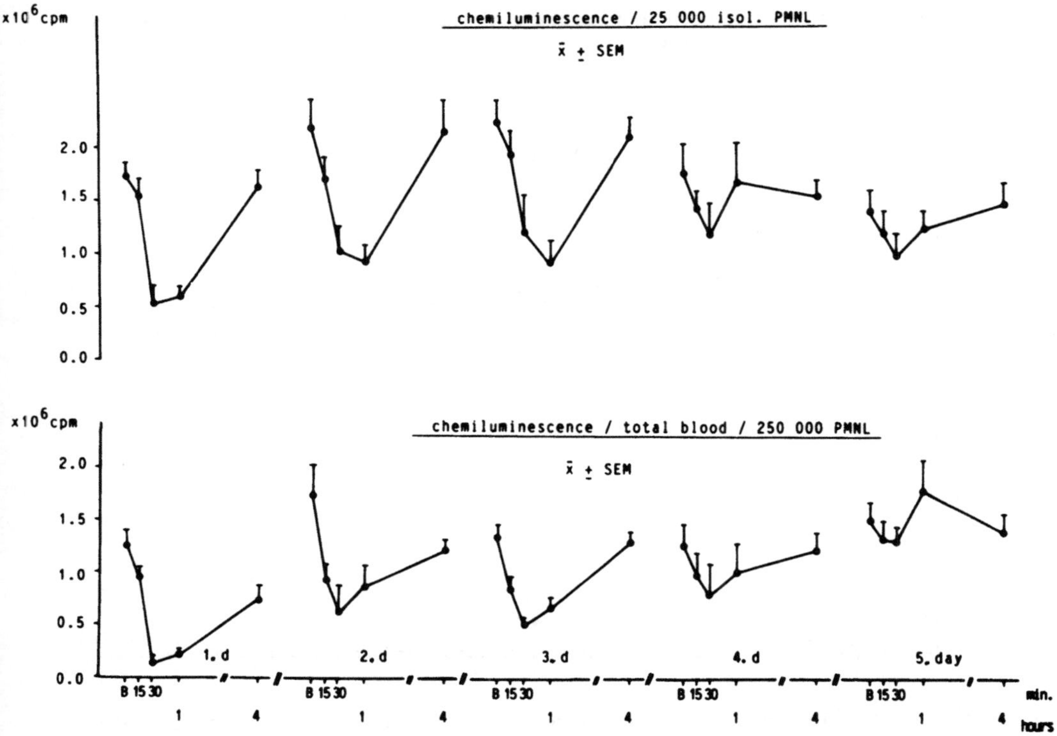

Fig. 4. The metabolic activity of PMNL decreased in recurrent endotoxemia

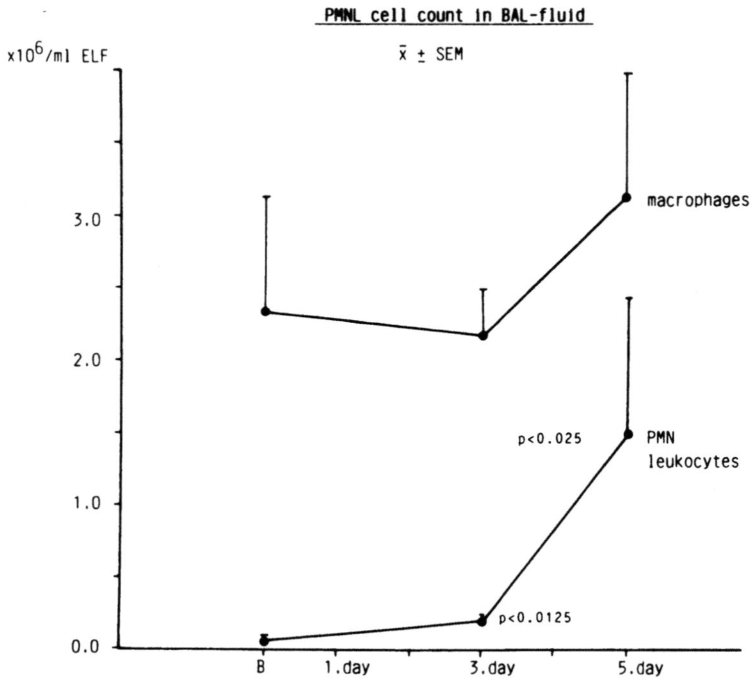

Fig. 5. Although the total cell count in the BAL increased, it was only the PMNL cell count which increased significantly

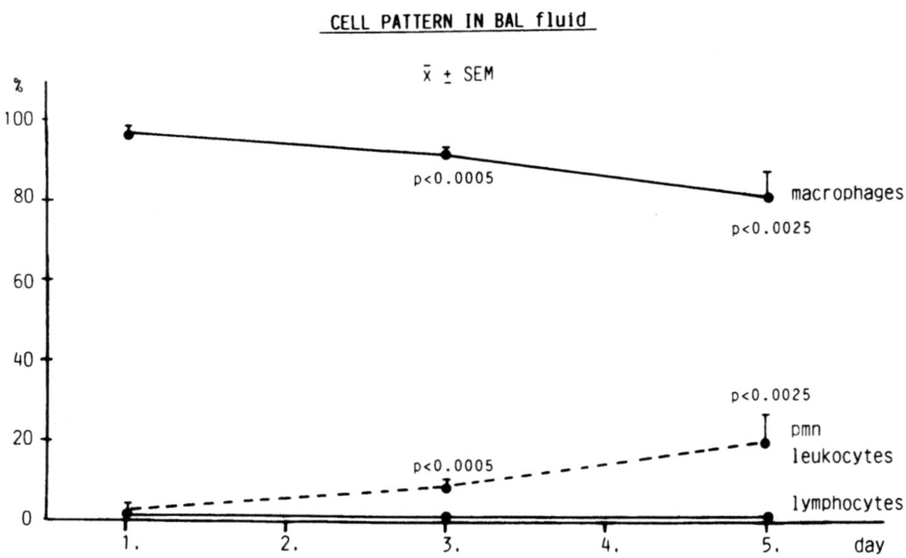

Fig. 6. The PMNL cell count in the BAL increased from a percentage of 1% at the baseline up to 25% at the end of study

The CL response could not be measured in these PMNL as it was not possible to isolate them accurately enough from the macrophages to get reliable results.

Protein and albumin concentration in the ELF increased only transiently over the 5-day period and did not change significantly from baseline values (Fig. 7). Therefore, the BAL/plasma protein ratio did not give any evidence for a protein flow into the alveolus, either.

Discussion

In the last few years, evidence has been mounting that the lethality of adult respiratory distress syndrome (ARDS) is not only due to hypoxia, but is also caused by hemodynamic instability and the failure of other organs apart from the lung [1]. In about 70% of ARDS patients, sepsis syndrome and pulmonary distress coincide [9]. Circulating endotoxin released from the ischemic splanchnic system in the presence of inadequate hepatic clearance (failure of the reticuloendothelial system, RES) is well recognized to be a mediator of sepsis syndromes [7] leading to both pulmonary and systemic hemodynamic responses.

The model of acute endotoxemia has frequently been used to simulate the cardiopulmonary effects which could be diagnosed in patients with ARDS or a sepsis syndrome. But after a single endotoxin injection, cardiopulmonary parameters returned to baseline after a few hours. Of main interest in those studies was the increase in the microvascular permeability, which now is

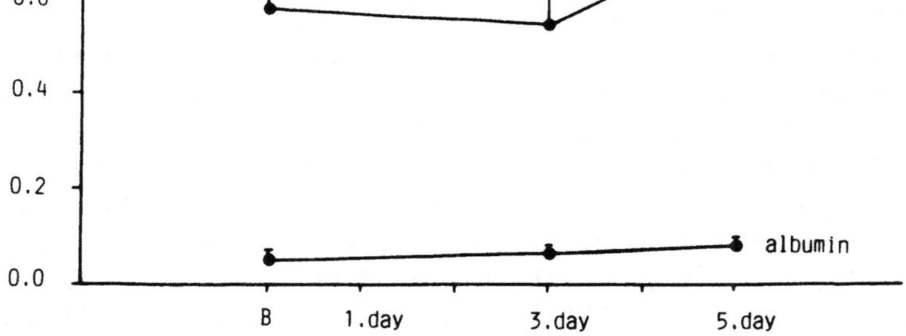

Fig. 7. The BAL/plasma ratio of protein and albumin did not change significantly

known to be due for the most part to PMNL [5, 6, 10, 20]. In order to simulate a more clinical situation, we chose a protocol of recurrent sublethal endotoxemia. We were mainly interested in the cellular and the pulmonary response to endotoxemia to determine the relationship between PMNL function and endothelial or epithelial permeability in the lung.

After the first endotoxin injection, we noted the characteristic hypodynamic state with a decrease in cardiac output and an increase in systemic vascular resistance (SVR). From the third endotoxin injection on, the systemic hemodynamics entered a hyperdynamic state with a significant increase in cardiac output and a decrease in SVR. Pulmonary artery pressure increased after each endotoxin injection and remained significantly elevated over the 5-day period, although less in degree on the last day. Previous studies [3, 14] have already shown that the pulmonary hemodynamics seem to be more dependent on plasma thromboxane levels, which had been reported to decrease in recurrent endotoxemia, than on circulatory regulations.

To evaluate microvascular permeability, we took protein clearance into consideration, as this parameter includes both the lymph flow and the lymph/plasma protein ratio [2, 19]. The characteristic response of protein clearance, i.e., a decrease within the first hour after endotoxin and a significant increase from the third hour on, could be noted only on the first day. Over the next 4 days, the protein clearance constantly returned to baseline values (Fig. 2). This would mean that after subsequent endotoxin injections the vascular permeability returns to normal again. As PMNL is supposed to play a major role in the damage to the vascular endothelium, the activity of PMNL is also expected to decrease over the 5-day endotoxemia.

The attenuation in the acute response of the PMNL cell count after each endotoxin injection already gives evidence of less PMNL activation, as the major reason for leukopenia is the increase in cellular adherence after stimulation. The decrease in cell recovery at the baseline of each day might be due to an exhaustion of PMNL release from the bone marrow [17]. The CL response gives more evidence of the decrease in PMNL metabolic activity over the whole time course. The significantly low baseline value on the fifth day and the only very modest decrease in the CL after the last endotoxin injection on this day might be due to the release of more and more unmature PMNL from the bone marrow. So the damage to the vascular endothelium depends on mature and maximally stimulated PMNL.

The permeability of the alveolar epithelium remains unaffected by the endotoxemia considering the BAL/plasma ratio of protein and albumin. For this barrier, we could not calculate a protein clearance as the constant transepithelial fluid exchange could not be measured. In contrast to the nondamaged epithelium, we found a significant increase in PMNL in the alveolus on the fifth day, at a time when even the endothelial permeability is normalizing. We therefore suppose that the PMNL in the alveolus are cells of subsequent released unmature PMNL populations which are penetrating the already damaged endothelium and the alveolar epithelium without causing any further damage by themselves [4].

In summary, we conclude that the three-compartment model combined with recurrent endotoxemia could be used to investigate epithelial and endothelial permeability abnormalities as they might occur in a sepsis syndrome. From our results a sepsis syndrome is not only characterized by a hyperdynamic state, but also by only little change in endothelial permeability and an exhaustion of PMNL function, which predetermines severe septic complications.

References

1. Bell RC, Coalson JJ, Smith JH, Johanson NR (1983) Multiple organ system failure and infection in adult respiratory distress syndrome. Ann Inter Med 99:293–298
2. Brigham KL, Owen PJ (1975) Increased sheep lung vascular permeability caused by histamine. Circ Res 37:647–657
3. Demling RH, LaLonde CC, Jin LJ, Albes J, Fiori N (1986) The pulmonary and systemic response to recurrent endotoxemia in the adult sheep. Surgery 100:876–883
4. Dwenger A, Schweitzer G, Regel G (1986) Bronchoalveolar lavage fluid and plasma proteins, chemiluminescence response and protein contents of polymorphnuclear leukocytes from blood and lavage fluid in traumatized patients. J Clin Chem Clin Biochem 24:73–88
5. Flick MR, Perel G, Staub NC (1981) Leukocytes are required for increased lung microvascular permeability after microembolism in sheep. Circ Res 48:344–351
6. Haslett G, Worthen G, Giclas P, Morrison D, Henson JE (1987) The pulmonary vascular sequestration of neutrophils in endotoxemia is initiated by an effect of endotoxin on the neutrophil in the rabbit. Am Rev Respir Dis 136:9–18
7. Jakob AI, Goldberg PK, Bloom N (1977) Endotoxin and bacteria in portal blood. Gastroenterology 72:1268–1272
8. Janoff A (1985) Elastase in tissue injury. Ann Rev Med 36:207–216
9. Montgomery AB, Stager MA, Carrico CJ, Hudson LD (1985) Causes of mortality in patients with the adult respiratory distress syndrome. Am Rev Respir Dis 132:485–489
10. Proctor RA (1985) Effects of endotoxin on neutrophils. In: Berry LJ (ed.), Cellular biology of endotoxin. Elsevier, Amsterdam, (Handbook of Endotoxin, vol 3 , Chap 12)
11. Regel G, Nerlich ML, Dwenger A, Seidel J, Schmidt C, Sturm JA (1987) Phagocytic function of polymorphnuclear leukocytes and the RES in endotoxemia. J Surg Res 42:74–84
12. Rennard SI, Basset G, Lecossier D, O'Donnel KM, Pinkston P, Martin PG, Crystal RG (1986) Estimation of volume of epithelial lining fluid recovered by lavage using urea as marker of dilution. J Appl Physiol 60:532–538
13. Shale DJ (1987) The adult respiratory distress syndrome – 20 years on. Thorax 42:641–645
14. Snapper JR, Bernard GR, Hinson JM, Hutchinson AA, Loyd JE, Ogletree ML, Brigham KL (1983) Endotoxemia-induced leukopenia in sheep: Correlation with lung vascular permeability and hypoxemia but not with pulmonary hypertension. Am Rev Respir Dis 127:306–309
15. Staub NC, Bland RD, Brigham KL, Demling RH, Erdmann AJ, Woolverton WC (1975) Preparation of chronic lung lymph fistulas in sheep. J Surg Res 19:315–320
16. Tate RM, Repine JE (1983) Neutrophils and the adult respiratory distress syndrome. Am Rev Respir Dis 128:552–559

17. Territo MC, Golde DW (1976) Granulocyte function in experimental human endotoxemia. Blood 47:539–544
18. Tono-Oka T, Ueno N, Matsumoto T, Ohkawa M, Matsumoto S (1983) Chemiluminescence of whole blood: a simple and rapid method for estimation of phagocytic function of granulocytes and opsonic activity in whole blood. Clin Immunol Immunopathol 26:66–75
19. Vreim CE, Snahall PD, Demling RH, Staub NC (1976) Lung lymph and free interstitial fluid protein composition in sheep with edema. Am J Physiol 230:1650–1653
20. Worthen GS, Haslett C, Rees AJ, Gumbay RS, Henson JE, Henson PM (1987) Neutrophil-mediated pulmonary vascular injury: synergistic effect of trace amounts of lipopolysaccharide and neutrophil stimuli on vascular permeability and neutrophil sequestration in the lung. Am Rev Respir Dis 136:19–28

Bacterial Toxins and Terminal Complement Complex: Significance for Lung Microvascular Injury

W. SEEGER, N. SUTTORP and H. NEUHOF

Introduction

Next to severe polytrauma bacterial sepsis is the most consistent factor associated with the adult respiratory distress syndrome (ARDS) [1–3]. Moreover, acute diffuse lung injury of different etiology is often complicated by nosocomial pneumonia [4, 5]. In experimental models, septic lung failure is mimicked by the application of lipopolysaccharide components of gram-negative bacteria (endotoxins), and plenty of detailed information is available on the mechanisms of lung injury by these agents. There is evidence for a critical role of circulating inflammatory cells, and activation of several humoral mediator systems [complement, arachidonic acid (AA) metabolites, reactive oxygen species, proteases] has been documented; this field has been reviewed recently by Brigham and Meyrick [6, 7].

Only very little information is available on abnormalities inflicted by "nonendotoxin toxins" in the pulmonary circulation. Both *Pseudomonas aeruginosa* and *Staphylococcus aureus* have become increasingly important pathogens in septicemia and septic lung failure [8]. These bacteria are known to liberate toxins capable of generating discrete transmembrane pores in vitro. Moreover, many strains of *Escherichia coli* elaborate a hemolysin, which similarly creates discrete transmembrane channels in target membranes of erythrocytes, but also of nucleated cells [9]. The significance of this cytolysin as a determinant of bacterial pathogenecity has been established in animal models and has been inferred from the high association of hemolysin production and severe organ infection as well as sepsis in human beings. We thus hypothesized that these toxins might create transmembrane aqueous channels in different cells of an intact lung, thereby allowing calcium flux and initiation of excessive arachidonic metabolism with adverse consequences in the pulmonary vascular bed. Moreover, there might be different metabolic

---

Department of Internal Medicine, Division of Clinical Pathophysiology and Experimental Medicine, Justus-Liebig-University, Klinikstr. 36, W-6300 Gessen, FRG

J.A. Sturm (Ed.)
Adult Respiratory Distress Syndrome

and physiologic effects for toxins from different sources. Therefore we started a series of experiments addressing the effects on lung tissue of three bacterial protein toxins: *S. aureus*, α-toxin, *P. aeruginosa* cytotoxin, and, *E. coli* hemolysin. Moreover, we extended the experiments to the terminal sequence of the complement system, known to create transmembrane pores in cell membranes with similar features to the bacterial exotoxins (C5b-8 and C5b-9 membrane complexes). In order to measure calcium kinetics and arachidonic metabolism as well as lung microvascular effects in response to these pore-forming proteins, we performed experiments in isolated, ventilated rabbit lungs, perfused, by recirculation, with Krebs Henseleit bicarbonate buffer [10, 11], and in cultured porcine pulmonary artery endothelial cells [12, 13]. These studies were intended to shed light on pathogenetic events induced by "non-endotoxin-toxins," which are frequently encountered in human disease but have been little studied to date, and by complement membrane complexes in lung tissue.

Staphylococcus aureus α-Toxin: Calcium Gating, Prostanoid Generation, and Acute Thromboxane-Mediated Pulmonary Vasoconstriction

Staphylococcus aureus α-toxin has long been considered one of the essential factors associated with staphylococcal pathogenicity [14]. The native toxin is secreted as a water-soluble 3S molecule with a molecular mass of 32000 daltons (α-toxin monomer). Füssle et al. [15] and Bhakdi et al. [16–17] demonstrated that upon contact with erythrocyte membranes the toxin monomers aggregate to form a hexamer. This hexamer is an amphiphilic ring-shaped complex, which becomes partially embedded within the lipid bilayer to generate an aqueous transmembrane pore with an effective diameter of 2–3 nm.

Fig. 1A–C Calcium dependence of prostanoid generation and vasoconstriction in rabbit lungs (**A, B**) and of the liberation of precursor AA in endothelial cells (**C**) after exposure to staphylococcal α-toxin. **A, B** The lungs were perfused with Krebs Henseleit buffer, containing 40 g/l hydroxyethylamylopectine as oncotic substance (*KHHB*), at a constant flow of 200 ml/min. The application of 5 μg α-toxin (corresponding to 40 ng/ml in a recirculating volume of 125 ml) causes pulmonary artery pressure (PAP) rise and release of TxB_2 and 6-keto $PGF_{1\alpha}$, the stable hydrolysis products of TxA_2 and PGI_2, after a short lag period. During perfusion with calcium-free buffer fluid, the administration of the toxin does not result in prostanoid generation or pressor response, though persistent potassium release (not given) indicates the formation of transmembrane pores. Changing the perfusion fluid to calcium-containing buffer, however, without a second application of the toxin, evokes instantaneous prostanoid generation and vasoconstriction. **C** Pig pulmonary artery endothelial cells preincubated with [^{3}H], AA for 16 h, and then washed 3 times with tracer-free buffer (Hanks buffer with 2.5 g/l albumin). Exposure of the labeled cells to α-toxin for 15 min results in a marked release of AA – given in deterioration per minute (dpm) × 10^3/250000 cells – strictly dependent on the extracellular calcium concentration, but independent of the extracellular magnesium concentration. [From 10, 12] ▶

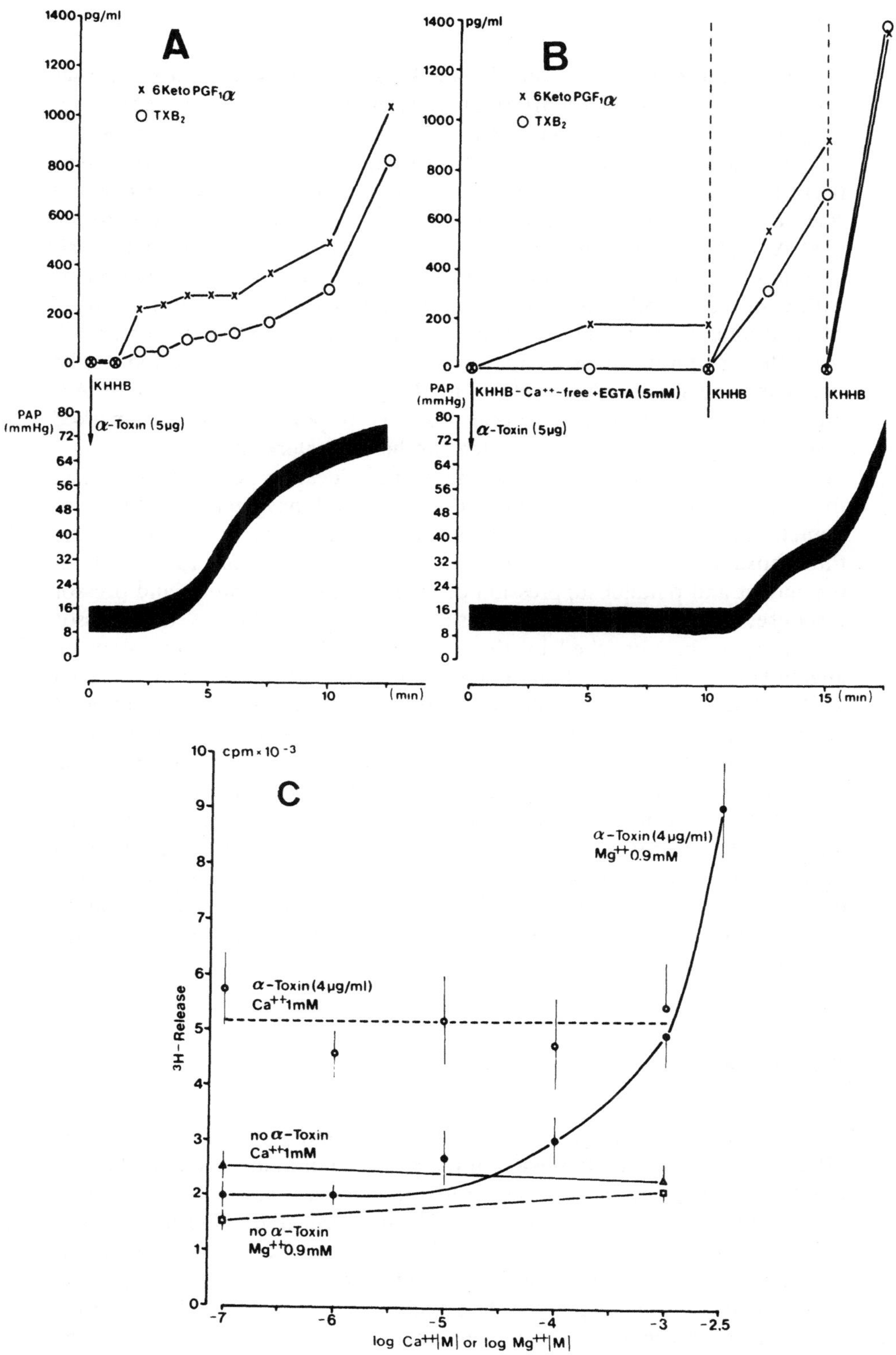
A
B
C
pg/ml
× 6 Keto PGF1α
○ TXB2
KHHB
α-Toxin (5µg)
PAP (mmHg)
KHHB - Ca++-free + EGTA (5mM)
(min)
cpm × 10-3
α-Toxin (4µg/ml) Mg++ 0.9mM
α-Toxin (4µg/ml) Ca++ 1mM
no α-Toxin Ca++ 1mM
no α-Toxin Mg++ 0.9mM
3H-Release
log Ca++|M| or log Mg++|M|

In concentrations between 4 and 40 ng/ml perfusate, α-toxin causes dose-dependent pulmonary artery pressor responses in isolated rabbit lungs (Fig. 1) [10]. The increase in vascular resistance starts after a lag period of 2–3 min and cannot be reversed by rinsing the vascular bed with fresh perfusion fluid. The pressor responses are accompanied by a dose-dependent release of prostanoids into the recirculating perfusion fluid; thromboxane (Tx) A_2 and prostaglandin (PG) I_2 were measured as their stable hydrolsysis products TxB_2 and 6-keto $PGF_{1\alpha}$. This finding is confirmed in experiments with cultured endothelial cells, where α-toxin dose dependently (0.1–8 μg/ml) and time dependently (5–30 min) induces the cleavage of precursor AA from the membrane phospholipid pool with subsequent generation of the dominant cell-specific AA metabolite PGI_2 [12]. The stimulation of AA metabolism by the staphylococcal toxin is responsible for the marked response in the isolated lungs, which can be characterized as thromboxane-mediated vasoconstriction: firstly, the toxin-induced pressure increase and the prostanoid release are inhibited by the cyclooxygenase inhibitor indomethacin, yielding superimposable dose-inhibition curves; secondly, the thromboxane synthetase inhibitors OKY-046 and imidazole cause a dose-dependent and parallel suppression of thromboxane generation and pressor response, whereas the PGI_2 release is unaffected; thirdly, the pressor response can be mimicked by the application of the stable thromboxane analog U-46619 in control lungs in the same range of concentration, in which TxB_2 is detected in the recirculating perfusion fluid after the administration of staphylococcal α-toxin. The vasoconstrictive potency of the toxin-induced thromboxane A_2 thus evidently surpasses the vasodilatory effect of the simultaneously generated PGI_2, resulting in net vasoconstriction.

What are the mechanisms by which the staphylococcal toxin exerts its lung vascular effects? From biochemical and pharmacologic studies, there is evidence that the sequence of events includes transmembrane pore formation, toxin-related calcium gating, calcium-mediated induction of phospholipolytic activities, and subsequent formation of cell-specific AA metabolites (see "Conclusion"; Fig. 7).

Pore Formation

In both the rabbit lungs and the cultured endothelial cells, the α-toxin effects are completely suppressed in the presence of neutralizing antibodies. Similarly, preformed hexamers of α-toxin, which are not longer capable of a membrane attack in erythrocytes [15], are ineffective. The native toxin monomers induce a marked release of K^+, but not of lactate dehydrogenase (LDH), in the isolated lungs, which is independent of the prostanoid generation and the pressor responses. This finding is compatible with the notion that discrete transmembrane aqueous pores might be generated also in the nucleated lung cells attacked by α-toxin, in analogy to its effect in erythrocyte membranes. This concept was directly proven by sieving experiments in the cultured endothelial cells: staphylococcal α-toxin increases the passive permeability of cell membranes for small molecules such as K^+, ^{45}Ca, and [^{3}H]-sucrose, but not for large molecules such as [^{3}H]dextran, [^{3}H]-insulin, and LDH. Thus toxin-related transmembrane aqueous pores are apparently formed in the endothelial cells, which correspond to those in erythrocyte membranes with an effective inner diameter of 2–3 nm. The absence of LDH release and morphologic criteria indicate that in the endothelial cells toxin insertion and pore formation evoke a biologic response below the threshold of overt cell damage.

Toxin-Related Calcium Gating, Calcium Dependence, and Stimulation of Phospholipolytic Activities

Prostanoid generation and vasoconstriction following administration of the staphylococcal toxin are strictly dependent on extracellular calcium; in a calcium-free medium, α-toxin is capable of inducing the primary membrane lesion (as indicated by K^+ release in rabbit lungs and by sieving experiments in the cultured endothelial cells), but prostanoid generation is absent in both models (Fig. 1). Re-addition of calcium in the isolated rabbit lungs without a second application of toxin induces an instantaneous burst of AA metabolite generation with concomitant marked vasoconstriction, and the endothelial PGI_2 formation is found to be strictly dose dependent on the extracellular calcium concentration but not the magnesium concentration. Moreover, in endothelial cells that are placed on ice after the primary toxin attack, a severalfold increase in passive ^{45}Ca uptake can be demonstrated: the time course of calcium flux antecedes that of AA liberation and PGI_2 formation in these cells. Collectively, these data suggest that the toxin-created transmembrane pores in the lung cells attacked by the staphylococcal protein serve as a (nonphysiologic) calcium bypass gate, allowing the flux of the bivalent cation along the high extracellular to intracellular gradient. Incoming calcium triggers various intracellular events, which include onset of AA cleavage and AA metabolism. The toxin-related calcium gating is thus distinctly different from the action of a calcium ionophore (such as A 23187 or ionomycin) or from the calcium shift following receptor occupancy and activation of receptor-operated (physiologic) calcium channels. The latter event, such as bradykinin-induced PGI_2 generation in endothelial cells [18, 19], can be inhibited by calcium-channel blockers, whereas different types of calcium antagonists do not interfere with the nonphysiologic α-toxin-related calcium flux and onset of AA metabolism. At the site of intracellular calcium action, however, α-toxin-induced and ionophore-induced calcium translocation appear to merge. The effect of both stimuli on AA liberation and formation of AA metabolites can be inhibited by TMB-8, an inhibitor of intracellular calcium function [20], in the rabbit lung and in cultured pulmonary endothelial cells. Additionally, calmodulin may be involved in the stimulus transmission pathway in both models: the generation of AA metabolites after application of α-toxin and the thromboxane-mediated vasoconstriction are inhibited by trifluoperazine and W-7, which are potent albeit not entirely specific inhibitors of (calcium)-calmodulin function [21, 22]. The calcium-induced or calcium-calmodulin-induced stimulation of phospholipases can be inhibited by mepacrine [23], an agent, which again is not monospecific, that suppresses prostanoid formation and thromboxane-mediated vasoconstriction in cultured endothelial cells and isolated rabbit lungs. The type of phospholipolytic activity that is stimulated after α-toxin attack (e.g., phospholipase A_2 or C) has not been further characterized.

Delayed Increase in Vascular Permeability upon Prolonged Exposure to α-Toxin

As described, acute thromboxane-mediated vasoconstriction is the predominant biophysical response to α-toxin in the isolated rabbit lungs. When this pressor response is blocked, e.g., by cyclooxygenase inhibition, a delayed, dose-dependent increase in vascular permeability emerges (Fig. 2). The underlying mechanisms have not been further elucidated; however, recent experiments revealed marked α-toxin-induced production of lipoxygenase products of AA. These characteristics recognized in the presence of cyclooxygenase inhibition thus show similarities to the *Pseudomonas aeruginosa*-evoked pulmonary response, described in the following section.

Pseudomonas aeruginosa Cytotoxin: Calcium Gating, Eicosnoid Generation, and Increased Lung Microvascular Permeability

Pseudomonas aeruginosa cytotoxin is an acidic protein with a molecular mass of 25 100 daltons, which is liberated independently of the lipopolysaccharide components (endotoxins) of this bacterium [24–26]. No enzymatic activities are attributed to this toxin, and it probably acts on target cell membranes to create small transmembrane aqueous pores. In cultured pulmonary artery endothelial cells, the pseudomonal cytotoxin attack shares many common features with the effects of staphylococcal α-toxin [13]: (a) sieving experiments applying labeled marker molecules demonstrate the formation of toxin-related transmembrane pores with an effective diameter of ~0.5–1.5 nm. This toxin attack induces the release of K^+ but not of LDH from the endothelial cells, i.e., the experiments were performed below the threshold of overt cell damage. (b) In concentrations between 10 and 60 μg/ml, *P. aeruginosa* cytotoxin evokes the cleavage of AA from the membrane phos-

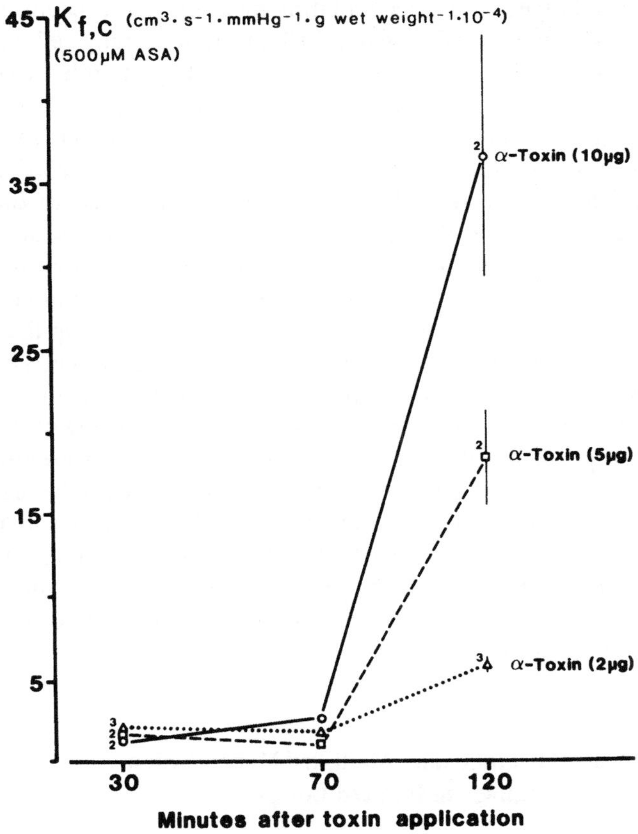

Fig. 2. Dose-dependent increase in rabbit lung capillary coefficient ($K_{f,c}$) by staphylococcal α-toxin. The experiments were performed in the presence of 500 μ*M* acetylsalicylic acid (*ASA*), thus preventing thromboxane-mediated alteration in microvascular pressure. Thirty and 70 min after toxin application, $K_{f,c}$ values are still at baseline levels. After 120 min, a dose-dependent severalfold increase in capillary permeability becomes evident (*n* indicates the number of experiments; means ± SEM are given). The α-toxin dose is admixed to perfusate volume of 150 ml

pholipid pool and the generation of PGI_2. This effect is strictly dependent on extracellular calcium but not magnesium. A severalfold increased passive uptake of ^{45}Ca along the high gradient from extracellular to intracellular calcium can again be demonstrated. The calcium flux antecedes the eicosanoid generation. (c) The ineffectiveness of different-type calcium channel blockers shows that the physiologic calcium channels are not involved in the toxin-related calcium translocation. The inhibitory potencies of TMB-8, W-7, and trifluoperazine correspond to those observed after staphylococcal α-toxin application in this model.

In analogy to the endothelial cell experiments, *P. aeruginosa* cytotoxin causes a marked release of K^+ into the perfusion fluid of isolated rabbit lungs

[11]. When the toxin is admixed in the recirculating medium at a concentration of 13 µg/ml over a period of 60 min, nearly 50% of the total lung cellular K^+ is liberated by this agent. This K^+ efflux is accompanied by the release of approximately 5%–7% of the total amount of lung cellular LDH. As in the cultured endothelial cells, the membrane attack by the pseudomonal toxin causes a severalfold increase in PGI_2 generation, detected in the recirculating perfusion fluid and in the bronchoalveolar lavage fluid. In contrast to the effects of staphylococcal α-toxin in the rabbit lungs, however, the pseudomonal protein causes only a slight increase in thromboxane formation and only a slight increase in pulmonary vascular resistance. The predominant biophysical response is an approximately fourfold rise of the capillary filtration coefficient ($K_{f,c}$) of the cytotoxin-treated lungs, which is followed by marked edema formation of the lungs after an initial lag period of ~20–30 min (Fig. 3). The increase in $K_{f,c}$ is not reversible upon rinsing of the vascular bed with fresh perfusion fluid, and it is accompanied by a greater than tenfold increase in the total protein content in the bronchoalveolar lavage fluid of the lungs at the end of the experiments [27]. The onset of vascular leakage is paralleled by a marked release of sulfidopeptide leukotrienes and leukotriene (LT)B_4 into the perfusion fluid (concentrations up to several nanograms per milliliter) and into the bronchoalveolar lavage fluid (Seeger et al., manuscript in preparation).

Escherichia coli Hemolysin: Thromboxane-Mediated Hypertension and Delayed Onset Vascular Leakage in Isolated Lungs

Escherichia coli hemolysin is secreted as a single-chain polypeptide of mol. wt. 107 000 [9]. Studies in erythrocytes and in planer lipid membranes have shown that the toxin generates discrete, hydrophylic transmembrane pores with marked selectivity of cations over anions and an effective inner diameter of approximately 2 nm. When hemolysin-forming *E. coli* bacteria are given to the perfusion fluid of isolated rabbit lungs, dose-dependent biophysical responses are encountered. In the concentration range of 10^4–10^7 *E. coli*/ml, there is a dose-dependent and time-dependent increase in pulmonary artery pressure. Further analysis of this pressor response showed that it is caused by the release of hemolysin into the recirculating perfusate. Accordingly, these pressor responses can be fully mimicked by application of the isolated hemolysin to perfusate free of *E. coli* bacteria. Low concentrations of this toxin in the perfusate (0.05–5 hemolytic units/ml, corresponding to approximately 5–500 ng/ml) caused a dose-dependent and time-dependent release of potassium, thromboxane A_2, and prostaglandin I_2, but not of LDH, into the recirculating medium, as well as a dose-dependent liberation of the prostanoids into the bronchoalveolar space [28, 29]. These events were followed by a dose-dependent pulmonary hypertension, and studies with different

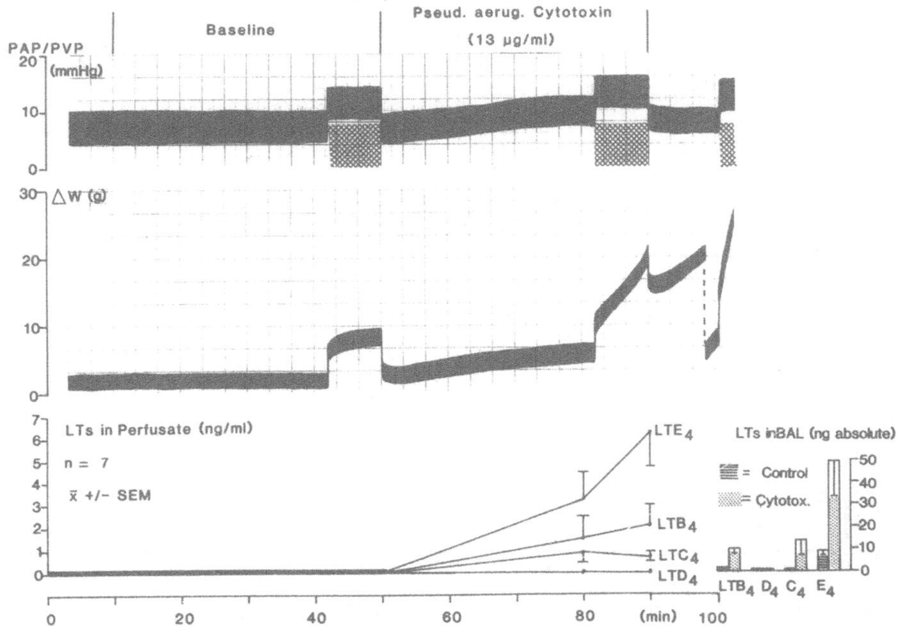

Fig. 3. Pulmonary artery pressure (*PAP*), lung weight gain (ΔW), and release of leukotrienes before and after admixture of *P. aeruginosa* cytotoxin to the recirculating buffer fluid (Krebs Henseleit buffer). *Shaded areas in the upper panel* indicate pulmonary venous pressure (*PVP*) elevations of 7.5 mmHg (two hydrostatic challenges). The *vertical lines* indicate exchanges of perfusion fluid. *P. aeruginosa* causes marked release of different leukotrienes (*LT*) into the recirculating perfusate and into the alveolar lining layer obtained by bronchoalveolar lavage (*BAL*) at the end of the experiment. After 30 min cytotoxin exposure there is a severalfold increase in microvascular permeability, as indicated by the steepness of the hydrostatic challenge-induced fluid filtration (weight gain)

inhibitors collectively indicated that the vascoconstrictor response was mediated predominantly by pulmonary thromboxane generation. The acute vascoconstrictor response to hemolysin-forming *E. coli* bacteria or to isolated hemolysin thus displays far-reaching similarities to the response to staphylococcal α-toxin in the same model.

In addition to the pressor response, hemolysin-forming *E. coli* bacteria elicited a protracted, dose-dependent increase in the lung capillary filtration coefficient, which was independent of the prostanoid-mediated pressor response and resulted in severe pulmonary edema formation (Fig. 4) [28, 29]. This increase in vascular permeability could again be fully mimicked by reapplication of isolated hemolysin to the perfusate of bacterium-free perfused lungs in the same concentration range, in which the toxin was noted to be liberated into the perfusate upon application of hemolysin-containing bacteria. Very recent studies showed that the onset of *E. coli* hemolysin-induced vascular leakage was again paralleled by the release of AA lip-

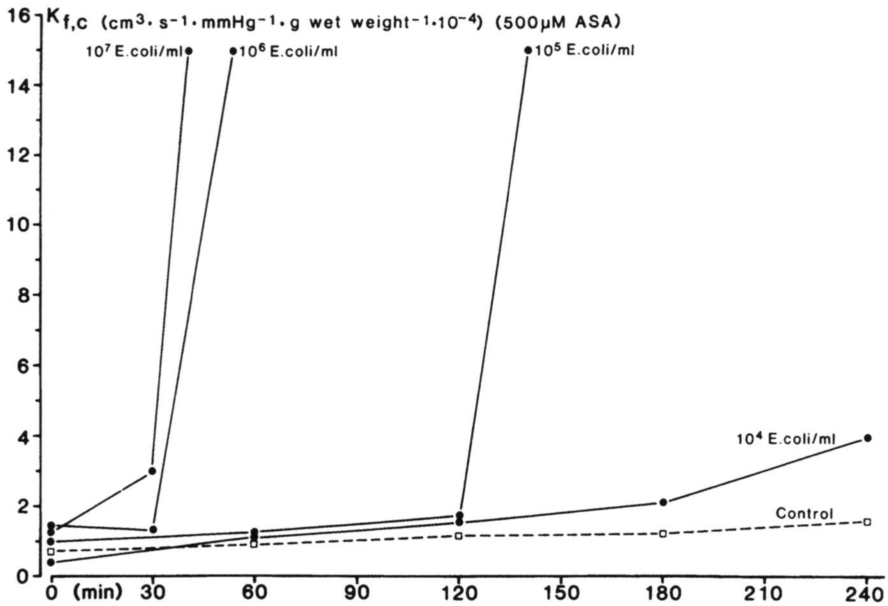

Fig. 4. Dose and time dependence of lung vascular leakage induced by hemolysin-forming *E. coli*. Different concentrations of *E. coli* were added to the perfusate, and the capillary filtration coefficient ($K_{f,c}$) was determined every 30–60 min. The experiments were performed in the presence of acetylsalicylic acid (*ASA*), in order to suppress hemolysin-induced thromboxane generation and thus to avoid an increase in microvascular pressure. The time and dose dependence of the $K_{f,c}$ increase is evident. *Each point* represents a mean of two to three independent experiments

oxygenase products into the recirculating medium and into the broncho-alveolar space. The characteristics of hemolysin-induced microvascular injury are thus similar to those noted after exposure to *Pseudomonas aeruginosa* cytotoxin and those encountered in the presence of staphylococcal α-toxin during cyclooxygenase inhibition (see above).

Local Complement Activation: Thromboxane-Mediated Vasoconstriction and Vascular Leakage in Rabbit Lungs: Mimicry of the Bacterial Exotoxin-Induced Pulmonary Effects

There is sound evidence for the involvement of complement in the pathogenesis of ARDS. Pulmonary lesions in this context have predominantly been ascribed to the generation of anaphylatoxins (C3a, C5a) with subsequent stimulation of granulocytes, pulmonary sequestration of these cells, and damage to lung endothelium by granulocyte-derived products [1, 6]. Being aware of the dramatic effects of pore-forming bacterial exotoxins in the lung microvasculature, we wondered whether similar effects might be evoked by the pore-forming terminal complement complex. We took advantage of the finding that rabbit cell surfaces spontaneously activate the human complement system, predominantly via the alternate pathway [30]. Admixture of small percentages of human serum to the perfusate of isolated perfused lungs was thus used as a tool to induce local complement activation. In these experiments, an immediate and dose-dependent pulmonary hypertension was again noted [31, 32]. Heat-inactivated serum, purified fluid face SC5b-9, and serum that had been activated with inulin in the absence or presence of a carboxypeptidase inhibitor all failed to elicit pressor responses. Both pressor response and prostanoid release were strictly dependent on complement factor C8, and evidence for C8-binding was obtained with the use of 125JC8 (Fig. 5). The pressor responses were paralleled by marked release of thromboxane A_2 and prostaglandin I_2 into the medium. Inhibitor studies collectively indicated that thromboxane A_2 was the predominant

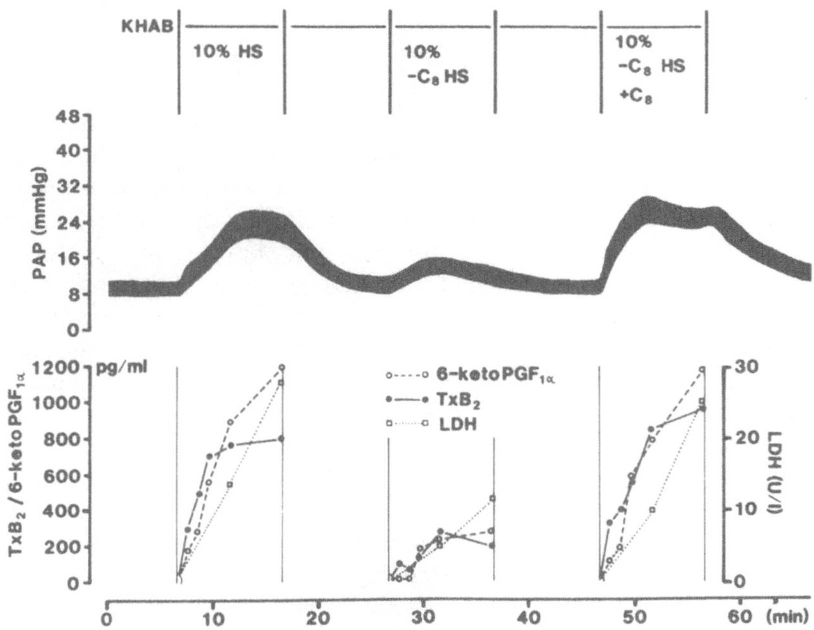

Fig. 5. C8/9 dependence of the pulmonary artery pressure (*PAP*) response as well as prostanoid and LDH release after admixture of human serum (*HS*; 10% v/v) the perfusate of isolated perfused rabbit lungs – example of one lung. Complement factor C8-depleted serum (−C8 HS) induced only a very moderate response compared with the initially applied whole human serum from the same serum pool (*HS*). Reconstitution of the depleted serum with purified C8 (25 μg/ml, final concentration) restored full activity, thus demonstrating the dependence of the vascular response on the terminal complement sequence. *Vertical dashes* indicate the changes of perfusion fluid; *KHAB*, Krebs Henseleit albumin buffer. [From 31]

vasoconstrictive agent. These data strongly suggest that in situ activation of complement in the rabbit lung vasculature with formation of terminal complement membrane complexes causes rapid thromboxane-mediated vasoconstriction, independent of circulating leukocytes, mimicking the biophysical effects of pore-forming bacterial exotoxins. Repetitive short-term application of human serum, with repeated exchange of perfusion fluid, evoked no major lung weight gain in the isolated lungs. Prolonged exposure to serum (40–80 min), however, without intermittent rinsing phases, evoked a delayed increase in the capillary filtration coefficient to maximally three- to fourfold values, with marked subsequent edema formation. Characteristics resembling the pulmonary effects of *Pseudomonas aeruginosa* cytotoxin, staphylococcal α-toxin, and *E. coli* hemolysin are thus encountered again.

Increase by Bacterial Exotoxins of the Permeability of an Endothelial Monolayer In Vitro

As already discussed, *S. aureus* α-toxin [12] and *P. aeruginosa* cytotoxin [13] are capable of stimulating the AA cascading in cultured pulmonary artery endothelial cells. Similarly, endothelial prostacyclin production is evoked by the induction of complement membrane complexes, using a specific antibody as trigger for complement activation [33]. We wondered whether, in addition to these metabolic alterations, biophysical responses are encountered upon exposure of the endothelial cells to the different pore-forming proteins. Cultured pulmonary artery endothelial cells were grown on a polycarbonate filter membrane and mounted in a modified chemotaxis chamber [34]. Filtration rates across the endothelial monolayers as well as the albumin-reflecting properties of this monolayer were registered. We observed that a continuous transendothelial pressure gradient resulted in a decrease of the filtration rate across the endothelial cell monolayer ("sealing") and in an increase in the reflection coefficient for albumin. *S. aureus* α-toxin (example given in Fig. 6) and *P. aeruginosa* cytotoxin increase the permeability of the endothelial cell monolayer for water and albumin dramatically. The increase in hydraulic conductivity and the loss of protein selectively were not dependent on endothelial cell eicosanoid metabolism. Morphologically, these changes in permeability were accompanied by the formation of gaps within the intercellular clefts. Thus, both toxins appear to increase transcapillary permeability by stimulating the endothelial cells to retract and to open a paracellular pathway for fluid exchange, independent of the arachidonate metabolism of these cells. Very recent studies demonstrated that a corresponding biophysical response could be evoked by the hemolysin of *E. coli* and by the induction of a local complement activation on the endothelial cell membranes, with formation of terminal complement membrane complexes.

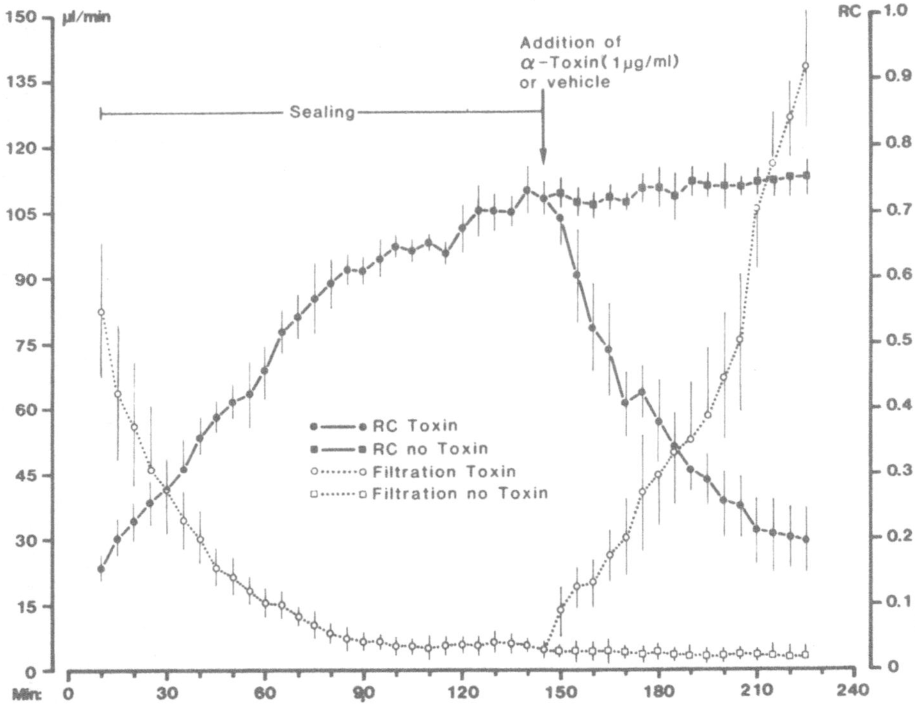

Fig. 6. Filtration rate across endothelial cell monolayer (in microliters per minute) and reflection coefficient (*RC*) for albumin of this monolayer during the sealing period and after addition of 1 µg/ml staphylococcal α-toxin. After application of a transendothelial pressure of 10 cmH_2O, there was an initial filtration rate of 80 µl/min and an RC of 0.2 of the monolayer system. During a 2-h control period, there was a sealing of the monolayer, i.e., filtration rate slowly decreased and reached a plateau of 4 µl/min and RC slowly increased and stabilized at 0.73. Addition of α-toxin to this sealed enothelial monolayer resulted in a substantial increase in filtration rate and in a dramatic collapse of albumin-reflecting properties of the endothelial monolayer. Control filters were stable throughout the entire experimental time. Data shown are means ± SEM of eight separate experiments. [From 34]

Conclusion

Summing up, it is obvious that all pore-forming proteins, the bacterial exotoxins staphylococcal α-toxin, *P. aeruginosa* cytotoxin, and *E. coli* hemolysin, as well as the membrane complexes of the terminal complement sequence, induce acute alterations in the pulmonary vascular bed (Fig. 7). The predominant short-term response is an increase in pulmonary artery pressure, accompanied by perfusion-ventilation mismatch due to irregular vasoconstriction. This pressor response is apparently evoked by the pore-forming proteins without the interaction of blood-derived inflammatory cells and humoral mediator systems, because the lungs were perfused with

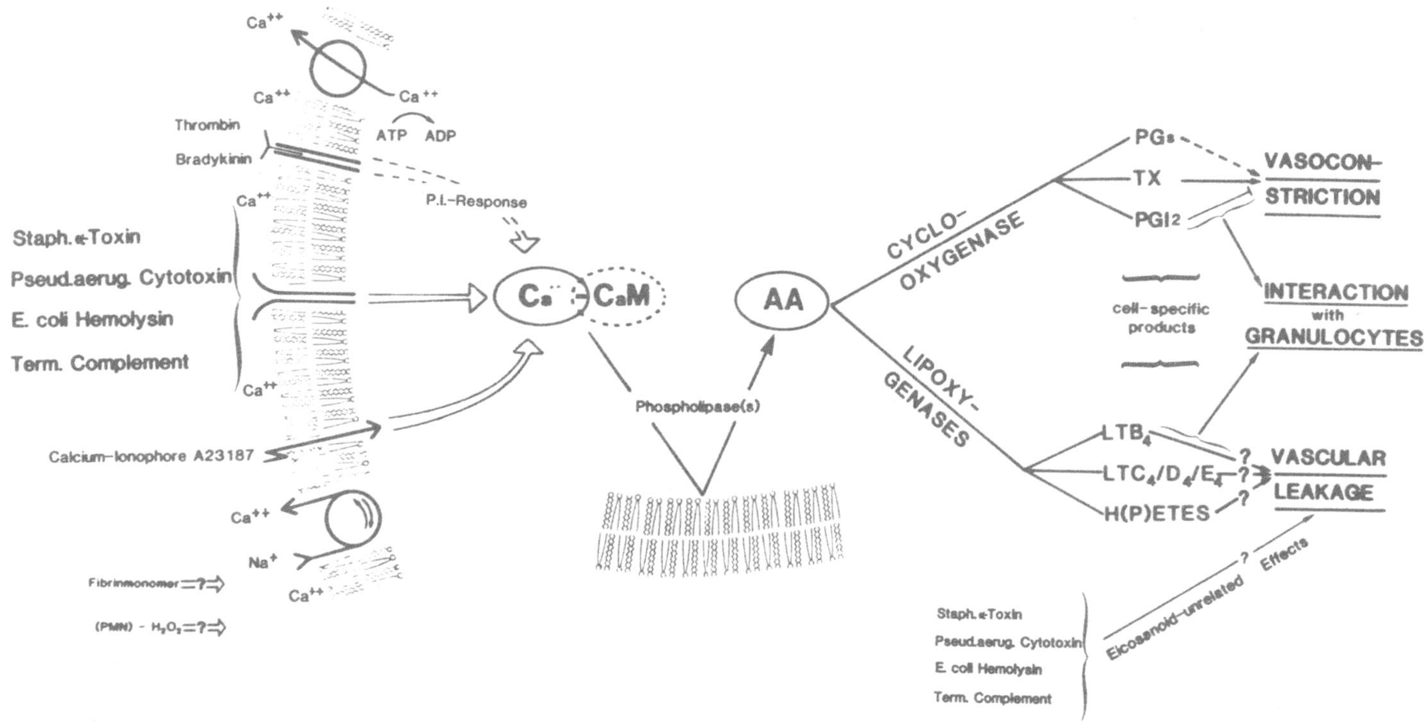

Fig. 7. Calcium gating, eicosanoid generation, and possible microvascular effects induced by pore-forming bacterial toxins and the membrane-attack complex of complement (*term. complement*). Calcium translocation was easily recognized after application of the synthetic calcium ionophore A 23187 and in the presence of receptor-operated stimuli [e.g., bradykinin or thrombin, probably linked to physiologic calcium channels and the "phosphatidylinositol (*PI*) response"]. Bacterial protein toxins and the membrane attack complex of the terminal complement sequence (C5b-9 or C5b-8) were capable of serving as (nonphysiologic) calcium bypass gates below the threshold of overt cell damage. Calcium flux and possibly calcium-calmodulin interaction stimulated phospholipolytic activities with subsequent cleavage of precursor arachidonic acid (*AA*). Cell-specific AA metabolites were generated. Among these, TxA_2 was the predominant mediator of toxin-induced vasoconstriction in rabbit lungs. Different AA-lipoxygenase products may be involved in an increase in lung microvascular permeability. Alternatively, vascular leakage following pore-forming proteins may be an eicosanoid-unrelated event. [52]

synthetic Krebs Henseleit buffer fluid. All experiments with inhibitors and receptor antagonists collectively indicated that the pressor response is, to a large extent, generated by the potent vasoconstrictive agent thromboxane A_2, which surpasses the vasodilatory effect of the simultaneously generated prostacylcin. No data are currently available on the effect of the pore-forming exotoxins as well as the terminal complement complex in lungs of other animals; however, there may be species differences concerning the predominant vasoconstrictive AA product, as recently reviewed [35]. Moreover, all bacterial exotoxins used in the present studies as well as the membrane complex of complement caused a delayed increase in the lung vascular permeability, resulting in the leakage of protein-rich edema into the pulmonary interstitium as well as the alveolar space. Alteration of lung surfactant function due to protein surfactant interaction with subsequent loss of lung compliance has been demonstrated as a consequence of bacterial exotoxin attack in this model [27]. As indicated in Fig. 3 for *Pseudomonas* cytotoxin, the increase in vascular permeability is accompanied by a marked release of AA lipoxygenase products into the recirculating perfusate as well as the bronchoalveolar space. The cause-effect relationship between vascular leakage and lipoxygenase product formation is, however, much less evident than that between thromboxane generation and vasoconstriction. In other words, it has to be asked whether the extotoxin- or complement-induced permeability increase is merely accompanied by or mediated by the generation of different lipoxygenase products including leukotrienes. This point is still unsettled. Administration of exogenous AA in high concentrations (1–6 mg AA/g lung weight) in isolated rabbit and dog lungs causes a severalfold increase in vascular permeability, which is reduced by lipoxygenase inhibitors, but not by cyclooxygenase inhibitors [36–39]. The smaller dose of 0.1 mg AA/g lung weight was, however, ineffective on vascular integrity in the lungs of these species [40, 41]. Application of exogenous AA or induction of the cleavage of endogenous AA by the calcium ionophore A 23187 in blood-free perfused rabbit lungs is known to cause a marked release of sulfidopeptide leukotrienes as well as LTB_4 into the perfusion fluid, as similarly noted after application of *Pseudomonas aeruginosa* cytotoxin in this model (LTs up to several nanomoles per milliliter perfusate) [42, 43]. Addition of exogenous LTC_4 or LTB_4 in even higher concentrations to the perfusion fluid of the lungs did not, however, mimick the AA-induced increase in rabbit lung vascular permeability [43]. This is in accordance with experiments in sheep, in which peptidoleukotriene administration did not significantly increase the pulmonary transvascular protein clearance [44], and with recent studies in salt-solution-perfused guinea pig lungs, in which LTD_4 administration did not effect $K_{f,c}$ [45]. Thus, marked induction of lung AA lipoxygenase metabolism appears to increase lung vascular permeability, but the products involved and the mechanisms of action are still unsettled. It may be possible that peptidoleukotrienes are effective on vascular integrity upon attack from the albuminal (interstitial) side, but not when released directly into the vascular space. Alternatively, non-leukotriene lipoxygenase products may be of major importance. It is an interesting recent finding in this context that 5-hydroxyeicosatetraenoic acid (HETE) and 15-HETE were noted to induce pulmonary edema, probably as a result of increased lung vascular permeability, in isolated perfused guinea pig lungs [46]. Moreover, cooperative eicosanoid synthesis, involving different pulmonary cells as well as pulmonary cells and sticking granulocytes, may be of major important. In recent studies in rabbit lungs, we demonstrated a marked shift of the leukotriene precursor LTA_4 from sticking granulocytes into pulmonary cells, predominantly endothelial cells, with resulting protentiation of peptidoleukotriene generation [47, 48]. Such transcellular precursor shifts, which may, moreover, be different whether occurring from the luminal or abluminal side of the endothelium, will further complicate the deciphering of the physiological significance of AA lipoxygenase metabolism in the lung microvasculature, in particular its impact on microvascular integrity. As an alternative possibility, eicosanoid-unrelated effects may be involved in the increase in lung vascular permeability of exotoxin and complement complex-exposed rabbit lungs. This has been demonstrated for the different exotoxins and the terminal complement sequence in endothelial cell monolayers, and the underlying mechanisms are currently under investigation.

Taken together, "non-endotoxin bacterial toxins" as well as membrane attack complexes of the complement system are capable of initiating the main features of the ARDS, i.e., vasoconstriction with resultant perfusion-ventilation mismatch and loss of vascular integrity with resultant leakage of protein-rich edema into the interstitial and intraalveolar space. However, many questions still remain open. What are the target cells of the toxins in the intact lung besides the endothelium, and what about the possibility that different "patterns" of toxin-attacked cells are responsible for variations in the metabolic (eicosanoid generation) and biophysical response to the different pore-forming agents? What about membrane repair mechanisms, which appear to have very rapid kinetics after the insertion of the terminal complement complex, but which are evidently very slow or even absent in face of the membrane attack by staphylococcal α-toxin and *Pseudomonas aeruginosa* cytotoxin? What additional effects must be expected if the simplified model of toxin-attacked blood-free perfused lungs is complicated by the presence of circulating inflammatory cells and humoral mediators? This question is particularly interesting with respect to the granulocytes, which themselves may be target cells of the pre-forming agents [49, 50], and which interact with lung cells in terms of cooperative eicosanoid metabolism (see above). Leukocytes are attracted to the lung tissue due to pulmonary leukotriene B_4 generation, and they may potentiate the vascular injury due to release of proteases (elastase) and oxidants. What "levels" of the different bacterial exotoxins can be expected under the conditions of sepsis, or which local concentrations will be achieved upon pulmonary tissue invasion by exotoxin-generating bacteria? Why should a local complement activation with resulting generation of membrane attack complexes be initiated under the conditions of ARDS? With respect to this question, it is an interesting finding that the complement system was noted to be activated at the "focus" of an exotoxin membrane attack, thereby amplifying the toxin-induced lesion [51]. Moreover, C3a in lavage fluids of severely traumatized patients was found to be increased severalfold in comparison to plasma levels (correction for alveolar lining fluid), thus suggesting a marked in situ complement activation in the pulmonary tissue. Besides its effectiveness on granulocytes, this C3a generation may indicate the insertion of membrane attack complexes in pulmonary cell membranes. Further studies, experimental and clinical, will be necessary to elucidate further the possible significance of pore-forming bacterial exotoxins and the membrane attack complex of complement for lung vascular and perivascular injury noted after severe polytrauma and under conditions of sepsis.

References

1. Fowler AA, Hamman RF, Zerbe GO, Benson KN, Hyers TM (1985) Adult respiratory distress syndrome. Prognosis after onset. Am Rev Respir Dis 132:472–478
2. Montgomery AB, Stager MA, Carrico CJ, Hudson LD (1985) Causes of mortality in patients with the adult respiratory distress syndrome. Am Rev Respir Dis 132:485–489
3. Petty TL (1985) Indicators of risk, course, and prognosis in adult respiratory distress syndrome (ARDS). Am Rev Respir Dis 132:471–472
4. Andrews CP, Coalson JJ, Smith JD, Johanson AG (1981) Diagnosis of nosocomial pneumonia in acute, diffuse lung injury. Chest 80:254–258
5. Bodey GP, Jadeja L, Elting L (1985) *Pseudomonas* bacteremia. Arch Intern Med 145:1621–1629
6. Brigham KL, Meyrick B (1984) Interaction of granulocytes with the lung. Circ Res 54:623–635
7. Brigham KL, Meyrick B (1986) Endotoxin and lung injury. Am Rev Respir Dis 133:913–927
8. Cruyz SJ (1985) New insights into the epidemiology, pathogenesis and therapy of *Pseudomonas aeruginosa* infections. Eur J Microbiol 4:153–155
9. Bhakdi S, Tranum-Jensen J (1987) Damage to mammalian cells by proteins that form transmembrane pores. Rev Physiol Biochem Pharmacol 107:148–223
10. Seeger W, Bauer M, Bhakdi S (1984) Staphylococcal alpha-toxin elicits hypertension in isolated rabbit lungs. Evidence for thromboxane formation and the role of extracellular calcium. J Clin Invest 74:849–858
11. Seeger W, Walmrath D, Neuhof H, Lutz F (1986) Pulmonary microvascular injury induced by *Pseudomonas aeruginosa* cytotoxin in isolated rabbit lungs. Infect Immun 52:846–852
12. Suttorp N, Seeger W, Dewein E, Bhakdi S, Roka L (1985) Staphylococcal alpha-toxin-induced PGI_2 production in endothelial cells: role of calcium. Am J Physiol 248:C127–134
13. Suttorp N, Seeger W, Uhl J, Lutz F, Roka L (1985) *Pseudomonas aeruginosa* cytotoxin stimulated prostacyclin production in cultured pulmonary artery endothelial cells: membrane attack and calcium flux. J Cell Physiol 123:64–72
14. Rogolsky M (1979) Nonenteric toxins of *Staphylococcus aureus*. Microbiol Rev 43:320–360

15. Füssle R, Bhakdi S, Sziegoleit A, Kranz T, Wellensiek HJ (1981) On the mechanisms of membrane damage by *Staphylococcus aureus* alpha-toxin. J Cell Biol 91:83–94
16. Bhakdi S, Füssle R, Tranum-Jensen J (1981) Staphylococcal alpha-toxin: oligomerization of hydrophilic monomers to form amphiphilic hexamers induced through contact with deoxycholate detergent micells. Proc Natl Acad Sci USA 78:5475–5479
17. Bhakdi S, Muhly M, Füssle R (1984) Correlation between toxin binding and hemolytic activity in membrane damage by staphylococcal alpha-toxin. Infect Immun 46:318–323
18. Whorthon AR, Young SL, Data JL, Barchowsky A, Kent RS (1982) Mechanism of bradykinin-stimulated prostacyclin synthesis in porcine aortic endothelial cells. Biochim Biophys Acta 712:79–87
19. Crutchley DJ, Ryan JW, Fisher GH (1983) Bradykinin-induced release of prostacyclin and thromboxanes from bovine pulmonary artery endothelial cells. Studies with lower homologs and calcium antagonists. Biochim Biophys Acta 751:99–107
20. Shaw JO (1981) Effect of extracellular Ca and the intracellular Ca-antagonist 8-(*N,N*-diethylamino)-octyl-3,4,5-trimethoxybenzoate on rabbit platelet conversion of arachidoinc acid into thromboxane. Prostaglandins 21:571–579
21. Roufogalis BD (1982) Specificity of trifluoperazine and related phenothiazines for calcium-binding proteins. In: Cheung WY (ed) Calcium and cell function. Academic, New York, pp. 129–138
22. Tanaka T, Ohmura T, Hidaka H (1982) Hydrophobic interactions of the calcium-calmodulin complex with calmodulin antagonists. Mol Pharmacol 22:403–407
23. Blackwell GJ, Flower RJ, Nijkamp FP, Vane JR (1978) Phospholipase A_2 activity of guinea pig isolated perfused lungs: stimulation and inhibition by antiinflammatory steroids. Br J Pharmacol 62:79–86
24. Lutz F (1979) Purification of a cytotoxin protein from *Pseudomonas aeruginosa.* Toxicon 17:467–475
25. Lutz F, Seeger W, Schischke B, Weiner R, Scharmann W (1983) Effects of a cytotoxic protein from *Pseudomonas aeruginosa* on phagocytic and pinocytic cells: in vitro and in vivo studies. Toxicon [Suppl] 20:35–38
26. Lutz F (1988) Interaction of *Pseudomonas aeruginosa* cytotoxin with plasma membranes from Ehrlich ascites tumor cells. Naunyn Schmiedebergs Arch Pharmacol 332:103–110
27. Seeger W, Stöhr G, Wolf HRD, Neuhof H (1985) Alteration of surfactant function due to protein leakage. Special interaction with fibrin monomer. J Appl Physiol 58:326–339
28. Seeger W, Henrik W, Neuhof H, Suttorp N, Bhakdi S (1989) *Escherichia coli* hemolysin causes thromboxane-mediated hypertension and vascular leakage in rabbit lungs. In: Schlag G (ed) Second Vienna Shock Forum. Liss, New York (in press)
29. Seeger W, Henrik W, Suttorp H, Bhakdi S (1989) Thromboxane-mediated hypertension and vascular leakage evoked by low doses of *Escherichia coli* hemolysin in rabbit lungs. J Clin Invest (in press)
30. Platt-Mills TAE, Ishizaka K (1974) Activation of the alternate pathway of human complement by rabbit cells. J Immunol 113:348–358
31. Seeger W, Hartmann R, Neuhof H, Bhakdi S (1989) Local complement activation, thromboxane-mediated vasoconstriction, and vascular leakage in isolated lungs. Role of the terminal complement sequence. Am Rev Respir Dis 139:88–99
32. Seeger W, Hartmann R, Neuhof H, Bhakdi S (1989) In-situ complement activation, pulmonary hypertension and vascular leakage in rabbit lungs — the role of the terminal complement copmplex. In: Schlag G (ed) Second Vienna Shock Forum. Liss, New York (in press)
33. Suttorp N, Seeger W, Zinsky S, Bhakdi S (1987) Complement complex C5b-8 induces PGI_2 formation in cultured endothelial cells. Am J Physiol 253:C13–21
34. Suttorp N, Hessz R, Seeger W, Wilke A, Koob R, Lutz F, Drenckhahn D (1988) Bacterial exotoxins and endothelial permeability for water and albumin in vitro. Am J Physiol 255:C368–376
35. Voelkel NF (1985) Species variations in the pulmonary responses to arachidonic acid metabolites. Prostaglandins 29:867–888
36. Seeger W, Walmrath D, Menger M, Neuhof H (1986) Increased lung vascular permeability after arachidonic acid and hydrostatic challenge. J Appl Physiol 61: 1781–1788

37. Seeger W, Wolf H, Stähler G, Neuhof H, Roka L (1982) Increased pulmonary vascular resistance and permeability due to arachidonate metabolism in isolated rabbit lungs. Prostaglandins 23:157–173
38. Seeger W, Radinger H, Neuhof H (1984) Increase in the capillary filtration coefficient in isolated rabbit lungs due to non-cyclooxygenase pathway of arachidonic acid. Microcirc Clin Exp 3:351
39. Littner MR, Kazmi GM, Lott FD (1984) Inhibition of cyclooxygenase production does not prevent arachidonate from increasing extravascular lung water and albumin in isolated dog lungs. Prostaglandins Leukotrienes Med 15:53–68
40. Townsley MI, Korthuis RJ, Taylor AE (1985) Effects of arachidonate on permeability and resistance distribution in canine lungs. J Appl Physiol 58:206–210
41. Selig WM, Noonan DF, Kern DF, Malik AB (1985) Pulmonary microvascular responses to arachidonic acid (AA) in blood versus Ringer's albumin perfused lungs. Fed Proc 44:1909
42. Schulz R, Seeger W (1986) Release of leukotrienes into the perfusate of calcium ionophore-stimulated rabbit lungs: influence of 5-lipoxygenase inhibitors. Biochem Pharmacol 35:183–193
43. Seeger W, Menger M, Walmrath D, Becker G, Grimminger F, Neuhof H (1987) Arachidonic acid lipoxygenase pathways and increased vascular permeability in isolated rabbit lungs. Am Rev Respir Dis 136:964–972
44. Noonan TC, Kern DF, Malik AB (1985) Pulmonary microcirculatory responses to leukotriene B_4, C_4, and D_4 in sheep. Prostaglandins 30:419–434
45. Greenberg GM, Henderson WR, Luchtel DL, Guest RJ, Albert RK (1985) Leukotriene D_4 induces bronchoconstriction but does not increase pulmonary vascular permeability after pulmonary artery injection in isolated perfused rabbit lungs (Abstr). Am Rev Respir Dis [Suppl A420] 131:A420
46. Burhop KE, Selig WM, Malik AB (1988) Monohydroxyeicosatetraenoic acids (5-HETE and 15-HETE) induce pulmonary vasoconstriction and edema. Circ Res 62:687–698
47. Grimminger F, Becker G, Seeger W (1988) High yield enzymatic conversion of intravascular leukotriene A_4 in blood-free perfused lungs. J Immunol 141:2431–2436
48. Grimminger F, Menger M, Becker G, Seeger W (1988) Potentiation of leukotriene production following sequestration of neutrophils in isolated lungs: indirect evidence for intercellular leukotriene A_4 transfer. Blood 72:1687–1692
49. Suttorp N, Seeger W, Zuker-Reimann J, Roka L, Bhakdi S (1987) Mechanism of leukotriene generation in polymorphonuclear leukocytes by staphylococcal α-toxin. Infect Immun 55:104–110
50. Seeger W, Suttorp N, Hellwig A, Bhakdi S (1986) Non-cytolytic terminal complement complexes may serve as calcium gates to elicit leukotriene generation in human polymophonuclear leukocytes. J Immunol 137:1286–1294
51. Bhakdi S, Tranum-Jensen J (1985) Complement activation and attack on autologous cell membranes induced by streptolysin O. Infect Immun 48:713–719
52. Seeger W, Suttorp N (1987) Role of membrane lipids in the pulmonary vascular abnormalities caused by bacterial toxins. Am Rev Respir Dis 136:462–466

Subject Index

GPSR Compliance

The European Union's (EU) General Product Safety Regulation (GPSR) is a set of rules that requires consumer products to be safe and our obligations to ensure this.

If you have any concerns about our products, you can contact us on ProductSafety@springernature.com

In case Publisher is established outside the EU, the EU authorized representative is:

Springer Nature Customer Service Center GmbH
Europaplatz 3
69115 Heidelberg, Germany

Batch number: 10723233

Printed by Printforce, the Netherlands